Honeybee Veterinary Medicine: *Apis mellifera* L.

Dedication

To my godson, Paul Sauvage, who wants to become a veterinarian.
May this path open many doors for him and lead to incredible discoveries.

To my friends, Lydia Vilagines and Christophe Roy, who have shared with me the honeybee veterinary adventure since 2007.
I have learned so much from your experience.

Honeybee Veterinary Medicine: *Apis mellifera* L.

Nicolas Vidal-Naquet

First Edition 2015, Reprinted 2018

Published by 5m Publishing
Benchmark House
8 Smithy Wood Drive
Sheffi eld S35 1QN
United Kingdom
www.5mpublishing.com
books@5mpublishing.com

ISBN: 978-1-91945-504-3

A CIP catalogue record for this book is available from the British Library.

Printed and bound in the UK by
CPI Anthony Rowe

Designed and typeset by
Forewords, Oxford

Before using any chemical treatment, prescribers and/or users must check legal posology, legal usage, legal withdrawal periods, and local regulation on veterinary medicine products (VMPs) and officinal drugs. The author and the publisher cannot be responsible for the prescription and/or use of treatments mentioned herein. The administration of drugs is the responsibility of the user and the prescriber. However, there is one main rule: **Never apply any treatment during honey flow.**

Contents

5 Parasitic diseases 109

Preface

For centuries *Apis mellifera* L., the honeybee, has been managed by humans, principally for honey production though today honeybees are also recognized for their crucial role as pollinators. Through pollination, honeybees play a major role in biodiversity, crop and orchard production and therefore in animal and human food security and livelihoods.

Honeybees face numerous diseases and threats: infectious diseases, parasitic diseases, pests and intoxications. The management of honeybee diseases has often been undertaken solely by beekeepers for their own beehives.

Uncontrolled international exchanges and trade have led to the spread of bee diseases. To face up to the challenges posed by this situation strong public- and private-sector components of veterinary services to manage the surveillance and control of honeybee diseases within their territories in close collaboration with beekeepers and technicians are of major importance.

The World Organisation for Animal Health (OIE, Office International des Epizooties), an intergovernmental organization established in 1924, with the current mandate to improve animal health, veterinary public health, and animal welfare worldwide, is dedicated to:

- ensuring transparency of the animal disease situation worldwide, including diseases transmissible to humans;
- collecting, analysing, and disseminating veterinary scientific information;
- providing expertise and promoting international solidarity for the control of animal diseases;
- guaranteeing the sanitary safety of world trade in animals and animal products;
- improving food safety from the farm to the abattoir;
- promoting animal welfare through a science-based approach;
- improving the legal framework and resources of national veterinary services.

Bee health and bee diseases have been addressed by the OIE since its establishment and continue to be an integral part of its mandate and activities. The OIE reaffirmed its commitment to the beekeeping sector by making bee health one of the priorities of its strategic plan for the years 2011–15. During this period, the OIE standards related to bee diseases, included in the *Terrestrial Animal Health Code* and the *Manual of Diagnostic Tests and Vaccines for Terrestrial Animals*, were or are in the process of being updated.

In 2014, the OIE *Bulletin 2*-2014 'Protecting Bees, Preserving our Future' pointed out the 'vital roles' of bees and the 'biological, agricultural, environmental and economic disaster' of the loss of bees as pollinators. The OIE also published in 2014 *Bee health and Veterinarians*, edited by Prof. Wolfgang Ritter, emphasising the asset veterinarians can be for the beekeepers.

In this context, *Honeybee Veterinary Medicine:* Apis mellifera *L.* written by Nicolas Vidal-Naquet, DMV and graduate in Beekeeping – Honeybee Medicine from the French Veterinary Schools of Nantes (Oniris) and Alfort, will provide further valuable scientific information to a wide readership, including veterinarians, veterinary officials, and practitioners involved in the beekeeping sector.

Dr Bernard Vallat
Director General, OIE

Foreword

The veterinary profession as we know it is just over 250 years old and originated in France to protect and heal mammalian livestock and working equids. Despite the long human history with honeybees and their propagation, veterinary medicine has had relatively little to do with this economically and culturally important domestic animal. This has now changed. We finally have a comprehensive book on honeybee medicine and management written by a veterinarian. And it seems quite appropriate that a French veterinarian, Dr Nicolas Vidal-Naquet, has written such a book.

While it is hard to quantify, or even imagine, the value of *Apis mellifera* to mankind, some financial estimates and comparisons can be made. It is estimated that the global impact of pollinating insects has a value of about €180 billion per year with most of the work being done by honeybees. Compare this to cattle at about €135 billion, pigs at €130 billion, and chickens at €105 billion. In fact nearly 10% of the world's agriculture relies on pollinating insects, with the most important impact being on fruits, oilseed crops, and vegetables.

This book, like a honeybee hive, is packed with richness in an organized and structured format. The author's systematic description of the honeybee, and the colony that he terms the 'super-organism', provides a strong foundation for the rest of the book. Chapters on specific diseases and clinical syndromes follow. These include environmental, viral, bacterial, fungal, and parasitic diseases that lead into sections on healthy beekeeping and clinical honeybee medicine.

The hundreds of text pages are richly illustrated with beautiful color images, helpful tables, informative charts and graphs, and easy-to-interpret original drawings by the author. The appendices are an important feature of this text and provide valuable information on honeybee biology and natural history, necessary supplies and equipment, sample collection protocols, and OIE notifiable diseases.

The timing for a comprehensive book on honeybee medicine could not be better nor could the author who has brilliantly accomplished this task. Dr Vidal-Naquet is a skilled veterinarian with nearly three decades of clinical experience, possesses a diploma in bee pathology, and is an expert apiarist with many years of hands-on proficiency and familiarity with his subject matter. This is a priceless combination that cannot be taught or learned from books or lectures. Like a delicate hive, this book was developed with passion, and nurtured with love.

Gregory A. Lewbart

Acknowledgements

This book on honeybee veterinary medicine could not have been completed without the help and support of many friends, colleagues, and associates in VetoAdom. My family was hopefully there.

I would like to thank first my mentors in honeybee pathology, Professor Monique L'Hostis, Dr Jean-Marie Barbançon and Dr M.-E. Colin, who developed graduate training in beekeeping and honeybee pathology for veterinarians at the French veterinary faculties of Oniris in Nantes and Alfort. They are the founders of honeybee veterinary medicine and practice in the frame of the 'One Health' principles. I thank and am very grateful to Dr Bernard Vallat (Director General of the OIE) and Professor Greg A. Lewbart (North Carolina State University) for their preface and foreword. Their contributions are a great honour for me.

I am very grateful to my friends and colleagues Lydia Vilagines (the best of us), Christophe Roy, and Claire Beauvais for their suggestions, advice, reviews, for the images they provided, and for encouragement when I needed this. Without their support, I am not sure this book could have been produced.

I would like to thank particularly my colleagues Dr Heike Aupperle and Professor Mariano Higes for their reviews, advice, and images.

Grateful thanks are also due to Magali Ribière, Marie-Pierre Chauzat, and Dr Stéphanie Franco (Anses Sophia-Antipolis), and to Quentin Rome and Claire Villemant (Muséum national d'Histoire naturelle, Paris) for their help and for the images.

My great thanks go also to Jon Zawislak, Instructor in Apiculture, University of Arkansas, Little Rock, for his fantastic figures of *Varroa destructor* and *Aethina tumida* life cycles, for his help, his very valuable advice, and his review of the chapter on *Aethina tumida*.

Sarah Hulbert, Senior Commissioning Editor at 5M Publishing, initiated this project. I am very grateful to her for this and for her support, assistance, and help throughout these two years. I am also grateful to the 5M Publishing editorial team and the fantastic work they achieved: Denise Power, Nick Allen, Jonathan Merrett, Alessandro Fratta Pasini, and Nicola Pickles.

Many thanks to Ian Molyneux (APHA) for his help with picture research. I would also like to thank Raymond Saunier (Beekeeping Union of Gironde, France) for pictures of the nests of the Asian hornet. I would like to thank also Nicolas Guérin for the drawings he produced for this book.

Finally, I am very grateful to my parents and my family for their support and for providing peaceful conditions in which I was able to write this book, in particular in Le Freyssinet in the French Alps.

Glossary

Alighting board A small projection or platform at the entrance of the hive.

Apiary Colonies, hives, and other equipment assembled in one location for beekeeping operations; bee yard.

Colony (honeybee colony) A group of individuals living together with biological, physiological, and behavioural characteristics. The colony must be considered as a super-organism with social features (eusociality), a complex organization, and mechanisms of homeostasis, reproduction and defence. The colony lives in the nest, where the brood is reared and where provisions are stored in wax combs.

Colony in good health Defining good colony health is not easy. However, a definition based on four points can be given:

- There is no clinical sign of disease.
- The reported brood/adult ratio is in line with the expected evolution of the colony and the time of year.
- There is foraging activity and production of honey and beebread.
- The total quantity of pollen and honey stored surrounding the brood is estimated to be in relation to the needs of the colony.

Colony weakening The definition of weakening is also quite elusive and difficult to comprehend. Weakening has been defined as 'a lack of strength of a beehive'. Weakening is linked to an unexpected decrease in bee population density and dynamics, associated with a decrease in colony activity compared with the expected seasonal activity and honeybee population. Weakening may be the consequence of a reduction of brood (surface and/or brood-comb frames) and/or of honeybee disorders and/or depopulation. Weakening is combined with a decrease or a cessation of honey production.

Colony mortality Colony mortality is defined as the death of the colony. However, a colony may also be considered dead if all the factors required for viability are missing (few bees, no brood, no queen, no food stored, etc.). The mortality of colonies may be characterized by the time of year but also by the rate of colony losses within an apiary: winter mortality of honeybee colonies 'is a normal annual seasonal phenomenon in apiaries' – depending on climate and region. A normal winter mortality of 5–15% is reported, but colony mortality during the beekeeping season is not a 'normal phenomenon in an apiary'.

Comb The wax portion of a colony in which eggs are laid, and honey and pollen are stored.

Comb foundation An artificial structure consisting of thin sheets of beeswax with the outlines of the cell bases of worker cells embossed on both sides in the same manner as they are produced naturally by honeybees.

Drifting The failure of honeybees to return to their own hive in an apiary (e.g. when the apiary contain many colonies). Drifting, along with robbing, is one means of pathogen transmission between colonies.

Foundation (wax foundation, embossed wax foundation) Thin sheets of beeswax embossed or stamped with the base of worker (or sometimes drone) cells on which bees will construct a complete comb (called a drawn comb); also referred to as comb foundation. It comes wired or unwired.

Frame A wooden rectangle, designed to hold brood and honeycombs, usually separated by a bee-sized gap in the hive body and the supers.

Hive The structure used by bees for a home.

Hive tool A flat metal device with a curved scraping surface at one end and a flat blade at the other; used to open hives, and pry apart and scrape frames.

Honeydew A material excreted by insects of the order Homoptera (aphids) which feed on plant sap. It contains almost 90% sugar, so is collected by bees and stored as honeydew honey.

Honey flow A time when nectar is plentiful and bees produce and store surplus honey.

Nucleus (nuc) A small hive of bees, usually covering two to five frames of comb, and used primarily for starting new colonies, or for rearing or storing queens.

Package bees A quantity of adult bees (usually 0.5–2 kg), with or without a queen, contained in a screened shipping cage with a food source.

Robbing Stealing of nectar, or honey, by bees from other colonies which happens when a weakened colony is unable to defend itself during a nectar dearth. Robbing, along with drifting, is one means of pathogen transmission between colonies.

Super A receptacle in which honeybees store honey; usually placed over or above the brood nest. It refers to hive bodies used for honey production (honey super).

Supersedure Rearing a new queen to replace the mother queen in the same hive; shortly after the daughter queen begins to lay eggs, the mother queen disappears.

Swarm The aggregate of worker bees, drones, and usually the old queen that leaves the parent colony to establish a new colony.

Winter cluster The arrangement of adult bees within the hive during winter (bees hanging together, forming a ball-like arrangement).

Introduction

> Or it could be that it was just the realization that treating cows and pigs and sheep and horses had a fascination I had never even suspected; and this brought with it a new concept of myself as a tiny wheel in the great machine of British agriculture. There was a kind of solid satisfaction in that.
>
> James Herriot,
> *All Creatures Great and Small*

This book, *Honeybee Veterinary Medicine:* Apis mellifera *L.*, has been written just as the apiculture sector is facing a major health crisis.

Honeybee colonies have a long history of human management and hold a special place in human life. If their more visible role is the production of honey, their major role is pollination: pollination of wild flora, with a crucial role in biodiversity, but also pollination of crops and orchards, with a fundamental role in food production. Eighty per cent of the 264 crop species cultivated in the European Union are reported to depend directly, totally or partially, on insect pollinators (including honeybees, bumblebees, wild and solitary bees), indicating just how fundamental they are to our existence (Chauzat *et al.*, 2013). Globally, the economic value of pollination is estimated to be €153 billion (Gallai *et al.*, 2008; Chauzat *et al.*, 2013) and the apiculture industry is of central importance to the world's agricultural economy.

The honeybee, *A. mellifera* L., has particular characteristics as a managed species. Firstly, the unit is the colony, which is considered as a super-organism, and not the individuals. Secondly, it is also the only managed species for which the farmer cannot control the food intake. The food resources of honeybees are the pollen and nectar of flowers and honeydew of plants they choose to gather. Thus, *A. mellifera* is totally dependent on the environment, and the management of the colonies is a challenge for the beekeeper, in particular in the face of the current health crisis.

For more than two decades, the apiculture health crisis has mainly been characterised by weakened and collapsed colonies leading to the impairment of pollination activity and honey production. There is quite general agreement on the causes of these health problems and colony losses which are thought to be linked to many stressors.

Awareness of the importance of honeybee colonies and other insect pollinators has lead worldwide governmental authorities (health, research, agriculture, etc.) to invest financial resources in particular to develop basic and diagnostic research but also epidemiological surveillance networks. The aims are to understand what is going on with honeybee colonies and other pollinators, the causes of their troubles, and how to control or mitigate these problems.

Because of the double role played by honeybees, i.e. in pollination and food production, honeybee health is a challenge for many sectors involving basic research and universities, and spanning the fields of industry, agronomy and agriculture: beekeepers of course, crop/orchard farmers, agronomic institutes, research and diagnosis laboratories, agricultural authorities, health authorities, official veterinarians, chemical and pharmaceutical industries, not forgetting non-governmental organisations and other environmental associations, and finally the veterinary profession (officials, researchers, practitioners).

For historical reasons, veterinarians and particularly practitioners have tended not to be greatly involved in honeybee health. If the veterinary profession and in particular practitioners have so far taken little interest in this managed species, many veterinarians in Europe are increasingly conscious of the stakes involved in the current health crisis. In France, a degree course was created in 2006 in order to train veterinarians in honeybee pathology. So far, approximately 120 French veterinarians have been trained and graduated, allowing an involvement of practitioners in the field. Other European countries, including Italy and Germany, have also instituted training for veterinarians in honeybee pathology. It must be recognized, however, that beekeepers tend not to be keen on seeking the help of a practitioner as is done in other husbandry sectors.

Nevertheless, the veterinary profession is involved in several aspects of the beekeeping sector (Vidal-Naquet and Roy, 2014):

- Official veterinarians are beekeepers' main interlocutors concerning notifiable diseases, suspected poisoning in colonies, and veterinary public health.
- Veterinarian researchers working in public laboratories and organisations, e.g European Union Reference Laboratory for Bee Health[1] (Sophia-Antipolis Laboratory), EFSA.[2]
- Lecturers and researchers in higher-education and research agronomic institutes and veterinary universities.
- Veterinarian pathologists and biologists.
- Veterinarians in the pharmaceutical industry producing veterinary medicines for bee diseases.
- Veterinarian practitioners.

Considering the health crisis facing the apicultural sector, veterinarian practitioners almost certainly ought to be associated with the health management of beekeeping farms in the same way as they are in other husbandries. This was implicitly recognised and supported by the OIE[3] in a book it published entitled *Bee Health and Veterinarians* (edited by Wolfgang Ritter) in 2014.

Veterinarians, and in particular practitioners competent in honeybee pathology, are trained and have professional experience in clinical examination, diagnosis, prophylactic methods, control of diseases, but also pharmacology and health management. Furthermore, as animal health professionals, veterinarians have the professional prerogative of being able to prescribe veterinary medicines. The veterinary profession is a part of the One World–One Health principles (FAO/OIE/WHO, 2009; One Health Initiative, 2014). The One Health principles are 'a worldwide strategy for expanding interdisciplinary collaborations and communications in all aspects of health care for humans, animals and the environment' (One Health Initiative, 2014). *Apis mellifera* is symbolic of the One World–One Health principles (FAO/OIE/WHO, 2009; One Health Initiative, 2014): it is a species dependent on the environment and is affected by a health crisis that is likely to impair human feeding, livelihoods, and welfare in the future.

As they are managing a food-producing reared species, using veterinary medicines and trading products of the hive (honey, pollen, propolis, wax, venom) as well as honeybees (queens, nuclei, package bees), beekeepers should consider veterinarians and, in particular

[1] European Union Reference Laboratory for Bee Health (Sophia-Antipolis Laboratory), Les Templiers, 105 route des Chappes, BP 111, F-06902 Sophia-Antipolis Cedex, France. The laboratory's main activities are wide-ranging, covering the major bee diseases (parasitic, bacteriological, and virological) as well as exotic diseases (insects and acari) which threaten the bee population. In accordance with the requirements of the European Commission, the Laboratory is also tasked with investigating the causes of bee colony poisoning incidents. https://eurl-milk.anses.fr/en/minisite/abeilles/eurl-bee-health-home.

[2] European Food Safety Authority, via Carlo Magno 1A, 43126 Parma, Italy. EFSA's role is to assess and communicate on all risks associated with the food chain. Since EFSA's advice serves to inform the policies and decisions of risk managers, a large part of its work is undertaken in response to specific requests for scientific advice. Requests for scientific assessments are received from the European Commission, the European Parliament, and EU Member States. http://www.efsa.europa.eu/en/topics/topic/beehealth.htm.

[3] OIE: World Organisation for Animal Health, 12 rue de Prony, 75017 Paris, France. One of the OIE's main missions is to ensure the transparency of the world animal health situation. www.oie.int.

practitioners competent in beekeeping and honeybee pathology, as an asset, especially given the problems that currently exist.

As already noted, colony losses, weakening, or collapse are considered to be a consequence of many stressors: environment and climate, intoxications, pathogenic agents (viral, bacterial, parasitic, pests), parasites and in particular the mite *Varroa destructor*, beekeeping practices, global apiculture trade and exchanges. Some of the diseases affecting honeybee colonies are notifiable diseases and pests to the OIE.

In European countries, the only veterinary medicines permitted for honeybees are those controlling *Varroa* infestation. Other kinds of medicines, e.g. antibiotics, are not allowed in the European Union but are permitted in other countries (e.g. USA and Canada). The safety of the products of hives depends on good practices concerning the prescription and use of veterinary medicines and drugs. It also depends on the residues of pesticides used on crops and orchards pollinated by bees.

Considering notifiable diseases and the associated mandatory health measures, and considering the potential risks of residues of medicines and pesticides in the products of hives, the honeybee sector, like other animal farming sectors, also raises question of veterinary public health, in which veterinarians must clearly play a central role (Vidal-Naquet and Roy, 2014). Thus, honeybee veterinary medicine has become a great challenge for the veterinary profession, in particular for practitioners.

Many books, basic research publications, and epidemiological surveillance studies are published each year on honeybee biology and physiology, honeybee health, and honeybee problems – all these are strong and fundamental sources of information and knowledge. This book has been written with the aim of presenting the diseases and health troubles found in honeybee colonies as a veterinary text because *A. mellifera* is a managed species. It aims to present a detailed overview of the veterinary medicine of the honeybee.

This is not a zoology and biology textbook; however, the first chapter aims to provide the main characteristics of the biology of *A. mellifera* which are of significance in the field of honeybee pathology. The subsequent chapters describe the intoxications, diseases, pests, and syndromes affecting honeybee colonies, following a standard veterinary pattern with the description of the disease, the causes (environment, human, chemicals, bacteria, viruses, parasites, fungus, pests), the pathogenesis, the epidemiological and transmission characteristics, the clinical signs, the diagnosis, the control and the prophylactic methods for dealing with diseases or problems occurring in hives. *Honeybee Veterinary Medicine* describes how to perform a clinical examination of a honeybee colony and a health audit of a honeybee farm. A chapter is also dedicated to essential sanitary beekeeping practices. The appendices of the book contain tables presenting biological data on honeybee colonies, the diseases which are notifiable to the OIE and to European countries, the methods of sampling, and a practical method for a health audit of an apiary.

Honeybee Veterinary Medicine has been written with the hope that it will be a valuable guide to veterinary students, veterinarians, professionals, and other stakeholders in charge of the medical care and welfare of honeybees.

References

Chauzat, M.-P., Cauquil, L., Roy, L., Franco, S., Hendrikx, P., and Ribière-Chabert, M. (2013) Demographics of the European apicultural industry. *PLoS ONE*, 8(11): e79018. doi:10.1371/journal.pone.0079018

FAO, OIE, WHO (2009) One World, One Health. Available at: http://www.oie.int/doc/ged/d6296.pdf (accessed 2 November 2014).

Gallai, N., Salles, J.M., Settele, J., and Vaissière, B. (2008) Economic valuation of the vulnerability of word agriculture confronted with pollinator decline. *Ecological Economics*, 68: 810–821.

One Health Initiative (2014) About the One Health Initiative. Available at: http://onehealthinitiative.com/about.php (accessed 2 November 2014).

Vidal-Naquet, N. and Roy, C. (2014) The veterinary profession: an asset to the bee-keeping sector. *Bulletin of the OIE*, 2014-2: 9–12.

1

Biology of *Apis mellifera* L.: from the individual to the super-organism

The honeybee, *Apis mellifera* Linneaus, 1758, is a social insect belonging to the order Hymenoptera. The social aspect of the honeybee is crucial for understanding this species, which comprises individuals living within a colony. The biology of *Apis mellifera* L. is the consequence of complex interactions between individual features and the relationship between adult honeybees (Figures 1.1 and 1.2). Understanding the biology of *A. mellifera* means understanding both individual and colony features and in particular social ones. The biology of *A. mellifera* and its particular characteristics are fundamental for beekeeping husbandry, and essential to understanding, diagnosing, and controlling honeybee colony diseases.

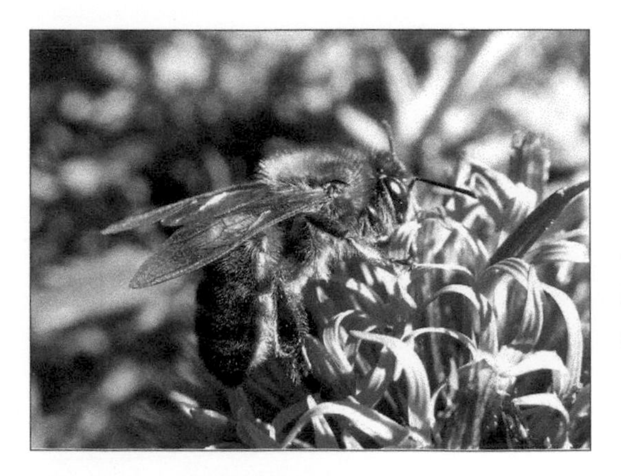

Figure 1.1 *Apis mellifera* L. is a social insect. Picture of an individual (outside worker/forager). (© Nicolas Vidal-Naquet.)

1 Taxonomy and natural history

1.1 Taxonomy

A bee is defined as any insect belonging to the order Hymenoptera and the superfamily *Apoidea.* Bees include both solitary and social species and are characterized by pollen-collecting structures on the hind legs or on the abdomen, and by sucking and chewing mouthparts for gathering nectar and pollen.

Apis mellifera L. (tribe Apini) is classified into the sub-family Apinae, with orchid bees (Euglossoni), bumblebees (Bombini), and stingless bees (Meliponinae) (Winston, 1987).

They belong to the phylum Arthropoda, the class Insecta, the order Hymenoptera, the superfamily Apoidea, and the family Apidae. The Apidae are characterized by a pollen basket on the third leg (on worker bees at least), and present

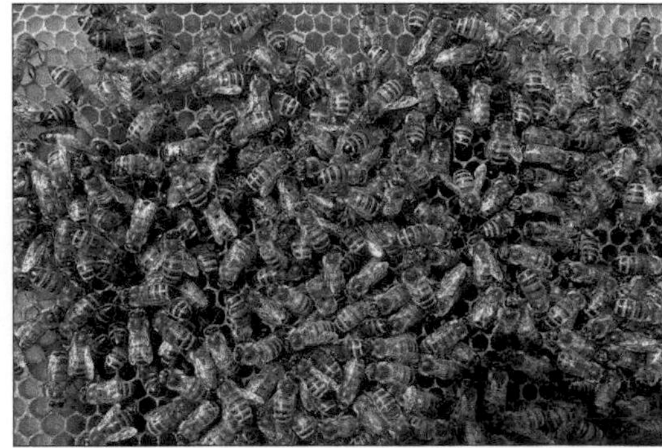

Figure 1.2 *Apis mellifera* L. is a social insect. Picture of a comb with nest worker bees and the queen. (© Nicolas Vidal-Naquet.)

a more or less developed social behaviour. The genus *Apis* is characterized by social behaviour, a perennial colony, and a nest built from wax in which immature forms (the brood) are reared and provisions (honey and pollen) are stored.

The genus *Apis* is the only member of the Apini tribe. *Apis* is considered to be represented today only by five to nine species according to taxonomists (Winston, 1987; Grimaldi and Engel, 2005). Taxonomic studies in the genus *Apis* and inside each species require DNA and mitochondrial (mt) DNA research (Engel, 1999a, b) in addition to morphological studies (wings veins, colour, pilosity, size) (Le Conte, 2006a). The honeybee found in western countries is *Apis mellifera* L. The Indian honeybee *Apis cerana*, the dwarf honeybee *Apis florea*, and the giant honeybees *Apis dorsata* and *Apis laboriosa* are eastern species. The other species, *Apis andreniformis, Apis nigrocinta, Apis nuluentis*, and *Apis koschewnikovi*, also live in Asia (Le Conte, 2006a).

Apis mellifera is very close to *A. cerana* in morphology and behaviour. However, the colonies of *A. mellifera* are larger than those of *A. cerana* (up to 100,000 bees vs. 7,000 bees) (Winston, 1987).

Of all these species, *A. mellifera* has the most interesting behaviour for rearing and apiculture. European strains of *A. mellifera* reared around the world are called European honeybees. African species of *A. mellifera* are called Africanized honeybees.

Colonies of European honeybee have been introduced throughout the world (and in Asia too). In managed colonies, processes of selection have been implemented by beekeepers to obtain favourable and optimal characters for apiculture – indeed, certain features are actively sought in beekeeping practice, including honey gathering, gentle behaviour, and non-swarming behaviour.

There are many variations of *A. mellifera*, defining in particular subspecies or strains (behaviour, colour, and size according to habitats, adaptation to local conditions, etc.) (Ruttner, 1988).

1.2 *Apis mellifera* L. natural history

Bees are thought to have appeared by divergence from sphecoid wasps about 100 million years ago (in the middle Cretaceous period). At the same time angiosperm plants became the dominant vegetation (Winston, 1987).

The evolution of angiosperm vegetation and the evolution of bees are believed to be linked: colour, odour, shape, excess nectar, and pollen attract bees, which became increasingly adapted to pollination over the millennia. Primitive bees were short-tongued, while more evolutionarily advanced bees have longer tongues. *Apis mellifera* is a long-tongued bee species (Le Conte, 2006a).

MtDNA studies suggest that the geographic origin of *A. mellifera* is the Middle East region (Garnery *et al.*, 1992; Le Conte, 2006a). There, the species is supposed to have divided into three branches: M, developing mainly in north and western Europe; C, developing mainly in southern Europe and the north Mediterranean sea; and A, developing mainly in Africa. MtDNA studies in *A. mellifera* species have confirmed these three mitochondrial lines:

- M (west Mediterranean);
- C (north Mediterranean);
- A (Spain, France, Algeria, Congo, Malawi) (Garnery *et al.*, 1992).

Within these branches, subspecies are defined that have their own morphological and behavioural features, allowing adaptation of *A. mellifera* to local environments. Studies on mitochondrial markers (mtDNA) and single-nucleotide polymorphisms (SNPs) may provide an explanation for the evolutionary lineages and hydridization, and enable us to understand the genetic profiles of the subspecies (De La Rua *et al.*, 2009).

1.3 *Apis mellifera* L. subspecies (Winston, 1987; Le Conte, 2006a; De La Rua *et al.*, 2009)

1.3.1 Main European subspecies

Apis mellifera mellifera is the dark honeybee of Europe (particularly distributed in northern

Europe and from France to Russia). These honeybees are medium to large with a relatively short tongue. Their dark-coloured body gives rise to their name: dark bee or black bee. *Apis mellifera mellifera* is adapted to its local environment. These honeybees are reported to present a relatively aggressive behaviour though are not likely to swarm. They are considered to be strongly resistant to cold weather. Because of their short tongue, they are not able to gather nectar in long corolla flowers (Winston, 1987). *Apis m. mellifera* is reported to be sensitive to brood diseases.

With the development of global apiculture and for a variety of beekeeping management reasons, in particular to improve honey production, to encourage hygienic and docile behaviour, and queen-rearing abilities but also because of the health crisis, beekeepers have selected and/or reared some strains and subspecies that are not necessarily adapted to local conditions. They are also often compelled to rear species 'foreign' to their environment, because of the health crisis in their apiaries and the difficulty of finding local *A. m. mellifera*. These 'foreign' subspecies and strains need certain conditions for rearing, in particular in the following generations (as in the case of the Buckfast honeybee described below). They may also hybridize with local black honeybees, which risks impairing the abilities of these local strains Currently, it seems that beekeepers are trying more and more, with the help of scientists, to rear local honeybee subspecies adapted to their local environmental conditions.

Apis mellifera ligustica is the Italian honeybee, also called the yellow bee. This is one of the most widely reared subspecies in beekeeping. These honeybees are medium shaped with long tongues, and are mostly 'yellow' or golden. They have gentle and high honey-gathering behaviours. They are not likely to swarm but seem more prone to robbing behaviour than other subspecies. They need more stock during winter because they overwinter in large colonies. It is a popular species in apiculture, and in particular in selection rearing.

Apis mellifera carnica, or the Carniolan bee, is distributed in middle and central–eastern Europe: the eastern Alps, Slovenia and the northern Balkans. These honeybees are large with long tongues. They are a dark bee that exhibits gentle behaviour (greatly appreciated by beekeepers). *Apis m. carnica* tends to swarm easily (Imdorf *et al.*, 2010). It is a honeybee adapted to cold winters, and overwinters in small clusters. *Apis m. carnica* is reported to be sensitive to nosemosis and acariosis.

Apis mellifera caucasica, the Caucasian bee, is a honeybee living from the Caucasus to the Black Sea. These honeybees are large with very long tongues. This dark grey bee tends to have a very gentle behaviour and does not tend to swarm. *Apis m. caucasica* is reported to be sensitive to nosemosis and acariosis in particular during overwintering.

Apis mellifera macedonia is distributed over Bulgaria, Greece, Romania, Ukraine, and Turkey. *Apis mellifera iberiensis* is the local bee living in the Iberian peninsula.

1.3.2 Main Eastern Europe and Middle East subspecies

Apis mellifera anatolica is distributed in Anatolia in Asia Minor. It is found mainly in Turkey and Iraq. It is a yellow bee (sometimes darkening) with an aggressive behaviour.

Apis mellifera syriaca, the Syrian honeybee, found in the Near East and Israel, is an orange-coloured bee. *Apis m. syriaca* is an aggressive bee adapted to the hot weather and very sensitive to cold.

Apis mellifera armeniaca (Armenia) and *Apis mellifera meda* (Iraq, Turkey, Iran) are also oriental subspecies.

1.3.3 Main African subspecies

The main distribution area of *Apis mellifera scutellata* is east Africa (Hepburn and Crewe, 1991). It is a small, yellow, very aggressive bee with a clear swarming and nest-absconding inclination. This honeybee was imported into Brazil in 1956 as part of a breeding programme to adapt the species to local environmental conditions (temperature in particular). Unfortunately, aggressive behaviour and a tendency to swarm and abscond (together with their ability to fly long distances) have been transmitted via this hybridization programme. The consequences are relentless migration from Brazil to the United States and dangerous, in some cases fatal, attacks on humans and animals (Mitchell, 2006).

Apis mellifera capensis lives in South Africa (Hepburn and Crewe, 1991). It is a gentle blackish honeybee. *Apis m. capensis* possesses some unique biological features: worker bees can lay down viable female diploid eggs. If reared in queen cells, these can become fertile queens. The Cape honeybee is adapted to the fynbos biome – the ecoregion that is characteristic of South Africa.

Apis mellifera adansonni lives over a large part of west Africa. Like *A. m. scutellata* it is a yellow, aggressive honeybee with a clear inclination to swarm and to abscond. *Apis mellifera sahariensis* lives in the northern Sahara and is adapted to large temperature fluctuations between –10°C and 50°C. *Apis mellifera intermissa* (Morocco, Libya, Tunisia) is very aggressive but adapted to local extreme conditions. *Apis m. major* (Morocco), *Apis m. lamarckii* (Sudan and Egypt), and *Apis m. nubica* (Sudan) are other African subspecies.

1.3.4 The Buckfast honeybee: a human-selected honeybee

Because of its large genetic variability, *A. mellifera* is adapted to many environmental conditions. Thus, beekeepers as well as queen breeders are always trying to improve the potential of honeybees for both economic and behavioural reasons: nectar and pollen gathering, royal jelly production, sensitivity to diseases, swarming tendency, docility, etc. (Le Conte, 2006a).

An 'artificial strain', the Buckfast honeybee, was 'created' in England. In the 1920s, honeybee colonies in the British Isles were being devastated by the endoparasitic tracheal mite *Acarapis woodi* (Beesource, 2014). A beekeeper monk at Buckfast Abbey (Devon, England), Brother Adam, decided to create a bee stock that could withstand this deadly disease. After travelling and learning about local bees in Europe and Africa, he created a strain of bees, largely from the Italian race, but adapted to the environmental conditions of the British Isles, with good foraging ability for nectar and pollen. Buckfast honeybees also have a lower tendency to swarm than many other varieties. The bees exhibit good house-cleaning and grooming behaviours and are reported to be resistant to *A. woodi*. This artificial strain of honeybee presents a docile behaviour and a quiet attitude on the frames. However, if left unmanaged for one or two generations, the Buckfast bee can revert to aggressive behaviour.

The Buckfast honeybee is very popular among beekeepers worldwide because of its docility and gathering ability.

2 The colony: definition and characteristics

Apis mellifera is a social insect. Individual features and a social organization characterize the biology of the honeybee colony. If one bee is an individual with its own characteristics, the colony is the unit. The colony must be considered as a super-organism with social features, a complex organization, and mechanisms of homeostasis, reproduction, and defence.

The colony lives in the nest, where the brood is reared and provisions stored. The nest is made up of hexagonal honeycombs built with the wax produced by the wax glands of the workers.

2.1 Features of the colony

The colony possesses the following features:

- The presence of three castes of individuals that exhibit various morphologies. A caste can be defined as a physically distinct individual or group of individuals specialized to perform certain functions within the colony. The three castes are: the queen, the only fertile female within the colony; the workers, which are

sterile females; and the drones (Winston, 1987).
- The brood, which is composed of developing juveniles also called immature forms (eggs, larvae, pupae) reared in hexagonal wax cells.
- Resources (honey, pollen) stored in hexagonal wax cells.

The colony is considered to be perennial. This means that once formed the colony continues from year to year, surviving through the winter; adults live together in the nest and are interdependent, unable to survive alone or isolated from the other honeybees.

The queen is in charge of reproduction and is the mother of all the workers (and drones) of the colony. During their lifespan the workers have successively different tasks, beginning with indoor tasks (cleaners, nurses, builders, etc.) and ending with outdoors ones (guards, foragers) (Winston, 1987). The drones are supposed to have only one task: fertilization of virgin queens.

The colony, as a super-organism, may divide into two colonies by swarming, allowing the species to spread.

2.2 Eusociality

The social organization of honeybee colonies (and other insects, in particular of the order Hymenoptera) is also called 'eusociality' (from the Greek *eu-* meaning 'good/real' + 'society'). Eusocial insects such as honeybees are mainly defined by four characteristics (Crespi and Yanega, 1995; Costa and Fitzgerald, 2005; Plowes, 2010):

- The adults live in a nest (the colony).
- There is a clear division of labour between sexual (queen, drones) and sterile individuals (workers).
- There is an overlap of adult generations.
- Adults (the workers) share the rearing of the brood (immature forms).

The order Hymenoptera is the largest group with social species. Some bees, wasps and ants are eusocial animals. The haplodiploid sex determination system (cf. section 10.3 below) may contribute to kin selection, favouring altruistic behaviour in this group (Winston, 1987).

3 The castes: morphology

Honeybees are insects with a head, a thorax, and an abdomen. As Hymenoptera, they have two pairs of wings, the forewings and the hind-wings, connected by a series of hooks (the hamuli). The well-developed mandibles of Hymenoptera allow capture of prey (hornets, wasps, ants) and/or nest shaping (honeybees). In all Hymenoptera, the maxillae and labium are united by a membrane and form a kind of tube that allows the aspiration of liquids (Winston, 1987).

Within the colony, the castes have their own roles:

- The queen ensures reproduction by positioning the eggs within the cells.
- The drones fertilize the virgin queens.
- The workers are in charge of the labouring tasks in the colony.

The following sections describe the anatomy of the three castes, beginning with the workers as the basic model. Then, the particularities of the queen and the drones will be described.

3.1 The workers

The workers (Figure 1.1) constitute the largest population in the colony (10,000 during the overwintering period winter to approximately 60,000 during the active season according to the strain, the strength, and the distribution range of the colonies) (Winston, 1987, Le Conte, 2006b).

The body of a worker is on average 15 mm long, with wings the length of the abdomen. It is divided into three segmented parts: the head, thorax, and abdomen. The body is supported by an exoskeleton. The main functions of the exoskeleton (cuticle) are to serve as a barrier to the outside medium, and to provide armour (mechanical protection), protection against dehydration, and muscle attachments.

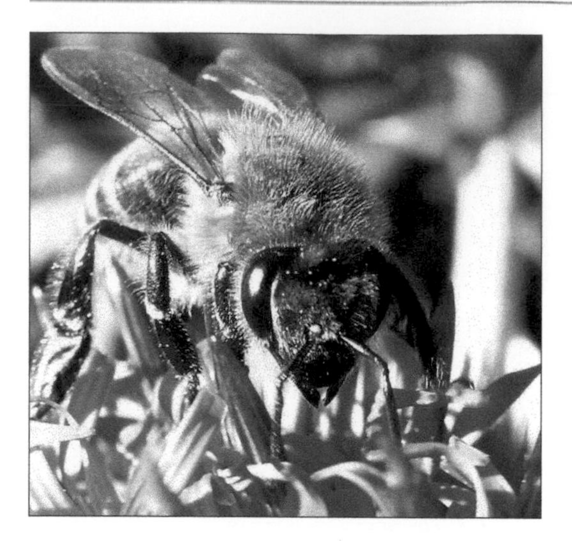

Figure 1.3 Photograph of a head of a worker honeybee showing the compound eyes, one of the three ocelli, the antennae, and one anatomical feature of the mouthparts: the mandibles. (© Nicolas Vidal-Naquet.)

3.1.1 The head

The head (Figures 1.3 and 1.4) allows ingestion, partial digestion of food, and feeding through well-developed mouthparts (long proboscis and mandibles) and food-producing and 'salivary' glands. The head also plays a major sensory role through the eyes (compound eyes and ocelli), antennae, and hairs.

Mouthparts: chewing and lapping (sucking)

The mandibles are adapted to chewing (e.g. wax) and the proboscis to sucking up nectar or honeydew (Figures 1.5 and 1.6). The mandibles are located on either the side of the mouth. They are strong and act like a pair of pliers. They play a major role in nest construction (manipulating wax and propolis), ingestion (pollen), feeding larvae and the queen, but also in cleaning, grooming, and fighting (Winston, 1987). A duct runs from the mandibles to the mandibular glands. The mandibular glands play a crucial role in particular in brood feeding, queen feeding, and, in the queen, in the secretion of pheromone (queen mandibular pheromone, QMP) (Dade, 2009).

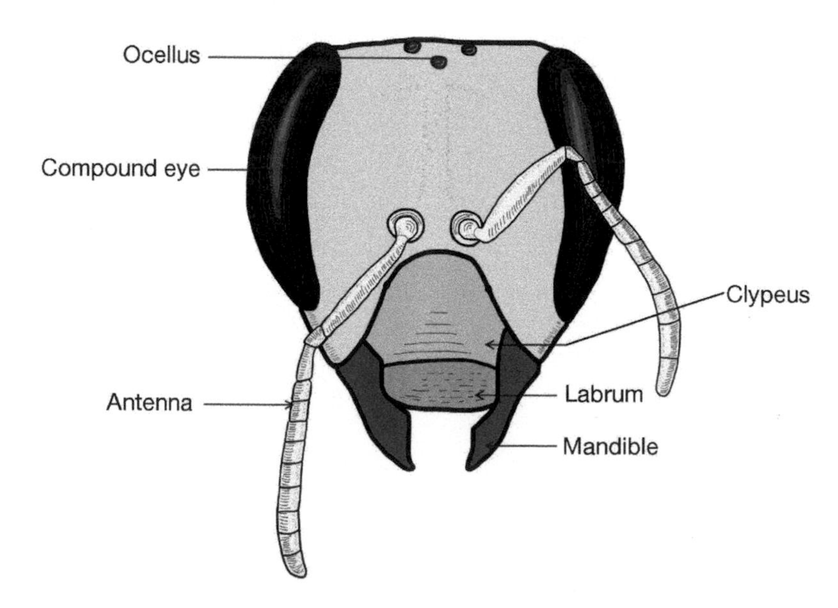

Figure 1.4 External anatomy (front view) of a worker bee. (© Nicolas Vidal-Naquet. Anatomy of the head (front view) redrawn from Snodgrass, 1910; Dade, 2009.)

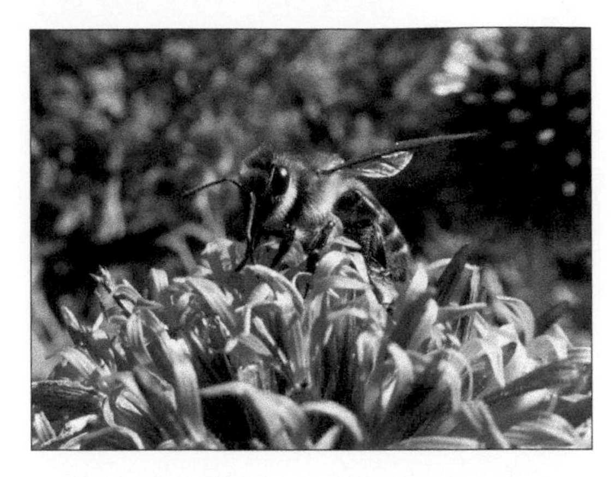

Figure 1.5 Picture of a forager bee presenting an extended proboscis sucking up nectar. (© Nicolas Vidal-Naquet.)

The proboscis is situated at the base of the mouth and is composed of the glossa, maxilla, labium, and flabellum parts. It functions like a straw, allowing liquid ingestion (nectar, honey, and water) but also trophallaxis, i.e. mouth-to-mouth transfer of food or other fluids among individuals within the colony. Liquid exchanges by trophallaxis occur between workers, workers and the queen, or/and workers and drones. When extended, the proboscis can reach 7.2 mm (Ruttner *et al.*, 1978; Winston, 1987).

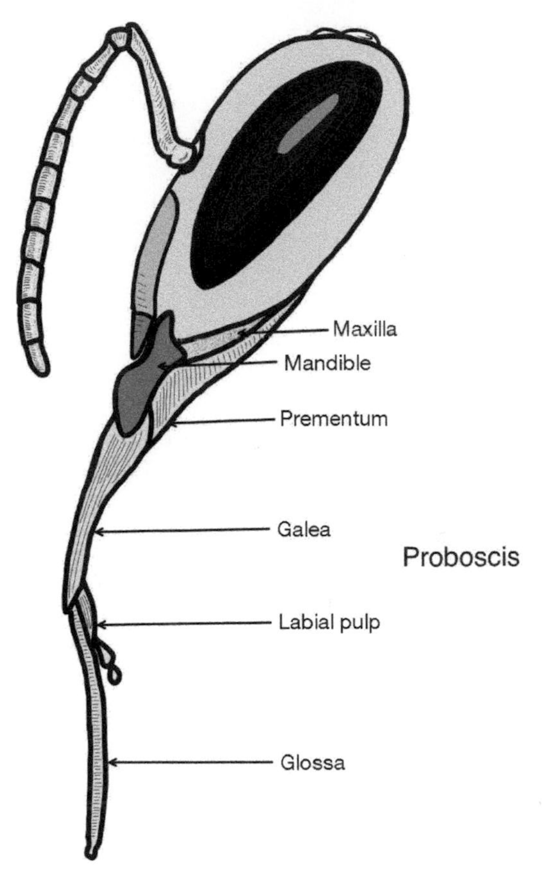

Figure 1.6 External anatomy (lateral view) of the head of a worker bee with the proboscis extended. (© Nicolas Vidal-Naquet, redrawn from Snodgrass, 1910; Dade, 2009.)

Sensory organs and the peripheral nervous system

Honeybees have two types of eyes, the compound eyes and the ocelli (Snodgrass, 1910; Winston, 1987). The compound eyes are composed of ommatidia. Each ommatidium has the structure of an eye, i.e. a transparent cornea, a crystalline cone, photoreceptor cells, and an optic nerve. Thus, each ommatidium provides the brain with a single picture element. The brain forms an image from these picture elements. Ommatidia are hexagonal in cross section, giving the compound eyes their typical aspect.

Three ocelli are disposed in a triangle at the front and top of the head. Ocelli register in particular light intensity and duration. At dusk, the ocelli estimate the level of increasing darkness, inciting foragers to return to their hives (University of Illinois, 2007).

The antennae are comprised of a ten-segment flagellum, a pedicel, and a scape attached at the base. They are involved in the smelling of volatile substances, in the sensory perception of vibrations and the movement of air, and in detecting sounds, temperature (the five terminal segments of the flagellum), and humidity (the eight terminal segments of the flagellum). There are seven types of sensory structures, known as sensilla, on the antennae (pits, plates, and hairs) (Winston, 1987). A sensillum is composed of one or more sense cells with a fibre connected to the central nervous system (CNS) and with a distal end in close connection with the cuticle. The sensillum structure is also characterized by one or two accessory cells and a structure issuing from the cuticle.

On the pedicel, the Johnston's organ is involved in the perception of changes in the position of the antennae and in measuring flight speed (by detection and analysis of vibrations of the antennae) (Heran, 1959; Winston, 1987; Dade, 2009).

3.1.2 The thorax

The thorax can be considered as the 'motor' of the honeybee, carrying the wings and the legs, and the associated strong muscles inside. The thorax is composed of three body segments merged with the first abdominal segment.

The legs

There are three pairs of legs, one per thoracic segment (Snodgrass, 1910). The terminal structures (claws and pad) of the legs are adapted for walking on horizontal and vertical surfaces. These structures also allow the bee to hang onto other bees (e.g. on combs, while swarming, or in a cluster). The legs also play a role in grooming as well as in packing and transporting pollen and propolis (Winston, 1987) (Figure 1.7).

The hairy brushes of the forelegs are used for head cleaning (removing pollen, dust, etc.). A further structure is used for cleaning the antennae: the antenna cleaner at the junction of the tibia and the basitarsus.

The hairy middle legs too are involved in cleaning, but also in the transfer of pollen and propolis from the first leg and the body to the hind leg.

The hind leg is adapted to the transportation of pollen and propolis back to the hive. The pollen basket, also called the corbicula, is situated on the outer surface of the tibia (Hodges, 1952; Winston, 1987). It is a polished cavity surrounded by a fringe of hairs, into which the pollen is placed in the form of a sticky ball. The pollen rake placed on the inner edge of the tibia, the pollen combs, and the pollen press situated on the inner surface of the basitarsus enable the pollen to be packed before transportation.

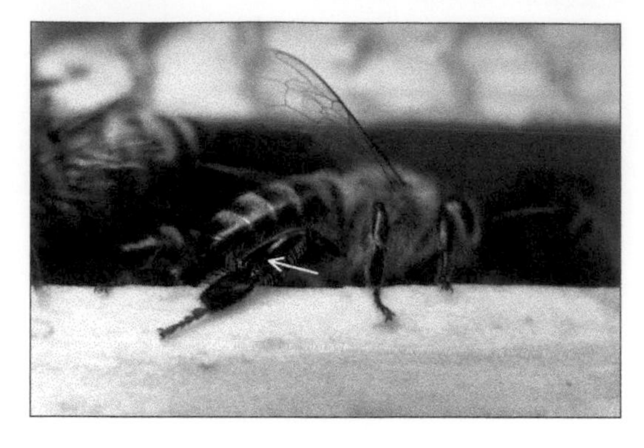

Figure 1.7 The legs of a honeybee *Apis mellifera*. The hind legs are adapted to transportation back to the hive of pollen or propolis in a structure called the corbicula or pollen basket (arrow). (© Nicolas Vidal-Naquet.)

Pollen is gathered from flowers actively by the proboscis and passively by the hairs of the body. The pollen is mixed with gathered nectar and salivary secretions and becomes progressively a sticky ball. The forelegs brush the proboscis and groom the head and thorax in order to collect the pollen. Then, in flight, the sticky substance is transferred to the middle legs and then to the hind legs where the pollen is stored as a sticky ball in the pollen basket.

The wings

There are two pairs of wings arising from the thorax. They are articulated with complex joints and hinges allowing a multitude of movements. The forewings are larger than the hind wings.

The front and hind wings can connect together by hooks, also called hamuli, in order to beat in synchrony during flight. The wing beating reaches a rate of over 200 cycles/second and the bee's average speed is around 24 km/hour (Winston, 1987).

The thoracic musculature is composed of longitudinal and vertical muscles and provides the strength and wing movements for the flight (Winston, 1987; Dade, 2009). These muscles, by their contraction, are also able to provide heat and to maintain a high temperature of 46°C within the thorax. During wintering, the contraction of these muscles serves to help maintain homeostasis in the winter cluster of the colony; the energy is provided by the honey ingested and stored in the stomach.

Flying muscles are essential for adult bees. In order to reach high wing-beat frequencies (which are limited by the refractory period of neural action potential), bees have so-called 'indirect' (also called 'asynchronous') flight muscles. These contract independently without receiving a new nerve impulse. These muscles move the wings indirectly through the deformation of the thoracic exoskeleton which transmits this power to the wings. Longitudinal muscles move the wings downwards. Dorsoventral muscles move the wings up (Heike Aupperle, personal communication, 2014).

3.1.3 The abdomen

The abdomen of the worker comprises nine segments, two of them being highly reduced (and associated with the sting of the worker or the reproductive organs of the queen or the drone) (Snodgrass, 1910). The abdominal segments or sclerites are constituted of two plates (dorsal and ventral) connected by membranes. This gives the abdomen the ability to dilate, which is important for nectar harvesting and carrying. The abdomen is usually hairy.

Wax glands are located on the inner side of the fourth to seventh sternites. There are four pairs of wax glands, producing beeswax for comb construction and cell capping.

The sting is a feature of the worker. It is an ovipositor adapted to defence. The sting consists of three parts: a stylus and two barbed slides (or lancets), one on either side of the stylus.

The sting is found in a chamber at the end of the abdomen, from which only the sharp-pointed shaft protrudes. The shaft is a hollow tube, like a hypodermic needle (Winston, 1987), and barbed so that it sticks in the skin of the victim. When the stinger is not in use, it is retracted within the sting chamber of the abdomen. The shaft is turned up so that its basis is concealed. The sting is connected to a venom gland and to glands that produce alarm pheromone.

After stinging, the worker bee loses its sting together with the venom gland, resulting in poisoning of the victim. The worker bee then dies.

Inside the abdomen, workers have an atrophied and non-functional reproductive system, which can produce eggs under certain conditions (e.g. in some cases following the death of the queen, when the colony is not able to rear a new queen).

3.2 The queen

Usually, the queen is unique in a colony and is the mother of all the workers and drones living in the colony. The (main) role of the queen is to lay eggs within the cells of the nest. The honeybee queen is always surrounded by a retinue of workers, known as the queen retinue (Free *et al.*, 1992). This retinue is composed of 6–10 workers (Allen, 1957), whose main role is feeding the queen by trophallaxis.

The queen is generally about 20 mm long, with a large abdomen and wings shorter than its body (Snodgrass, 1910).

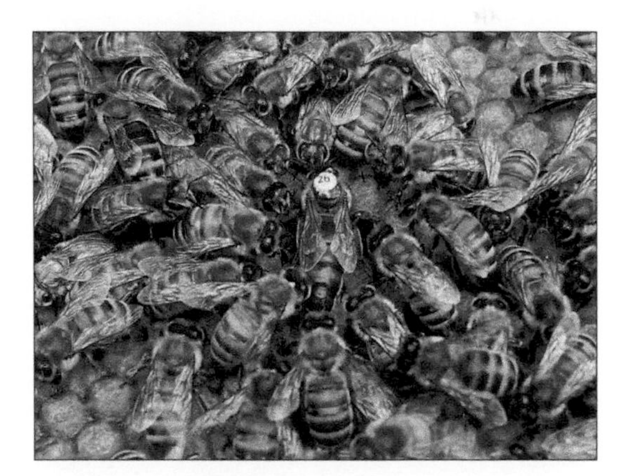

Figure 1.8 The queen presents a larger abdomen and smaller head and wings. In this picture, the queen is surrounded by the retinue of workers. In a managed colony the queen is marked by painting a colour on her thorax as a record of the year of her birth and to make it easier to find her. (© Nicolas Vidal-Naquet.)

The head of the queen is small, and her eyes poorly developed. The proboscis is shorter than those of the workers. On the thorax, the three pairs of legs are similar, and lack a pollen-collecting structure.

The abdomen is large, with a developed reproductive system inside. There are no wax glands.

The reproductive system of a queen consists of two large pyriform ovaries composed of 150–180 ovarioles which produce the eggs (Winston, 1987; Dade, 2009). The eggs pass through the ovaries into the oviducts. The oviducts open into the vagina and the bursa copularis, through which the eggs travel before being laid in cells. A spermatheca opens into the vagina via a duct and an opening valve. The spermatheca is a spherical sac and can hold up to seven million spermatozoa in a mated queen (Dade, 2009). Spermatozoa are stored for the lifetime of the mated queen until used for fertilization. Fertilization occurs when the valve opens and releases spermatozoa as the eggs are on their way through the vagina.

The honeybee queen has a curved and smooth stinger firmly attached to the abdomen. The queen does not die after stinging because the sting is smooth and can be retracted after use. A larger poison sac than in workers is present in the sting apparatus. The queen stings rivals in some circumstances. The queen may fly in some circumstances such as the nuptial flight (when virgin) and during swarming (section 13 below).

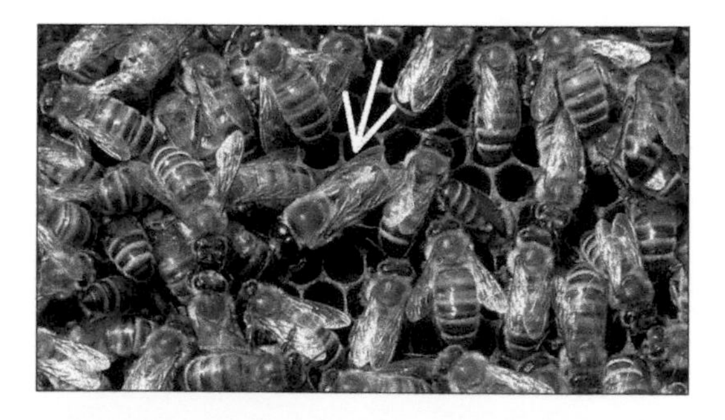

Figure 1.9 The body of the drone is stocky, and the wings cover and extend past the abdomen. The compound eyes are well developed and join behind the occiput. (© Nicolas Vidal-Naquet.)

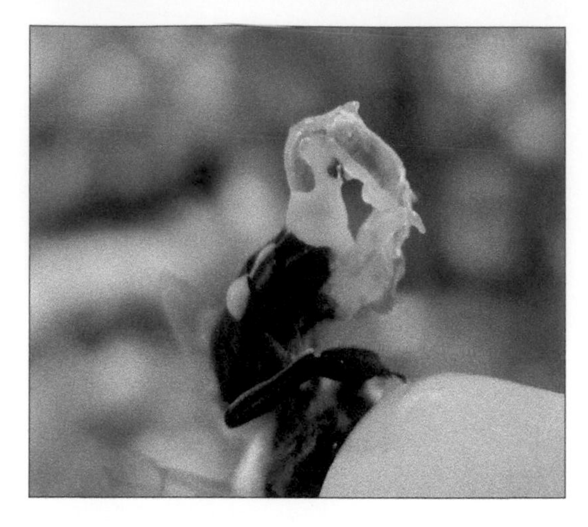

Figure 1.10 Endophallus (shown here everted by manual pressure). (© Nicolas Vidal-Naquet.)

3.3 The drones

The drones are mainly present in spring and autumn. The body is stocky, about 19 mm long, with wings covering and extending past the abdomen (Figure 1.9). On the head, the compound eyes are more developed than those in the other castes and join behind the occiput. The compound eyes have more facets than those of the workers. Otherwise, the proboscis is short, and the mandibles small (Snodgrass, 1910; Winston, 1987).

The three pairs of legs are similar and lack a pollen-collecting structure. The thoracic muscles of drones are thicker and stronger than those of workers.

Drone anatomy is adapted to flight and to mating with the queen. The drone genital organ consists in a large internal and evaginable endophallus (Figure 1.10). The spermatozoa are produced in the testes and stored in the seminal glands. The spermatozoa are ejaculated along with mucus produced by the mucus glands. When mating, the drone penis is everted and ejaculation occurs. Drones die after mating, since much of the endophallus remains in the queen (Winston, 1987).

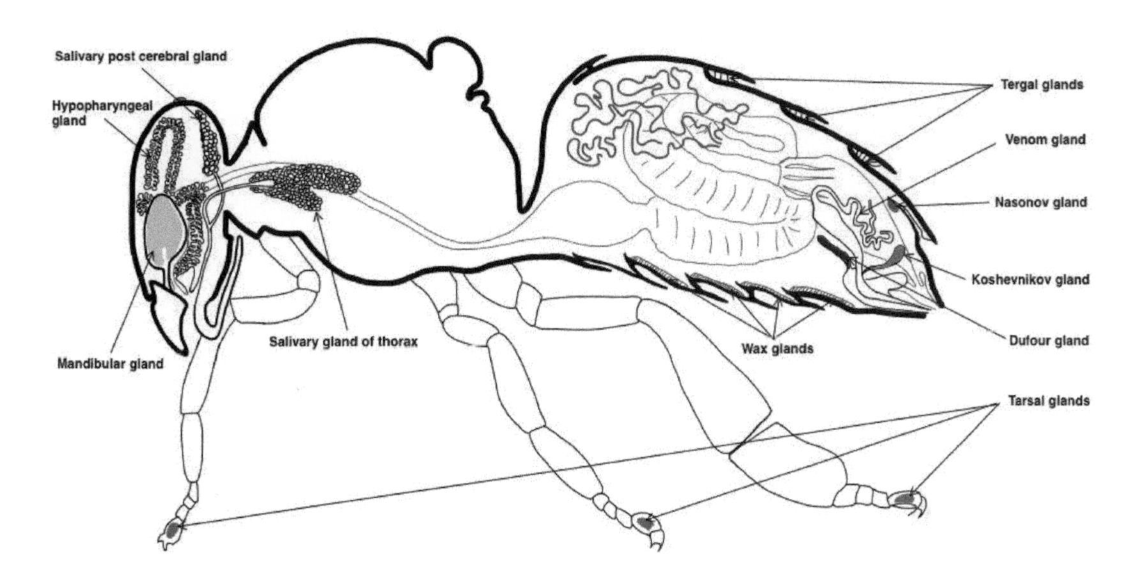

Figure 1.11 Glands of the honeybee. The main glands of the worker honeybees (salivary, food processing, wax, pheromone, and venom glands). (Redrawn by Nicolas Vidal-Naquet. Adapted from Snodgrass, 1910; Goodman, 2003; Bortolotti and Costa, 2010; Tofilski, 2012.)

4 Digestive tract and metabolism

The digestive tract allows digestion of nutrients. In workers, the crop, also called the honey stomach, plays a major role in liquid storage and transportation. In addition, the digestive tract plays a significant role in the social life of the colony, in particular by the means of its associated glands, i.e. the salivary glands, hypopharyngeal glands, and mandibular glands, which are involved in food gathering, food storage, feeding of the brood and the queen, and the secretion of pheromones.

4.1 Food-processing glands

The food-processing glands are the salivary, hypopharyngeal, and mandibular glands (Figure 1.11).

The salivary glands are located in the posterior part of the head (postcerebral gland) and in the thorax (thoracic salivary gland). They are connected to the mouth via a common duct. The thoracic labial gland seems to play a role in digesting and moistening solid food, i.e. pollen. The postcerebral glands produce an oily secretion containing in particular hydrocarbons and imaginal disc growth factor 4. These secretions are important for softening wax, lubricating mouthparts, and provide a source of hydrocarbons for the cuticle (Tofilski, 2012).

The main role of the hypopharyngeal and mandibular glands is to feed the brood and the queen.

The hypopharyngeal glands are located within the sides of the head. The secretion of the hypopharyngeal glands is rich in proteins, lipids, and vitamins. The secretion is an important component of the larval food. It is also involved in feeding the queen, the drones, and the young workers. The hypopharyngeal glands also secrete enzymes involved in the transformation of nectar into honey (glucose oxidase, invertase) (Winston, 1987).

The mandibular glands of workers also play an important role in brood and queen food secretion, in particular in secretion of royal jelly. In queens, the mandibular glands are well developed, secreting a complex chemical

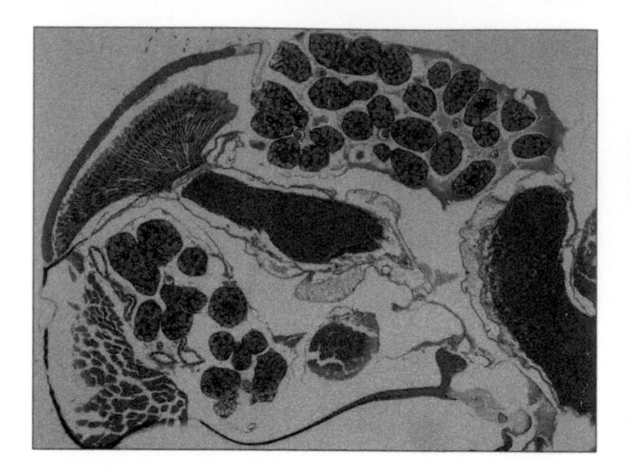

Figure 1.12 Worker bee, adult. Horizontal cut through the head showing the hypopharyngeal gland, sections of the compound eye and the brain (HE 40×). (© Heike Aupperle.)

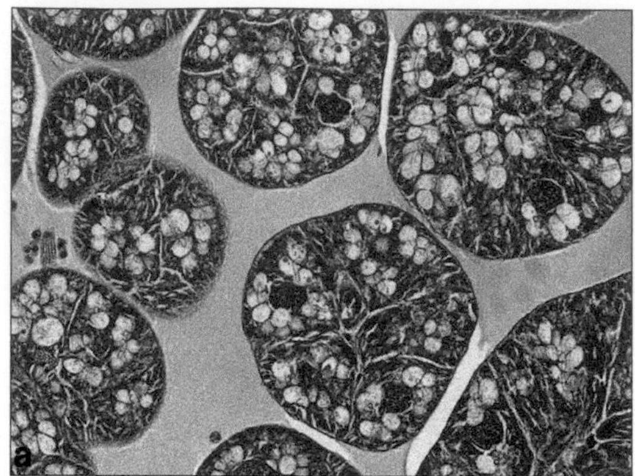

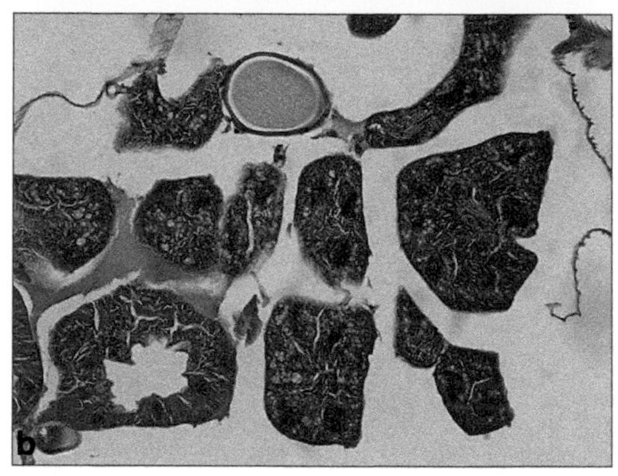

Figure 1.13 Worker bee. The hypopharyngeal gland in nursing bees (day 7) shows large and active lobuli (a) – in contrast to small and inactive lobuli in forager bee (b) (HE 400×). (© Heike Aupperle.)

pheromone known as queen mandibular pheromone (QMP).

In workers, the activity and the development of the hypopharyngeal and mandibular glands depend on age, food quality and quantity, the presence of the brood, but also on environmental and chemical (e.g. pesticides) factors (Heylen *et al.*, 2011; Hatjina *et al.*, 2013). Some pathogenic agents may impair the secretion of food-producing glands. The hypopharyngeal glands are well developed in young bees in particular when nursing. In older bees (foragers), the glands are likely atrophied as their role is less important (Figures 1.12 and 1.13).

The age-dependent development of the food-producing glands is a major feature of the worker bee's life (brood-rearing stage) and of colony life. The age dependence of the wax glands is also a significant factor in the life of the colony (sections 9–12.1.4 below). This age dependence is one of the main characteristics of the social features of the honeybee colony and of the sharing of the tasks within the nest.

4.2 Digestive tract and excretory system

In workers, the digestive tract begins with a long oesophagus connecting the mouth to the crop, located within the abdomen (Figure 1.14). The crop or honey stomach is expandable, and its volume increases when it is filled with nectar, water, or honey, in particular during foraging or before swarming. The abdomen expands when the crop is full thanks to the membranes connecting the sclerites. In the crop, nectar and water are stored for transportation back to the nest, and honey is stored as an energy source before a flight or before swarming (Winston, 1987).

After the honey stomach comes the proventicular valve and then the midgut, also called the ventriculus. The proventricular valve allows most of the liquid (i.e. nectar, honey, or water) to remain within the crop. Digestion

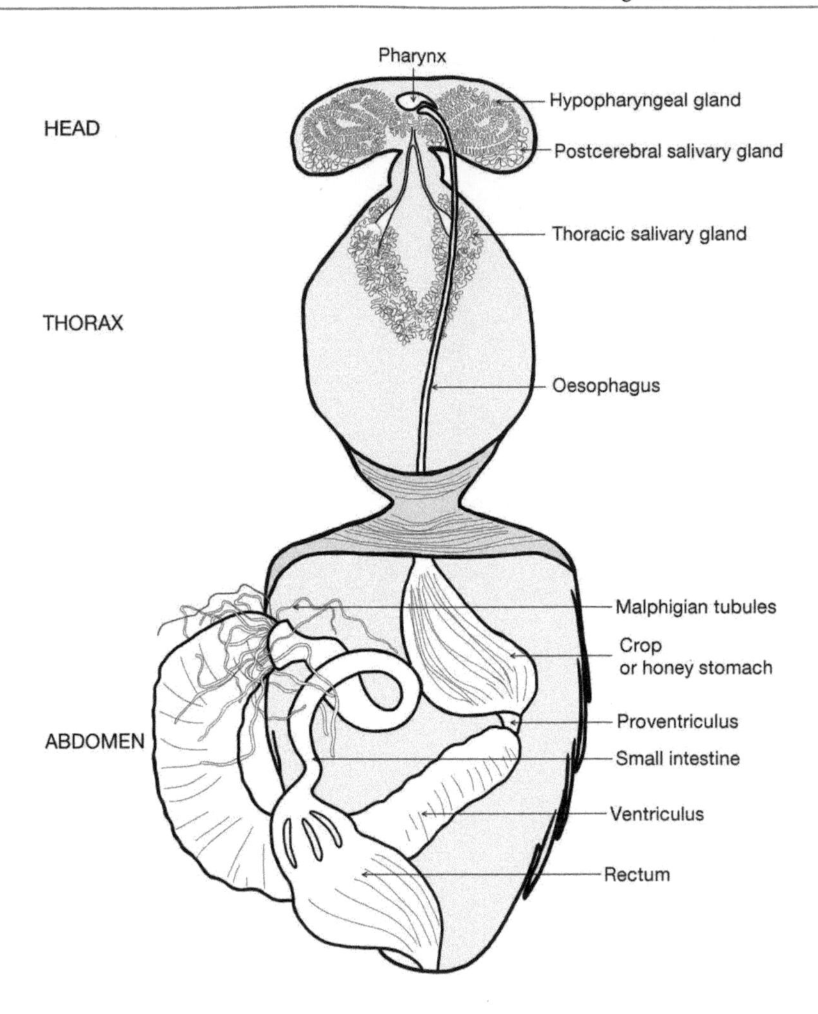

Figure 1.14 Anatomy and dissection: dorsal view of the digestive tract. (Redrawn by Nicolas Vidal-Naquet. Adapted from Snodgrass, 1910; Dade 2009.)

takes place in the midgut. One of the histological features of the midgut is a porous non-cellular membrane between the epithelium and the lumen: the peritrophic membrane or matrix (Figure 1.15). The peritrophic matrix is composed of regularly arranged chitin microfibrils and specific proteins embedded in a proteoglycan matrix. The functions of this membrane are improvement of digestion, protection against mechanical and chemical damage, and as a barrier to pathogenic agents (Lehane, 1987).

Finally, the waste from digestion is evacuated via the rectum. Defecation usually does not occur in the hive or in the nest but during a cleansing flight, in particular after wintering. The rectum can expand significantly, in particular during overwintering when the honeybees stay within the hive. If defecation occurs in the hive, it is usually a sign of a diseased colony (e.g. dysentery, amoebosis or nosemosis).

The Malpighian tubules open into the terminal digestive tract. Liquid waste (including nitrogenous waste, potassium ions, water, urate ions, sugar, amino acids) is excreted by diffusion through the walls of the tubules (urea, amino acids) or via active pumps (ions) after absorption by the Malpighian tubules from the haemolymph.

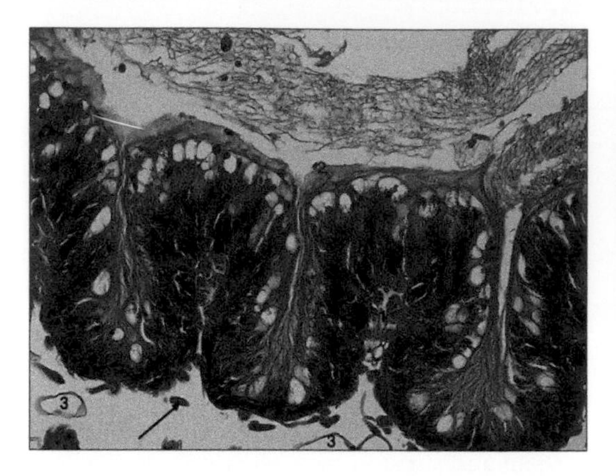

Figure 1.15 Worker bee, adult. In the lumen of the midgut, layers of the peritrophic membrane (2) are present. Stem cells (1) are located in the niches of the epithelial folds. In the periphery, a thin layer of slender myocytes (arrow) and some tracheae (3) are visible (HE 200×). (© Heike Aupperle.)

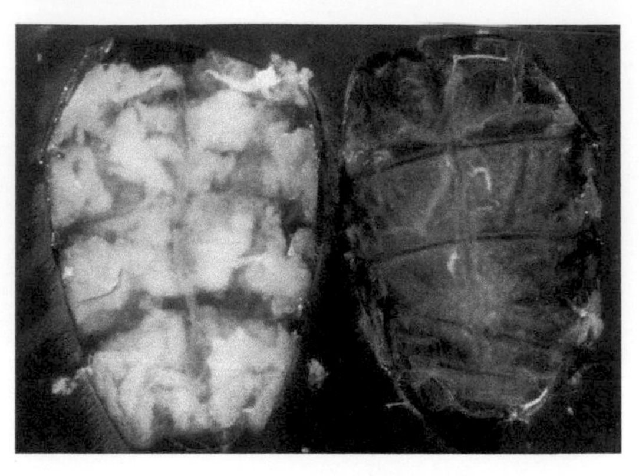

Figure 1.16 Fat bodies of a winter worker (left) and of a summer worker (right). Note the well-developed fat bodies in winter bees, allowing in particular amino acid and lipid reserves for overwintering. (Photograph courtesy of Station de Recherche Agroscope Liebefeld-Posieux. © Station de Recherche Agroscope Liebefeld-Posieux ALP. Imdorf *et al.*, 2010.)

4.3 Fat bodies

The fat bodies are a layer of conspicuous cells concentrated on the roof and the floor of the honeybee abdomen (Figure 1.16) (Winston, 1987). These fat bodies are the main organ responsible for the intermediate metabolism of nutrients in honeybees, and are involved in the metabolism of proteins, lipids, and carbohydrates (Chan *et al.*, 2011). Most of the proteins found in the haemolymph are synthesized in the fat bodies. The fat bodies provide a source of proteins during long non-feeding periods, e.g. overwintering.

Another role of these fat bodies is to store and release glycogen and lipids according the needs of the honeybee's metabolism. Lipid metabolism is essential for growth and reproduction, and adipocytes can store a large amount of lipid reserves. Thus, the fat bodies, as a source of lipids, also provide some of the energy needed during extended non-feeding periods (Arresses and Soulages, 2010).

This tissue is in particular responsible for the synthesis of vitellogenin, a female-specific 180 kDa protein (Wheeler and Kawooya, 1990) which plays major roles in reproduction of the queen, social organization, lifespan, immunity, and hibernation (Amdam *et al.*, 2004; Antúnez *et al.*, 2009). The next paragraph is dedicated to this crucial glycoprotein.

If the fat bodies play a major role in the storage and release of fat, glycogen, and protein, in particular during metamorphosis and wintering, they also play an important role in detoxification. Detoxification mechanisms are the consequence of several enzymes, in particular the mixed-function oxygenase (MFO) system also called cytochrome P450-linked microsomal oxidases, but also glutathione transferases, carboxylesterases, and epoxide hydrolases (Gregorc *et al.*, 2012). However, in honeybees, these enzyme-coding genes are reported to be relatively deficient compared to other insects (Claudianos *et al.*, 2006).

To compare with vertebrate animals, fat bodies are to the honeybee what both adipose tissues and liver are to vertebrates (Chan *et al.*, 2011).

In worker bees during the productive season, the fat bodies are more developed within the abdomen of inside (nest) bees than in the abdomen of forager bees. On another hand, in winter workers, which are long-lived bees, the fat bodies are well developed (Imdorf *et al.*, 2010) (Figure 1.13). During this period, the fat bodies are the only source of lipids and proteins for the bees and the colony, while the stored honey provides the carbohydrate resources. Thus, fat bodies must be well developed for an optimal overwintering. In managed colonies, the beekeeper must ensure that his beekeeping practice encourages well-developed fat bodies.

4.4 Vitellogenin, a potential indicator of colony health?

Vitellogenin is a female-specific phospholipo-glycoprotein yolk precursor found in all oviparous species (Amdam *et al.*, 2003). In *A. mellifera*, vitellogenin is found in both queens and sterile workers. This protein is synthesized by the fat bodies (Amdam *et al.*, 2012), and plays a central role in reproduction and in the social life of the colony.

In the queen, after 3 days of life and throughout the rest of her life, the vitellogenin represents up to 70% of the protein found in the haemolymph. It is transported to the ovaries, and plays a major role in oogenesis (Amdam *et al.*, 2003; Roma *et al.*, 2010).

In worker bees, the synthesis of vitellogenin begins about 10 hours before emergence. In the haemolymph of workers, vitellogenin is detected at lower levels than in the queen. Vitellogenin is the main storage protein in honeybee workers (Fluri *et al.*, 1977).

During the first 7 days of the adult workers' life (when their tasks are nursing and brood-rearing), vitellogenin may reach up to 40% of the haemolymph protein. At this time, the protein is used to produce brood food in the hypopharyngeal glands of the nurses (Amdam *et al.*, 2003, 2004).

The synthesis of vitellogenin decreases progressively during their lifetime and ends approximately 20 days after the last moult before emergence (Engels, 1987; Piulachs *et al.*, 2003). Vitellogenin has been shown to inhibit the onset of foraging activity (Nelson *et al.*, 2007). When the level of vitellogenin decreases, foraging activity begins. At the same time, the level of haemolymph juvenile hormone (JH) increases (Nelson *et al.*, 2007; Bomtorin *et al.*, 2014). JH and vitellogenin probably work together in a feedback relationship (Guidugli *et al.*, 2005; Nelson *et al.*, 2007; Bomtorin *et al.*, 2014).

Thus, vitellogenin and JH are involved in the social regulation of the colony, acting on the division of labour, foraging onset, and foraging specialization. Furthermore, vitellogenin is reported to be involved in the regulation of the lifespan and survival process of the workers (via oxidative stress resilience and cellular immunity) (Amdam *et al.*, 2012).

In temperate climates, before the over-wintering period, when brood rearing stops, vitellogenin is accumulated in long-life winter workers (Amdam *et al.*, 2004). Long-life workers possess well-developed fat bodies compared to short-life bees (Figure 1.13) (Imdorf *et al.*, 2010). In winter, the only food resource is honey; pollen is not available. The proteins stored in the fat bodies are the only source of amino acids for the workers and the colony. They are also the source of amino acids for brood production when hibernation ends but blossoming has not yet started again (Amdam *et al.*, 2004).

Considering all these important features, in particular in short-life and long-life workers, vitellogenin can be related to the strength of the bees and the colony, but also to the lifespan of honeybees, in particular in winter bees. Thus, the level of vitellogenin and/or expression of the gene *vitellogenin* may potentially be considered as indicators of colony and bee health and honeybee lifespan, especially long-lived workers, and may in the future be extended beyond research and prove of interest for practical evaluation of colony health (Amdam *et al.*, 2004; Nelson *et al.*, 2007), as follows:

- In the case of parasitic disease, e.g. varroosis or other weakening disease, measuring the level of vitellogenin in winter bees may potentially predict bee lifespan and thus the ability of the colony to overwinter in good condition. Indeed, it has been shown that workers

infested during the pupal stage present lower vitellogenin levels than non-infested workers (Adam *et al.*, 2004).
- In the case of the examination of colonies in the autumn, measuring the level of vitellogenin can help to evaluate the nutritive state of the colony before hibernation (Otis *et al.*, 2004).

Unfortunately, at this time, there are no normal values known or defined for bees or standard methods of measurement in veterinary practice. Otis *et al.* (2004) found on average 60 μg/abdomen in winter bees (60-day-old bees), with a large range (10–200 μg/abdomen).

In the research sector, vitellogenin level and especially *vitellogenin* gene expression are currently being evaluated (Otis *et al.*, 2004; Nelson *et al.*, 2007). However, according to Dainat *et al.* (2012), vitellogenin expression does not seem to be a 'viable predictive marker' of honeybee colony collapse during winter.

Vitellogenin has the potential to become an interesting field of investigation for honeybee veterinary medicine and practice as a factor used to evaluate colony strength in certain circumstances. Further research is needed to establish the veterinary use of this marker.

5 Respiratory and circulatory systems

In insects, an extensive tracheal system, with 10 pairs of spiracles, provides oxygen to the various organs. Two large respiratory sacs are located in the abdomen and smaller ones in the head and thorax. The sacs and tracheas ramify into smaller tubes, terminating in a single cell (Snodgrass, 1910; Winston, 1987). The haemolymph does not play an important role in gas transport.

At rest, respiration occurs passively by diffusion. During flight, bees pump their abdomens to increase gas exchange and expand the air sacs of the trachea like bellows, resulting in greater gas exchange.

The circulatory system is 'open', consisting of a dorsal heart and aorta to assist in haemolymph circulation. This system serves to transport nutrients from the midgut to body cells but also transports proteins, lipids, and carbohydrates around the organism. The circulatory system also brings metabolic waste material from the cells to the Malpighian tubules.

6 Immune system and mechanisms of protection and defence

The mechanisms of defence in the honeybee occur at both the individual and the colony level.

6.1 At the individual level

At the individual level, the cuticle and the peritrophic membrane are the first physical barriers to pathogens and parasites. Secondarily, the haemolymph (via the immune response) plays a major role in immunity.

The immune response to pathogens is characterized by a cellular immune response, e.g. encapsulation and phagocytosis (phagocytic haemocyt), as well as a cellular-free defence mechanism.

Haemocytes are involved in defence against fungal and bacterial infections (Gliński and Buczek, 2003; Scientific Beekeeping, 2014). Three primary classes of immune-related haemocytes (plasmatocytes, crystal cells, and lamellocytes) are generally present in insects and likely to occur in the honeybee (Evans and Spivak, 2010).

Enzymes (e.g. lysozyme, kinases), antimicrobial peptides (apidaecins, abaecins), and polypeptides (e.g. hymenoptaecines) found in the haemolymph of honeybees provide antibacterial protection (Casteels, 1990, 1993).

Honeybees, like other insects, possess four major and interconnected pathways for responding to pathogen exposure: the Toll, Imd, Jak/STAT, and Jnk pathways (Theopold and Dushay, 2007). Antimicrobial peptide (AMP)-encoding genes are regulated by the Toll and Imd pathways (De Gregorio *et al.*, 2002). The Jak/STAT-dependent humoral factors (thioester-containing proteins, Tot peptides) are produced by the fat bodies in response to a septic injury. The Jak/STAT pathway seems to be involved in cellular responses, including haemocyte proliferation and differentiation (Agaisse and Perrimon, 2004). The Jnk pathway represents one of the mitogen-activated protein kinases primarily activated by cytokines and by exposure to environmental stress (Weston and Davis, 2007).

These pathways consist of proteins that recognize signals from invading pathogens, proteins that modulate and amplify this recognition signal, and effector proteins or metabolites directly involved in parasite inhibition (Evans and Spivak, 2010).

6.2 At the colony level

The colony as a super-organism presents defence features, which effectively constitute a colony-level immune system. The mechanisms of protection and defence of honeybee colonies involve the following behaviours:

- Grooming behaviour between bees.
- Hygienic behaviour (Spivak, 1996), which is a specific type of general nest hygiene. In the honeybee, hygienic behaviour is defined as a collective response by adult bees to the presence of a diseased and parasitized worker brood.
- Necrophoric behaviour, also called 'undertaking' (Evans and Spivak, 2010), which consists of the removal of dead adults from the nest.
- Modifications of the nest environment play a role in the defence of the colony against pathogens, parasites, and pests. For example, the collection of propolis used as a mechanical and antiseptic barrier in the nest is a way to fight intruders and pests.
- Nest defence behaviour by the workers is one of the main mechanisms to protect the colony against predators. Honeybees have developed several defence behaviours depending on the threat and predator.

7 Temperature regulation

Honeybees are heterothermic, but regulation of body temperature seems to be possible, in particular in foragers when flying (Cooper *et al.*, 1985).

The social organization of the honeybee enables homeostasis in the colony. There is a relatively constant temperature and humidity inside the nest. Wild colonies build their nests in places chosen to be suitable for overwintering. In apiculture, the role of the beekeeper is to maintain optimal conditions to allow the colonies to maintain homeostasis all year long (food, water, and hives location during wintering must all be taken into consideration).

In winter, the temperature inside the cluster allows bees to survive this challenging period.

In summer when the temperature is too high, cooling the colony is important. Water plays a crucial role in this homeostasis in particular on hot days by evaporative cooling (Kovac *et al.*, 2010).

The thermoregulation of the colony is a real challenge in cold areas during winter. When the temperature falls below 14°C, the workers cluster together. Inside the winter cluster, thermal stability is achieved together with a high core temperature (approximately 20–35°C), and a high humidity level. The lower the temperature, the smaller and more compact the winter cluster becomes. The heat transfer in the cluster seems to be the consequence of heat conduction between bees (Watmouth and Camazine, 1995). At the individual level, the heating is the consequence of thoracic muscular contraction by the workers (Stabentheiner *et al.*, 2003). Honey is the source of energy and workers move in the cluster to the stored honey and feed periodically.

When the temperature is too high, nest cooling becomes necessary. Indeed, temperatures above 36°C are dangerous for the brood, causing death and abnormalities (Winston, 1987). Colonies seem to be able to maintain the temperature under 36°C even if the outside temperature is much higher. Cooling the nest is the consequence of ventilation by workers fanning their wings

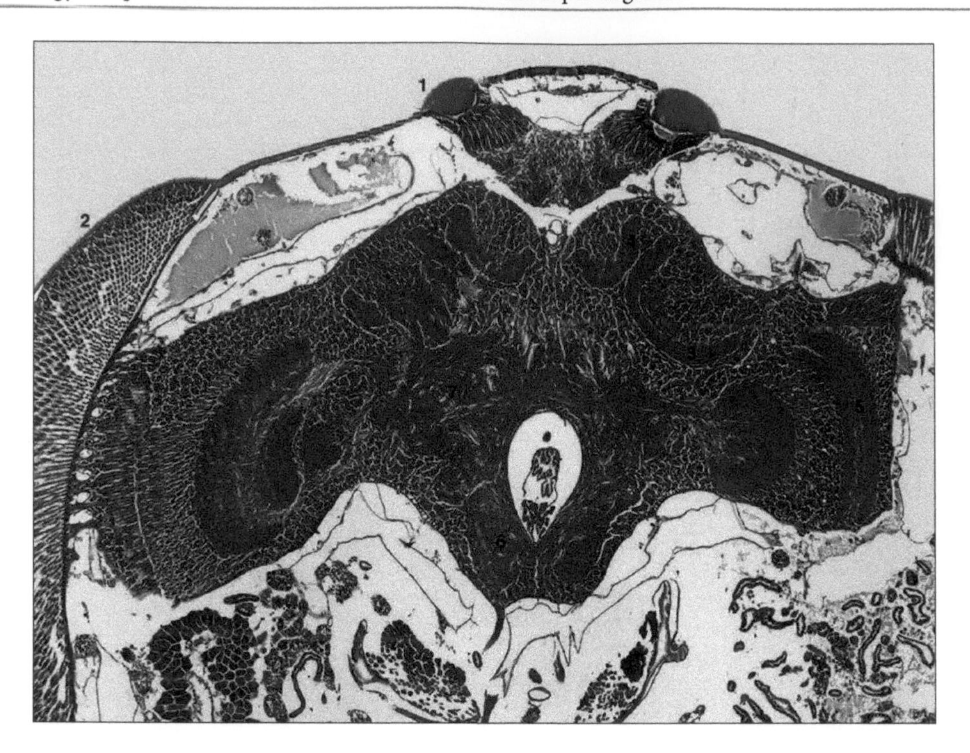

Figure 1.17 Queen, just emerged. The cross-section of the head shows simple (ocelli) (1) and compound eyes (2). The brain is surrounded by tracheal sacs. The following brain regions are recognizable: 'mushroom bodies' with the lateral (3) and medial (4) calyces, medulla (5), antennal lobes (6) as well as protocerebral lobe (with alpha and beta lobes) (7) (HE 40×). (© Heike Aupperle.)

inside the nest and at the entrance, but also due to the use of water spread in puddles on capped cells (Winston, 1987).

8 Nervous system

The nervous system of the honeybee is complex and adapted to the environment. It is composed of the central nervous system (CNS) and the peripheral nervous system (PNS).

The CNS comprises the brain and seven ganglia forming the ventral chain. The brain comprises three cephalic ganglia: the protocerebrum, responsible for vision and composed of two large optic lobes innervating the thousands of units of the compound eyes (Dade, 2009); the deutocerebrum, the centre for olfaction, innervating the sense organs of the antennae; and the tritocerebrum, which is smaller, and innervates the lower part of the head, in particular the labrum involved in taste (Figure 1.17).

In the protocerebrum are located the corpora pendunculata, or mushroom bodies, containing groups of nerve cells connected to the optic and antennal lobes and other parts of the nervous system by nerve fibres (Dade, 2009). They play a major role in coordination.

The ventral chain of the CNS is composed of seven ganglia. Two large ganglia are located in the thorax and five in the abdomen. The first one is the suboesophageal ganglion innervating the mouthparts and the salivary glands. The ganglia of the ventral chain innervate the thoracic and abdominal segments and the related organs, including the legs, the wings, and the sting apparatus.

The PNS enables relationships with other bees and the environment. It consists of the sense organs (cf. section 3.1.1 above).

As in other insect and mammalian brains, neurons in the honeybee brain and CNS use many neurotransmitters. Thus, acetylcholine, glutamate, gamma-aminobutyric acid (GABA), serotonin, octopamine, and other neuropeptides are present. The major excitatory neurotransmitter in the CNS is acetylcholine. GABA and glutamate are the main inhibitory transmitters in the CNS through ligand-gated chloride channel receptors (El Hassani *et al.*, 2008).

Neurotransmitters, in particular glutamatergic neurotransmission, are involved in honeybee learning and memory. Honeybee memory is characterized by short-term memory, middle-term and long-term memory (Hammer and Menzel, 1995). This allows relationships and communication between workers, in particular when finding a resource location (e.g. flowers, honeydew plants) and sharing the information with other workers (Lindauer, 1959; von Frisch, 1967). Memory also allows homing behaviour by enabling the bees to use landmarks.

This neuroregulation may be affected by the use of pesticides, in particular insecticides that are neurotoxic.

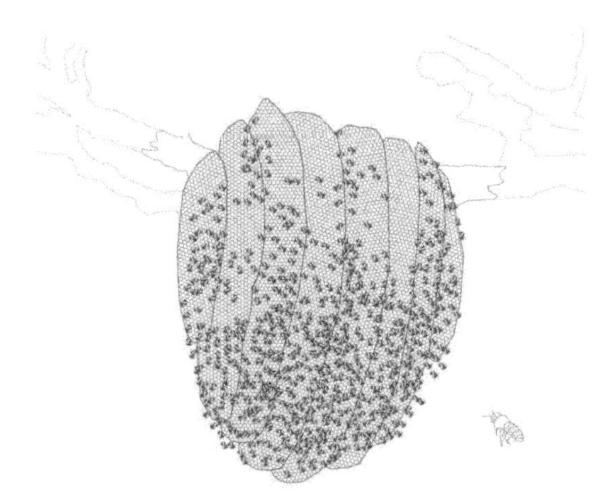

Figure 1.18 Feral nest architecture with the usual arrangement of the combs (inside a cavity of a tree for European species, sometimes hung on tree branches). (© Nicolas Guérin.)

9 The nest structure

9.1 Feral colonies

In the wild, a swarm of *A. mellifera* choses a nest site to build its colony within a cavity based on a number of characteristics, linked to the volume, the nature of the entrance, how exposed the site is, the height above the ground, the dryness, or the dampness. The sites preferred are usually visible (so as to serve as a landmark for the bees), and relatively insulated from wind, rain, and sun. The bees also avoid damp and draughty sites even if they may limit those disadvantages by using propolis. The entrance needs to be sufficient to allow ventilation in summer and to protect the colony from the rigours of winter.

The construction of the combs proceeds quickly once the site has been chosen in order to store pollen and honey and rear the brood. The nest is composed of several vertical combs; each comb has hexagonal cells on both sides. The combs are parallel and separated by an exact distance (Figure 1.18) (Winston, 1987).

Each hexagonal cell is built horizontally in a slightly oblique position (angled up at about 13%) with an upward aperture in order to retain the larvae and prevent the outflow of honey. In European *A. mellifera* strains there are 857 cells worker brood cells and 520 drone brood cells per 10 cm^2 (Winston, 1987). The worker cells are 5.2–5.4 mm in diameter and the drone cells are 6.2–6.4 mm in diameter. African *A. mellifera* strains cells are smaller.

The typical structure of a comb during the season may be described as follows (Figure 1.19):

- In the upper and peripheral part of the comb, honey and pollen are stored. In the peripheral combs of the nest, mainly honey and pollen are stored.

- The central part of the comb is devoted to the development and rearing of the brood. The worker brood occupies a large central zone; the drone area, when it is present (in spring and sometimes in autumn), is usually on the edge of the worker brood (or of the comb).
- Queen cells may appear on the edge of the comb in the case of swarming or in the central zone of the comb in the event of re-queening by supersedure or after the death of the queen. In such cases, only one cell will produce a new queen.

9.2 Managed colonies

Hives for managed colonies must provide the honeybees with the features of a feral nest, allowing the bees to live, rear broods, and store food (Figure 1.19). Hives must also allow a practical, rationalised, and adapted management for beekeeping practices. The location of the hives must be chosen considering the features needed for honeybee nests.

Modern beekeeping began in 1850 with a hive built by Langstroth, with wood frames regularly spaced within a body hive (Figure 1.20) (Winston, 1987; Philippe, 2007). The bees build their combs in the frames, which the beekeeper is able to remove for examination without damaging the nest architecture.

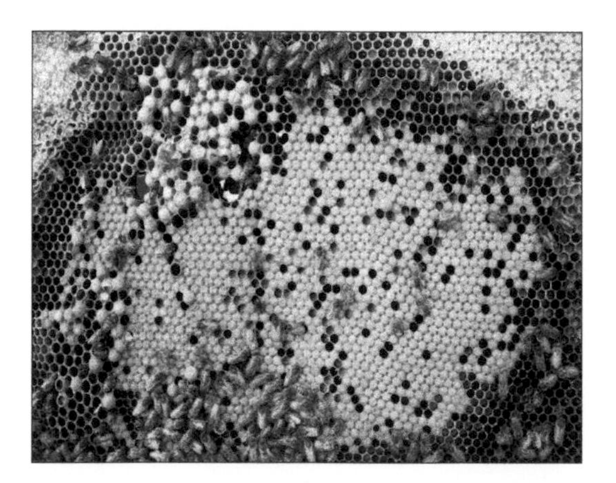

Figure 1.19 Typical aspect of a brood comb in a frame of a managed colony. The worker brood occupies a large centre part. The large cells on the upper left part of the brood are the drone brood with larger cells. Around the brood is stored the uncapped beebread, and around the beebread, the honey cells capped with a white wax. (© Nicolas Vidal-Naquet.)

Wax foundations have been developed as a base for the cells. The foundation is created from beeswax, pressed into thin flat sheets, each one embossed with an imprinted pattern of (worker-sized) cell bottoms. The wax foundation is wired within the frame (Philippe, 2007).

Thus, frames with brood combs may be easily examined. Honey frames can be removed from the honey supers for extraction. (A super is a receptacle in which honeybees store honey; it is usually placed over the hive body.) The frames may be reused year after year, according to good beekeeping practices. The hives can also be easily moved from place to place (migratory beekeeping) for pollination and to produce monofloral honey (lavender, etc.).

Much in the way of new material and techniques appear year after year. At this time, there are many models of hive (Langstroth, Dadant, Warré, Voirnot, etc.) (Philippe, 2007). Wood is still the standard material used for hives, though plastic hives and frames are now used by some beekeepers. Even the wax foundations can be replaced by similarly printed plastic sheets, which offer some advantages such as easy cleaning and disinfection.

10 Reproduction: drones, queen, and brood development

Reproduction and brood rearing usually occur between spring and autumn.

10.1 Mating the queen

Honeybee colonies are considered protandrous. This means that they produce drones before the emergence of virgin queens in spring. Colonies also produce drones in late summer, as well as some virgin queens, following the summer swarming peak (Winston, 1987).

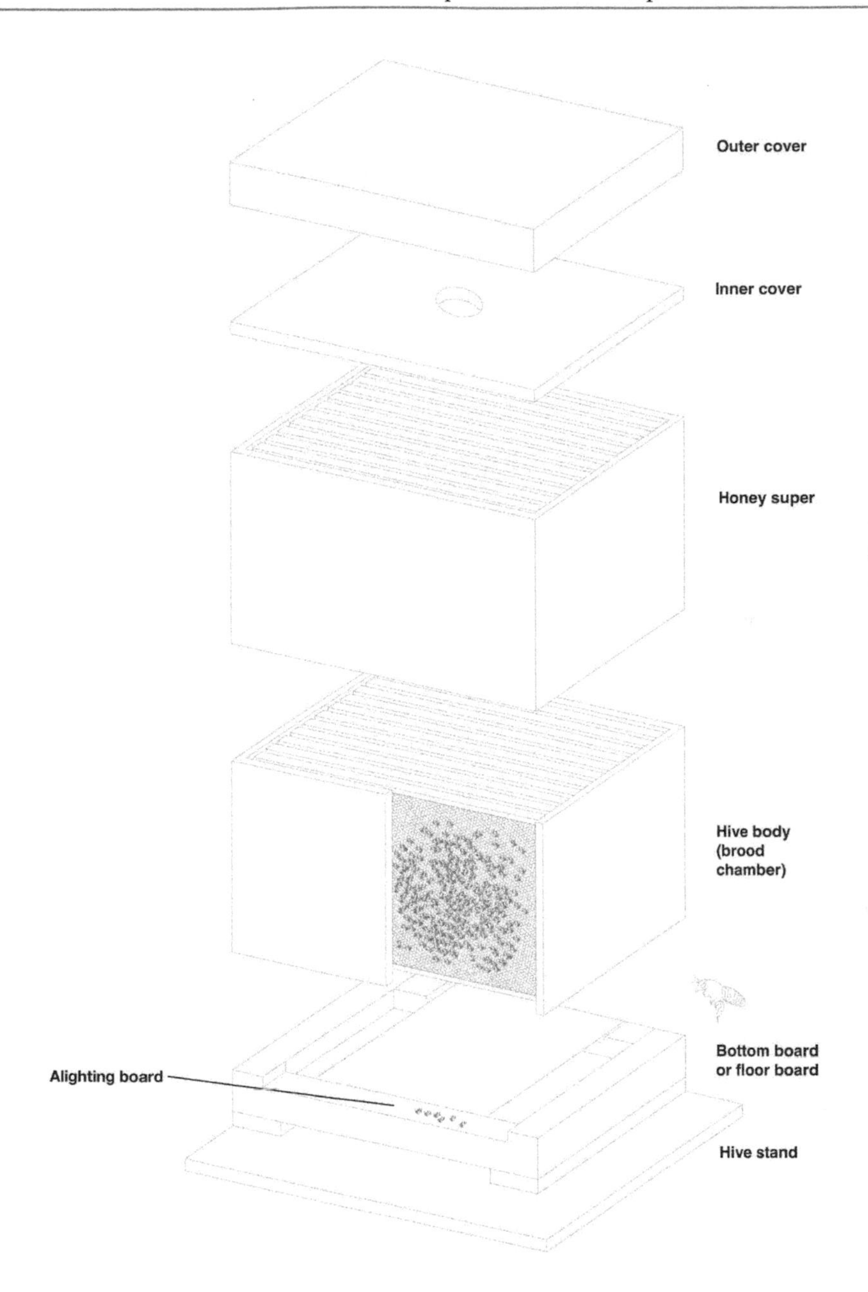

Figure 1.20 Typical architecture of a hive with removable frames. (© Nicolas Guérin.)

The queens only mate in one period of their life. Sometime between 5 and 13 days after emerging from the cell, a virgin queen performs short orientation flights (Philippe, 2007). The orientation and mating flights generally occur in mid-afternoon and on a sunny day.

The queen flies to a congregation area where the drones have already arrived. The congregation area is at least 12 km from the original colony of the queen and drones. The reasons underlying the selection of this area are not well known, but these areas usually seem to be protected from the wind, and surrounded by more than 1 hectare of open ground (Ruttner and Ruttner, 1966; Winston, 1987). The choice of congregation area seems to depend on geographical, meteorological and chemical (i.e. bee pheromone) factors. QMP (cf. section 12.2.1 below) plays a major role in attracting the drones.

Mating occurs in flight and is rapid and 'explosive'. The endophallus of a successful drone becomes lodged in the queen's vagina and is then torn from its body – a signal that mating of the queen has occurred (Winston, 1987; Philippe, 2007).

This drone then falls and dies. After the transfer of the spermatozoa into the spermatheca, the queen removes the evaginated male genital system and mates again; on average 7–17 subsequent copulations take place (Winston, 1987). If this number is not reached, two or three mating flights can occur. This mating period occurs only once at the beginning of the queen's life. The queen stores enough spermatozoa to lay eggs for between two and five years (Remolina, 2007; Rueppell *et al.*, 2007).

10.2 Ovipositioning

Fertilized queens initiate ovipositioning between 2 and 23 days (usually 2–4 days) after the beginning of the mating flights (Philippe, 2007; Woyke and Jasinski, 2008; Texas A&M University, 2014). Before laying the eggs, the queen opens a valve in the spermatheca duct to allow fertilization of the egg at her discretion by releasing a tiny quantity of sperm.

10.3 Sex determination in the honeybee: haplodiploidy

There are three castes of honeybees: queens, workers, and drones. The first differentiation is male versus female. Haploid males and diploid females characterize the differentiation of sex in honeybees, as in other Hymenoptera and some other insects.

The diploid queens and workers have 2 × 16 chromosomes and the haploid drones have 16 chromosomes. Fertilized eggs become females (diploid individuals) and non-fertilized eggs give rise to haploid males (parthenogenesis) (Winston, 1987; Le Conte, 2006b).

The queen controls the release of spermatozoa when laying and can 'decide' whether an egg will develop into a male or a female. The 'decision' is the consequence of the larger size of drone cells compared to worker cells. Before laying an egg, the queen measures the cell size with her forelegs and then oviposits the egg, opening the valve of the spermatheca if it is a smaller worker cell, allowing fertilization. If it is a larger one, the spermatheca will not release spermatozoa and the egg will be laid and develop without fertilization (Winston, 1987).

Sex determination in *A. mellifera* is controlled by a single-gene sex locus called the complementary sex determiner (*csd* gene) with 6–19 alleles (Page, 1980). Females are diploid and heterozygous on this sex locus.

If one diploid individual is homozygous at this *csd* gene, it will be a diploid male. Diploid male larvae do not survive. The workers find and remove them from the cells and eat them (cannibalism); otherwise they become 'non-functional' drones (Winston, 1987).

10.4 Development of the brood

Development of the immature forms occurs within the cells (Le Conte, 2006b), and proceeds through four stages: egg, larva, pupa, and then adult or imago. Because the honeybee is a social insect living in a perennial colony, certain adults, the nurse workers, are in charge of the brood rearing. Many interactions between adults and the brood occur (Winston, 1987). The development of the brood and the quality of adults emerging depend on multiple factors, including rearing, temperature, nutrition, behaviour of the workers, and strain. These factors are therefore also significant for managing colonies in order to produce strong and healthy adults.

The larval stage is the period of feeding and nursing by the nurse workers. The larva develops in weight and size. At the end of this stage, workers cap the cell and the larva spins its

Table 1.1 Brood development characteristics of the three castes

QUEEN	EGG	LARVA	PUPA	
	3 days	5.5 days	7.5 days	
		ROYAL JELLY		
WORKER	EGG	LARVA	PUPA	
	3 days	6 days	12 days	
		WORKER JELLY		
DRONE	EGG	LARVA	PUPA	
	3 days	6.5 days	14.5 days	
		DRONE JELLY		
	←LAYING		CAPPING OF THE BROOD CELL	EMERGENCE OF ADULT

cocoon and turns into a pupa. The pupal stage is a period of metamorphosis, during which the brood changes into an adult. The imago emerges from the wax-capped brood cell. Six moults occur from the egg to the adult (Wendling, 2012). While the egg stage always lasts 3 days, the larval and pupal stages of the three castes have their own duration characteristics (Table 1.1).

10.4.1 Eggs

The queen oviposits an egg at the centre of a cell, gluing the egg to the cell floor with a mucous strand. The egg oviposited is positioned vertically but over the following 3 days progressively lays down on the floor of the cell. One egg is laid per cell (Figure 1.21) (Winston, 1987). Eggs are white, pearly, short cylindrical structures, rounded on both ends, and measuring 1–1.5 mm × 0.5 mm. Egg incubation lasts 3 days (Le Conte, 2006b).

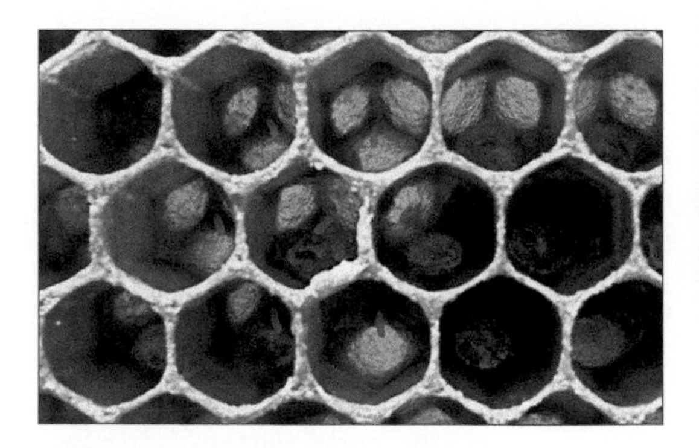

Figure 1.21 One egg is oviposited per cell by the queen. (© Nicolas Vidal-Naquet.)

10.4.2 Worker brood development (duration: 21 days after ovipositioning) (Figure 1.22)

The worker brood represents the main brood in terms of size reared in the nest or the managed colony. Its rearing is of crucial importance to the strength, the life, and the production of the colony.

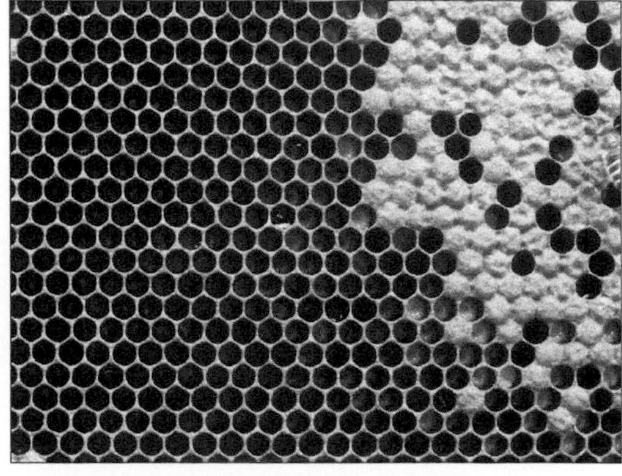

Figure 1.22 Worker brood: uncapped cells with eggs and larvae. Capped brood containing pupae. (© Nicolas Vidal-Naquet.)

The worker larval stage lasts 6 days before capping. Larvae are frequently visited by workers (feeding, nursing, inspection of the cell) and are fed with worker jelly secreted by the food-processing glands of the nurses. The composition of this jelly changes after the third day and mandibular gland secretion decreases.

The capped stage begins when the cell is closed by workers with wax and propolis. At this time, the larvae spin their cocoon and turn into pupae. The capped brood stage lasts 12 days. Thus, from egg-laying to the emergence of the worker bee takes 21 days.

In workers, the development of the genital tract produces atrophied ovaries. Only 2–12 ovarioles remain within the residual ovaries after the larval and pupal stages (Piulachs *et al.*, 2003). The ovarioles of workers may in some circumstances produce unfertilized eggs (e.g. in queen-less colonies that are unable to rear new queens).

Summer workers live for 4–8 weeks, while winter workers can live for 20 weeks in order to allow the colony to survive through the winter period (Remolina, 2007; Rueppell *et al.*, 2007).

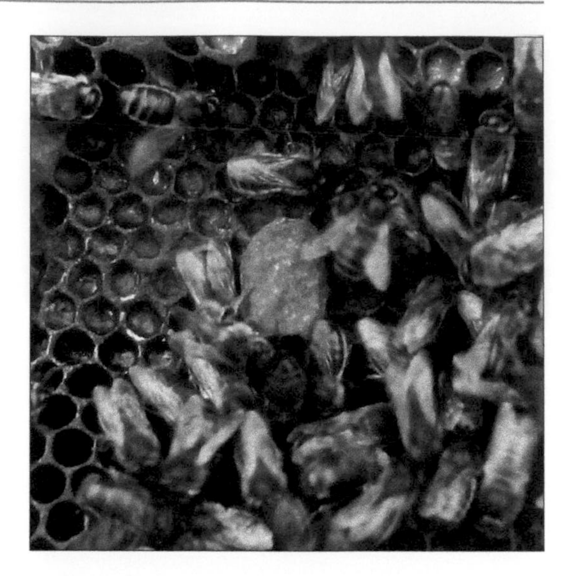

Figure 1.23 Uncapped queen cell. (© Nicolas Vidal-Naquet.)

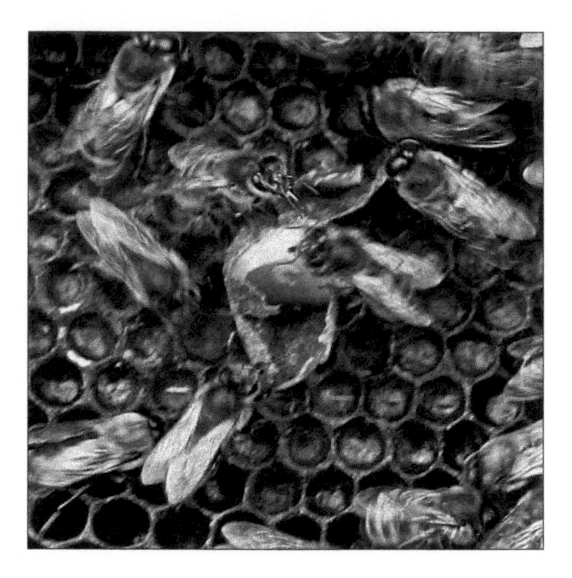

Figure 1.24 Young larvae lying in a pool of royal jelly within the queen cell. (© Nicolas Vidal-Naquet.)

10.4.3 Drone brood development (duration: 24 days after ovipositioning)

The drone larval stage lasts 6.5 days. Drone cells are larger than those of workers, and are often placed on the edge of the worker brood. Drone jelly seems to be quite different to worker jelly. Drone larvae receive more jelly probably because drones are larger than workers. The capped brood stage lasts 14.5 days, and therefore from the laying of the egg to the emergence of the drone takes 24 days (Winston, 1987).

10.4.4 Queen brood development (duration: 16 days after ovipositioning) (Figures 1.23 and 1.24)

The queen cells, also called cups, are oval-shaped, prominent, vertical, and open at the bottom. The future queen larvae are fed with royal jelly and nurses visit them at least 10 times more frequently than they do the worker larvae.

During the first 3 days of larval life, the quality and quantity of the royal jelly is enhanced (containing secretions of mandibular and hypopharyngeal glands). Determination of caste between workers and queen is mainly based on nutritional factors (cf. Chapter 1, Section 11). Stimulation of juvenile hormone secretion by the corpora allata of the queen larva is increased (Wirtz and Beetsma, 1972; Rembold *et al.*, 1974).

The protein royalactin within the royal jelly has been shown to play an important role in the dimorphism between worker and queen. Royalactin is reported to increase the level of juvenile hormone in larvae, increasing the body size and decreasing the developmental time (Kamakura, 2011). Throughout most of the larval stage of queens, a high level of juvenile hormone is synthesized, resulting in quite complete development of the ovariole anlagens. Thus, the ovaries of adult queens contain up to 180 ovarioles (Piulachs *et al.*, 2003). On the contrary, as noted above, in workers only 2–12 ovarioles remain within the residual ovaries after the larval and pupal stages (Piulachs *et al.*, 2003).

Following the third day, and until brood capping, the queen larva will receive a stable composition of royal jelly. At the end of the larval stage, the queen larva begins to spin a cocoon, and workers cap the cell just before the pupal stage. The larval stage before capping lasts 5.5 days. Then, the larva becomes a pupa, and a virgin queen emerges 7.5 days after metamorphosis, i.e. 16 days after the egg is deposited.

Emergence occurs after the workers have consumed the external part of the brood cell cap. The following day, the queen cuts the cap with her mandibles, pushes it away, and exits the cell.

Although queens can live as long as 5 years, after about 2 years their fertility declines, and in managed colonies they should be replaced in order to keep the colony as healthy as possible.

11 Nutrition

The three castes and their larval stages have different nutritional needs and resources (Winston, 1987). Honey (and honeydew honey) and stored pollen are respectively the colony's source of carbohydrates and lipids/proteins. Pollen is also the main source of minerals and vitamins.

A honeybee colony needs water to thermoregulate the hive by evaporative cooling in the case of high temperature, to maintain a certain moisture level within brood cells to protect eggs and larvae, to dilute stored honey, and for the consumption of nurse workers to produce brood food for feeding the larvae (Haydak, 1970; Winston, 1987; Kovac *et al.*, 2010). Water is not stored and permanent access is crucial. A lack of water seriously impairs colony health. In managed colonies, the beekeeper must ensure a constant supply of water is available for the bees.

11.1 Honey

Honey is a product of the nectar secreted by the nectariferous glands of flowers gathered by foragers. Another type of honey, called honeydew honey, can be produced by the transformation of honeydew, a carbohydrate-rich liquid secreted by aphids and some other scale insects that feed on plant sap. Honey is stored in the honeycombs (Figure 1.25).

After nectar or honeydew has been gathered while foraging, its transformation begins inside the crop of the forager bee. When the forager comes back to the hive, the nectar is transferred to nest workers by trophallaxis (mouth-to-mouth feeding). In the honey stomach, the nectar

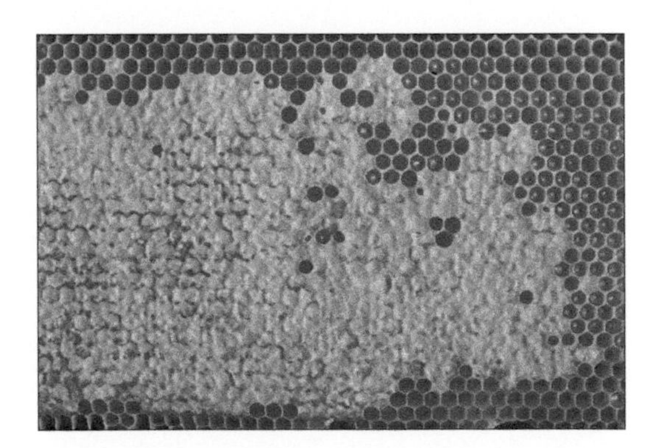

Figure 1.25 Honeycomb. The honey is stored in the cells. After being transformed (enzymatic action and evaporation), the nectar and the honeydew are stored as honey within capped cells. (© Nicolas Vidal-Naquet.)

continues to be transformed by enzymes – notably diastase, invertase and glucose oxidase – secreted by the hypopharyngeal glands. These enzymes convert sugars into simple carbohydrates, which are more digestible by honeybees. The enzymes also play an antiseptic role, protecting the honey from bacteria in particular.

The nectar is then placed into cells where its enzymatic transformation continues. Fanning workers begin to ventilate the transformed nectar to evaporate water. When the enzymatic action is complete and the water content is less than 20%, the nectar has been transformed into honey. The cell is then capped with white wax secreted by building workers.

The composition of honey is on average 38% fructose, 31% glucose, and some other di- and tri-saccharides (Donner, 1977).

A honeybee colony needs honey to provide carbohydrates during the beekeeping season (in managed colonies) but also to overwinter. In temperate climate areas, it is usually considered that a colony needs 20 kg of honey to overwinter. In northern USA and Canada, colonies are reported to need more than 40 kg to survive the overwintering period (October–April) (Beesource, 1978).

The annual honey yield may vary according to, in particular, resources, climate, beekeeping practices, and crop factors.

11.2 Pollen

Pollen is the honeybees' source of protein; it also provides lipids, vitamins, and minerals. The nutritive value of pollen is very diverse according to the flower species. Thus, diversity of flowers is necessary to accrue all the elements needed by the honeybees (amino acids, lipids, minerals, vitamins, etc.).

When visiting flowers, the forager retains grains of pollen with its hairs. The bee then cleans its body with its legs, and passes the pollen from its forelegs to its hind legs, where it is stored for the flight back to the hive as a sticky ball (mixed with nectar and food-processing gland secretions) in the pollen basket situated on the hind legs (Figure 1.26). The residual pollen grains trapped on the hairs of the honeybee can pollinate flowers; this is the adaptation of bees to pollination of the angiosperm (and of the angiosperm to the bees).

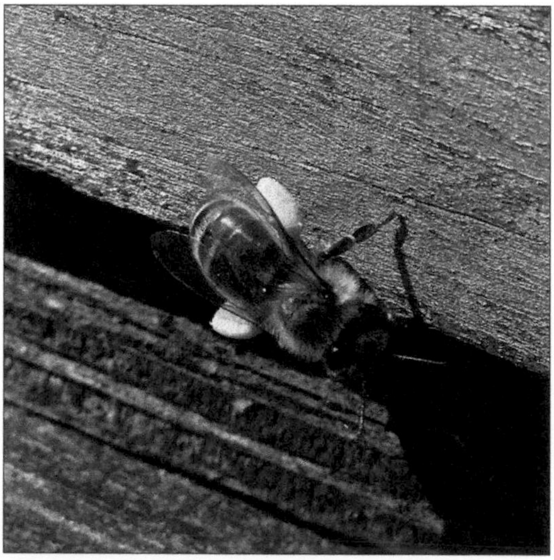

Figure 1.26 Forager coming back to the hive with sticky balls of pollen in the pollen baskets. (© Nicolas Vidal-Naquet.)

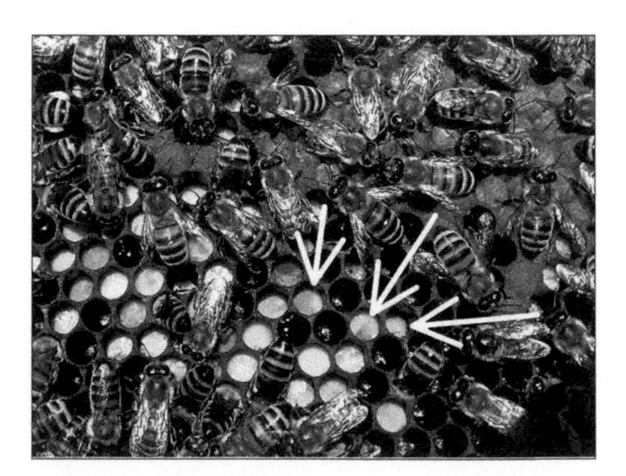

Figure 1.27 Beebread. Beebread is stored in uncapped cells. The colour of the beebread may vary due to the diversity of the flowers visited by foragers. During one flight foragers visit only one species of flower. (© Nicolas Vidal-Naquet.)

Inside the colony, nest workers take charge of the pollen, beginning digestion and preventing germination. Symbiotic microbes play a major role in protecting the stored pollen from spoilage (DeGrandi-Hoffman *et al.*, 2012). This symbiotic action begins while foraging. Bacteria and fungi are added to the pollen with nectar in the sticky ball, lowering the pH and initiating a fermentation process. This process converts the pollen into a long-term storage form called 'beebread' in uncapped cells (Figure 1.27). The roles of these symbiotic microbes seem to be important to honeybee health. Therefore, the use of antibiotics or fungicides (as treatment within the hive or on crops as pesticides) is reported to endanger the balance of symbiotic microbes in the colony and may impair colony health (Yoder *et al.*, 2012). Beebread can, in some respects, be compared to silage (fermented stored fodder) for feeding ruminants.

11.3 Feeding behaviour of adult bees

The food of the workers is composed of honey and pollen (beebread). The basic nutritional requirements of the workers depend on their activity and the activity of the colony. When nursing, workers need a high level of nutrients in order to feed the brood and the queen. In winter, honey is necessary to ensure a carbohydrate supply; at the beginning of spring and during the honey flow, honey and pollen are necessary.

Young drones are fed by workers with a mixture of brood jelly, pollen, and honey. Later, they are able to feed by themselves in the honey cells, in particular before the mating flight.

Queens are fed brood food by the worker nurses. They seldom feed themselves on honey within the colony. Isolated queens may feed on candy (when exchanging or trading queens, they are often sent with their retinue in boxes along with some sugar for food). Feeding duration and nutrient supply quantity depend on the queen's laying rate (Winston, 1987).

11.4 Feeding behaviour of larvae

Larvae are fed with brood food, also called jelly (royal jelly, worker jelly, or drone jelly), produced by the food-producing glands of the nurse workers.

The hypopharyngeal and mandibular glands produce the main components of the brood food and are well developed by the time the workers are at the nursing stage. Proteins, carbohydrates, lipids, vitamins, minerals, and of course water are required to produce the larval jelly. The proteins in larval jelly contain all the essential amino acids necessary for the development of honeybee adults (Haydak, 1970). Lipids are also necessary. 10-Hydroxy-2-decenoic acid (10-HDA) and 24-methylene cholesterol produced in the mandibular gland seem to be involved in growth and development (Winston, 1987). Carbohydrates are of major importance in development. The difference in composition between worker jelly and royal jelly, but also the higher rate of feeding of queen larvae explains the caste differentiation between the diploid eggs.

The brood food is provided as soon as the egg hatches.

The worker larvae food brood changes on the third day after hatching. For the first 2 days, the worker jelly consists of a blend of hypopharyngeal and mandibular secretions, in a ratio of 3:1 or 4:1 (Haydak, 1970). The mandibular portion then decreases and the jelly is mainly composed of hypopharyngeal secretion. At this time, both the quantity and quality of proteins decrease (Winston, 1987). Honey and pollen become a part of the jelly (the pollen is a yellow component in the jelly). The addition of honey has an important dilution effect (Haydak, 1970). The food requirements of worker larvae are not well known. If underfeeding occurs, dwarf adults can emerge from cells. The quality and quantity of worker jelly are fundamental to producing 'strong' workers (Winston, 1987). Underfeeding (weak colonies, diseases, starvation, etc.) adversely affects the worker brood.

The nutritional composition of drone brood food (drone jelly) is not well known. Drone larvae receive much more food during their growth and development than worker larvae do (Haydak, 1970).

Queen larvae are reared in special vertical oval-shaped cells. Throughout the larval stage, an abundance of royal jelly is supplied by nurse bees to feed queen larvae (Figure 1.22). Even after capping, some jelly remains in the cell. Royal jelly contains much higher levels of mandibular secretions than the jelly fed to other castes. Royal jelly has two components: white (mandibular secretions) and clear (hypopharyngeal secretions), in a ratio of 1:1 (Jung-Hoffman, 1966; Haydak, 1970). The mandibular secretions and high levels of sugars are the main characteristics of royal jelly. The quality of the royal jelly, and in particular the presence of the protein royalactin, induces the secretion of juvenile hormone in the female larvae corpora allata and the development of a diploid egg into a queen, stimulating in particular the development of ovarioles within the ovaries and the growth of the body (Winston, 1987; Kamakura, 2011).

12 Organization and communication within the colony

The colony must be considered as a super-organism organised with the queen in charge of laying eggs and workers in charge of all tasks in the nest. The drones' only role seems to be mating virgin queens.

12.1 Age polyethism: the division of labour among worker bees (Winston, 1987; Le Conte, 2006b)

During their lifetime workers undertake many jobs in a quite defined order. This temporal division of labour is also termed age polyethism. The first tasks undertaken are inside the nest (cleaning, nursing, comb building, etc.); then, when workers become older, the tasks are mainly outside tasks (guarding, foraging). The lifespan of summer workers is on average 25–30 days (Winston, 1987). As their tasks change with time, the glands of the workers develop according to the corresponding task. Thus, in nurses, food-processing glands are well developed but decline when it is the turn of other tasks to be performed. In comb-building workers, wax glands are at their peak of processing; thereafter, these glands become atrophied.

In winter, the main task of all the winter bees is to allow the colony to go through winter and survive the cold. Their role is also to rear the brood of the new generation of workers in the following spring. The life span of winter workers is 2–6 months, depending on the region.

These task and temporal divisions of labour is one of the explanations for the organization of the colony.

12.1.1 Cleaning

After emerging, and on average for the first 2 days thereafter, the adult bees serve as cleaners, removing the remains of the larvae and pupae from the cells. After emergence, cells are quickly cleaned, allowing the queen to oviposit within them again. The adult bees also remove all kinds of debris, e.g. moult skin, pollen, capping, diseased or dead larvae and adult bees (Figure 6.5).

12.1.2 Brood and queen nursing

On average, from 3 to 16 days of age workers inspect larval cells and feed larvae. This is the nursing task. At this age, the hypopharyngeal and mandibular glands are well developed, allowing the secretion of royal and worker jelly. Inspections of larval cells are frequent, allowing nurses to adapt the quality and quantity of brood food to the larval age.

At the same time, nurses are tending the queen. Feeding is adapted to the laying activity: the more the queen lays, the more workers feed her with royal jelly.

12.1.3 Food handling and storage

Stockers (on average, days 10–15 of life) store nectar and pollen. The nectar is transmitted to the storing bees by the forager via trophallaxis. The worker exposes the nectar repeatedly to the air (evaporation) with her mouthparts. This is also a stage when enzymes are added to the nectar. The nectar is then stored in the cells and the fanning workers continue the drying process until nectar contains less than 18–20% water.

The pollen is directly stored as beebread by foraging bees in cells and manipulated by workers with honey and saliva before pushing it to the bottom of the cell.

12.1.4 Comb building

At about the same age, workers (comb-builders) produce small wax scales from four pairs of ventral abdominal hypodermal wax glands (Snodgrass, 1910). These secreted wax scales are initially colourless, becoming opaque after mastication by the worker bee. The wax of the honeycomb is nearly white, but becomes progressively more yellow or brown.

Secretion is maximal when the glands are well developed in 2-week-old workers. Wax is produced via the metabolism of honey and is composed of around 300 different substances (hydrocarbons, monoesters, diesters, free acids, and hydroxypolyesters). Younger comb-builders are in charge of capping cells while older builders are in charge of comb construction.

Combs are built by workers, which transfer the wax scales with their third legs to the catching and kneading mandibles. In both wild nests and managed hives, combs are built vertically. The comb-building of the nest begins on the upper side and portions are joined afterwards at different points of the developing nest (or hive). The cells are hexagonal, and orientated on average 13–15° from the horizontal, preventing the honey from flowing out. The hexagonal shape is the most economical use of space and resources and allows bees to accommodate the maximum number of larvae with minimal wax production (Réaumur, 1734–1742). Cellular uniformity results from the sensory and gravity receptors of the bees.

12.1.5 Fanning

Ventilation is the first outside job the workers undertake. Fanning workers are on average 18 days old at the peak of this job period; however, workers of any age may ventilate if necessary.

Fanning plays many roles: cooling, evaporating water from nectar, and controlling humidity and carbon dioxide levels within the nest. Fanning occurs at the entrance of the nest (or the hive), but also near the honey cells inside.

12.1.6 Guarding

On average from the age of 12–25 days, some workers become guards for a few hours, defending the colony against predators and robbing bees. At the entrance to the hive, guards, when faced with a potential danger, secrete an alarm pheromone from their mandibular glands, inspect the situation, and take a defensive posture. Workers have a sting, allowing defence and attack if required. Nest defence is the consequence of the guards recognizing and alerting the other workers of the colony. Workers sting predators and then die, losing their stinger within the prey.

Another strategy of defence is 'behavioural fever'. Workers group together in a ball and collectively raise the temperature to at least 45°C around a predator such as a hornet (Evans and Spivak, 2010). This is the way used by some Asian honeybee species to fight *Vespa velutina*, the Asian hornet that invaded France in 2005 (Figure 7.13).

There is a great variability in defence behaviour according to strain and subspecies but also according to weather, colony size, etc. (Winston, 1987).

12.1.7 Foraging

Foraging begins around the 21st day after emergence and lasts 4–5 days. This is the last task workers perform before dying. The efficiency of foraging behaviour is due to the division of the task between scout and foraging workers. Scout honeybees are in charge of discovering sites and recruiting forager bees. Nectar and pollen are brought back to the nest respectively in the crop and in the pollen basket or corbicula.

Each forager makes 10–15 trips a day, and visits between one and 500 flowers of the same species during each trip. This specificity is favourable to pollination. Trips are generally less than 3 km long around the nest or hive but bees have been reported to fly up to 10 km. This ecologically successful activity allows a large panel of workers to take advantage of floral diversity and vice versa.

Foragers also gather water, which is crucial for the colony. Some honeybees in the colony specialise in water gathering (Lindauer, 1952; Robinson *et al.*, 1984). As previously noted, water plays a crucial role in temperature modulation within the individuals and the colony. Water is not stored, so there is a permanent need for a source near the hive.

12.1.8 Plasticity and adaptation

Plasticity and even reversibility are reported to be possible in this temporal division of labour (Lindauer, 1952; Winston, 1987). Thus, when necessary, young workers can become foragers earlier than normal. For example, if there is a lack of foragers (e.g. due these being killed, or rendered unable to return to the hive during foraging as a result of poisoning), inside workers can quickly turn into foragers.

Another feature of the temporal division of labour is reversibility. An older worker can return to being an inside worker. Thus, in the case of trouble, such as a lack of nurses or foragers, the colony is able to adapt to the situation because workers are able to do the different tasks at any age (Lindauer, 1952; Winston, 1987).

Mitochondrial RNA (mtRNA) expression within the brain is reported to play a role in the regulation of behavioural plasticity of the honeybee (Greenberg *et al.*, 2012).

12.1.9 Winter workers

Overwintering is a highly risky period for a colony. Colonies and winter workers must be strong enough to go through the winter; winter workers, which have a long lifespan, are essential to a colony's survival through the winter months. Winter workers ensure in particular thermoregulation of the nest. At the end of winter, these long-life winter bees become nurses and/or foragers and rear the new brood, producing the first generation of spring workers. This allows the colony to develop a new period of honey flow. Overwintering mainly depends on the strength and lifespan of winter bees. The role of their fat bodies, the only source of proteins and lipids during overwintering, is crucial. Carbohydrates are provided only by the honey stored in feral colonies. Carbohydrates are fundamental to maintaining homeostasis within the colony in winter. In managed colonies, if all the honey stored has been removed from the hive for trade, the beekeeper has to substitute it by a feeding carbohydrate supplement (e.g. candy).

12.2 Communication between bees

The organization and life of the colony is not only the sum of individual roles but involves also complex interactions between bees. Communication between individuals and castes and orientation are essential conditions of social insect colonies such as *A. mellifera* (Winston, 1987). Thus, for example, orientation allows foragers to find food and water resources, and communication allows them to share information with their nest mates and recruit other forager bees.

Communication between honeybees can involve chemicals, dance, or sound (Maschwitz, 1964; von Frisch, 1967; Towne, 1985; Free, 1987; Blum, 1992). Much scientific work has been done on this subject, in particular by Karl von Frisch, who won the Nobel Prize for his work on the dance of the honeybee (von Frisch, 1967).

12.2.1 Chemical communication: pheromones

Many pheromones are involved in communications between honeybees within the colony. Honeybees possess 15 documented glands producing these chemicals (Free, 1987; Blum, 1992). At least 18 chemicals have been described as pheromones (Winston, 1987). In honeybees, pheromones are produced by queens, workers, and probably drones (Figure 1.11), and are involved in mating, alarm, cohesion, recognition of the colony, inhibition of queen rearing, etc.

Queen pheromones

The main queen pheromone is queen mandibular pheromone (QMP), which plays several roles in reproduction (Winston and Hugo, 1991; Blum, 1992; Pankiw, 1998). Chemically, QMP is very diverse, containing at least 17 major compounds (Slessor *et al.*, 1990; Winston and Hugo, 1991). QMP is distributed throughout the colony. The first bees involved in this transfer are the retinue workers, who lick the queen, and the pheromone is then spread to other workers of the colony (Bortolotti and Costa, 2010).

The functions of QMP are (Bortolotti and Costa, 2010):

- Formation of the queen retinue.
- Inhibition of queen-rearing by the colony.
- Social behaviour and cohesion of the colony – QMP allows workers to recognise the queens and inhibits ovarian development in workers.
- Stimulation of worker activities, such as comb building, brood feeding, guarding, and foraging.
- Stimulation of Nasonov pheromone release.
- Attraction of drones and mating behaviour by virgin queens (sexual pheromone role).
- Formation and maintenance of the swarm cluster – QMP attracts workers to the swarm, stabilizing the swarm and helping swarm movement to a new nest site (Winston, 1987).

Under natural conditions, at the end of her life, the queen secretes less QMP, loses hairs, and her wings become indented. This phenomenon will induce the replacement of the queen by supersedure.

The queen possesses other pheromone glands:

- The glands of Arnhart situated on the tarsus produce a tarsal gland pheromone, also called the footprint pheromone. This secretion is deposited by the mated queen on the comb and inhibits the building of queen cells by workers (Bortolotti and Costa, 2010).
- The Dufour's gland produces a pheromone linked to reproduction and ovipositioning.
- The tergal glands (situated between the tergites of the abdomen) secrete a pheromone involved in drone copulation; this pheromone also inhibits queen rearing and ovarian development in workers.

Worker pheromones

Workers emit a range of pheromones, including the following:

- Alarm pheromones. These are involved in guard behaviour. One alarm pheromone is released by the Koschevnikov gland when a honeybee stings another animal. This pheromone then stimulates other bees of the colony to behave defensively (sting or charge) (Koschevnikov, 1899; Free, 1987). A second alarm pheromone is released by the mandibular glands and is used to discourage potential enemies and robber bees.
- Dufour's gland pheromone. The Dufour's gland opens into the dorsal vaginal wall, and secretes a pheromone that allows workers to distinguish between eggs laid by the queen, which are attractive, and those laid by workers in particular circumstances, e.g. when the colony is queenless (Oldroyd *et al.*, 2002; Dor *et al.*, 2005).

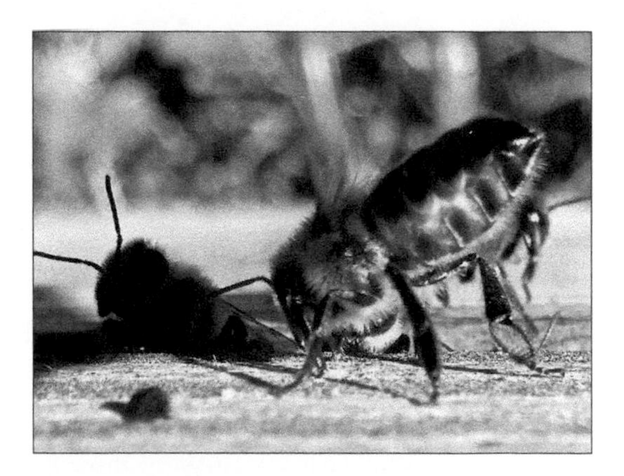

Figure 1.28 Worker bee releasing Nasonov pheromone (typical attitude). (© Nicolas Vidal-Naquet.)

- Nasonov gland pheromones (Figure 1.28), composed of seven chemicals, principally geraniol. The pheromones play a major role in orientation, and are used in diverse situations including guiding foragers back home, during swarming, marking the new nest entrance after swarming, and forage marking. Nasonov pheromones also play an important role in foraging for water and are released to mark the water site in order to guide water foragers (Williams *et al.*, 1982; Winston, 1987; Schmidt, 1999).
- Footprint pheromones involved in, among other things, orientation, foraging, brood recognition and egg marking are also emitted. Other pheromones are emitted by worker bees.

Drone pheromones

Drones seem to produce pheromones from their mandibular glands. These chemicals are reported to be involved in attracting flying drones, and in attracting the queen to the congregation area (Winston, 1987).

The brood is also a pheromone producer. The roles of brood pheromones are brood recognition, stimulating foraging behaviour, and inhibiting ovarian development in workers (Free, 1967; Scott, 1986; Winston, 1987).

12.2.2 Dances of honeybees

In 1788, Spitzner, and later Unhoch in 1823, observed a worker dance within a colony. In 1973, the Nobel Prize was given to Karl von Frisch who described the dances of the honeybee as a 'bee language' (von Frisch, 1953, 1967, 1969).

Three kinds of dance have been described: the round dance, the waggle dance, and the dorso-ventral abdominal vibrating dance (DVAV dance). Dancing occurs within the hive, on the comb surface, and near the entrance. These dances give information in particular on foraging sites to workers but also regulate foraging activity and when swarming occurs. Workers follow the dancer to obtain the information.

- In a colony, a round dance is the simplest dance – it does not give information on the distance and/or the direction, but only informs bees of a nearby source of nectar (within 15 m). When a scout bee discovers a source of nectar, it returns to the hive and conveys this information to foragers via the round dance. Honeybees take into account the 'nutritional value' of the resource: the longer and more vigorous the dance, the higher the sugar concentration.
- A waggle dance (a figure-of-eight dance), performed by scout bees, indicates a food site more than 100 m from the hive. It informs foragers of the direction and distance of the site, as well as the quality of the food there. The bees dance in a direction determined by the angles between the sun, the resource site, and the hive; the distance to the resource is given by the speed of the dance; and the food quality is indicated by the amplitude of the waggles.
- The DVAV dance is characterized by a worker vibrating its abdomen dorso-ventrally while grabbing another worker or the queen (Winston, 1987). The role of this dance is to regulate foraging and swarming.
- Other dances exist, in particular, a dance to help the colony choose a new site during swarming.

12.2.3 Acoustic communication

Piping and tooting are sounds made by queens (Winston, 1987; Kirchner, 1993). Tooting is a sound emitted by the first virgin queen upon emergence, when there are several queen cells. This sound is reported to prevent the other queens from emerging. A piping sound (tooting + quacking) is usually made when there is more than one queen in a hive. It is postulated that this piping is a form of 'battle cry', announcing to competing queens a willingness to fight. Workers also emit and are sensitive to sounds.

Reproduction, the temporal division of labour, and communications between bees all serve to regulate the colony and explain why a colony is regarded as a super-organism.

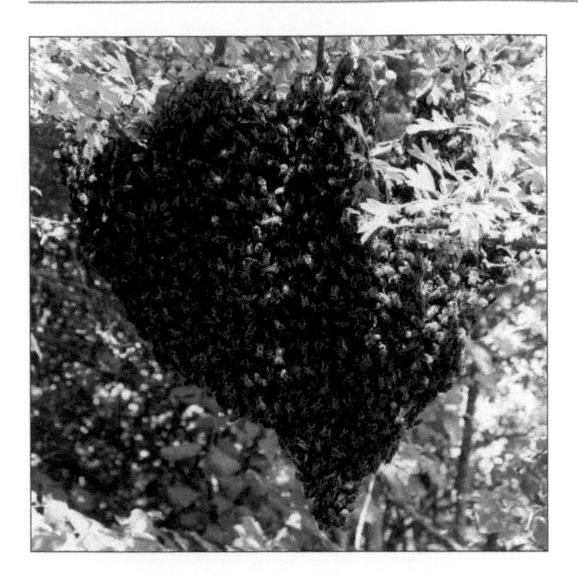

Figure 1.29 A swarm of a honeybee colony attached to a branch of a tree. A location to build a new nest will be search by scout bees. (© Nicolas Vidal-Naquet.)

13 Swarming and supersedure: division of the colony and replacement of the queen

The colony, as a perennial super-organism, is able to divide by swarming and to rear a new queen in case of reproductive failure or death of the queen in order to continue its life.

13.1 Swarming

Swarming allows the division of the colony and the perpetuation of the species (Winston, 1980, 1987; Villa, 2004). Swarming usually occurs when the colony population is maximal. An excess of brood and an overcrowded colony are thought to be the main causes of swarming, but other causes are possible (e.g. inherited factors and resource abundance) (Winston, 1987).

The main cause of these colony changes is reported to be a reduction in QMP transmission. This leads workers to build up queen cells and to begin to rear queen larvae. With the development of queen cells, the queen stops laying eggs, usual hive activities are also stopped, and the colony becomes highly excited. After filling their crops with honey, a group of workers and the mother queen, together with tens of drones, fly out of the hive. This group builds up a swarm, usually on a branch of the tree where the parent nest resides (in feral honeybee colonies) or near the parent hive (Figure 1.29). Then, the swarm moves to a new location found by scout bees (e.g. in a tree trunk, between a window and a shutter). In the parent colony, the remaining workers rear queen cells and a worker brood. A queen will lay eggs about one week after swarming. In some cases, 'after-swarms' may follow the first one (Winston, 1980, 1987). In temperate countries, swarming usually occurs when the worker population reaches a peak, in mid-spring (May and June). However, swarming period and swarming behaviour depend on the climate, the region, the subspecies, and the strain of honeybee.

If swarming is the way of colony division in the wild, in apiculture natural swarming poses a risk as it may weaken the colony for a while. On another hand, swarming offers an opportunity for beekeepers, and indeed, this biological process can be used to divide colonies and maintain or increase livestock by producing artificial swarms.

In the case of swarming, it is reported that queen cells are mainly located on the edge of the frame or comb. However, it seems that 'swarm cells' may also be located elsewhere on the frame.

13.2 Supersedure

Supersedure is another method by which the colony can replace its queen. This happens when the queen becomes unreproductive through age, injury, or sickness. The process of supersedure requeening is initiated by a decrease in QMP level within the colony (Butler, 1957; Winston, 1987). In colonies superseding their queens, several queen cells are built and several future queen larvae are reared. At the same time the queen continues to lay eggs until the emergence of a new queen. After the emergence of a virgin queen and her mating, the old queen will usually be killed.

Supersedure can be used as a beekeeping practice to replace the queen. For example, by clipping off one of the middle or posterior legs of the queen, she will be unable to place her eggs accurately at the bottom of the brood cell. The workers will detect this failure and will then build supersedure queen cells to replace the queen.

Both supersedure and swarming are queen-replacement and queen-rearing mechanisms. Large colonies seem to replace their queen more often by supersedure than by swarming (Winston, 1987). Swarming provides a way to divide the colony and for the honeybee to perpetuate the species.

Supersedure queen cells are reported to be located mainly in the centre though sometimes at the fringe of the brood nest.

13.3 Emergency queen cells

In the event of the sudden death of the queen (accidentally or following a disease), workers will rear worker eggs or very young worker larvae (a few hours old) with royal jelly. The workers then build emergency queen cells around the chosen eggs and larvae. However, these 'emergency queens' are usually smaller and less prolific, especially if the queen is raised from a larva that is 'too old'.

14 Colony life cycle

The different steps that determine the development and the dynamics of the colony on an annual basis define the colony life cycle (Vidal-Naquet, 2009). This cycle can be evaluated by examining the brood area in the combs and/or by the quantity of workers in the colony.

The cycle follows the laying activity of the queen and the presence of the brood (Le Conte, 2006b).

According to the seasons, the colony has either summer or winter workers. The first summer workers emerge in spring and summer and participate in the development of the colony and the preparation for wintering by gathering resources that will be stored in the combs. Their lifespan is on average 5–6 weeks. The second group of workers appears at the end of the summer and/or the beginning of autumn,

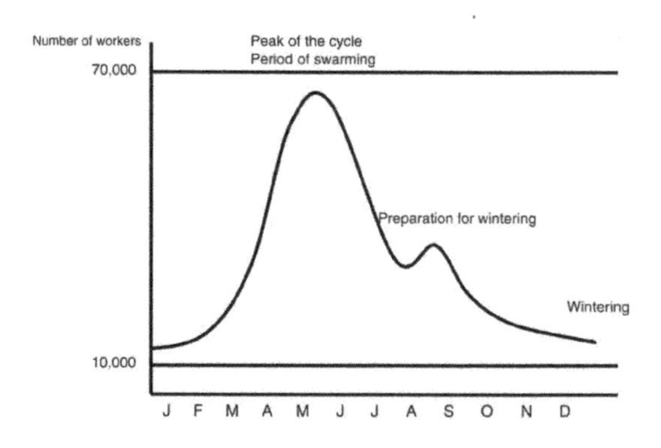

Figure 1.30 Typical life cycle of a honeybee colony in a temperate climate. The dynamics of the bee population, showing the main peak in June with the emergence of summer workers during the height of flowering, and a second peak in August/September with the emergence of winter workers in preparation for overwintering. (Adapted from Le Conte, 2006; and OIE Terrestrial Manual, 2014.)

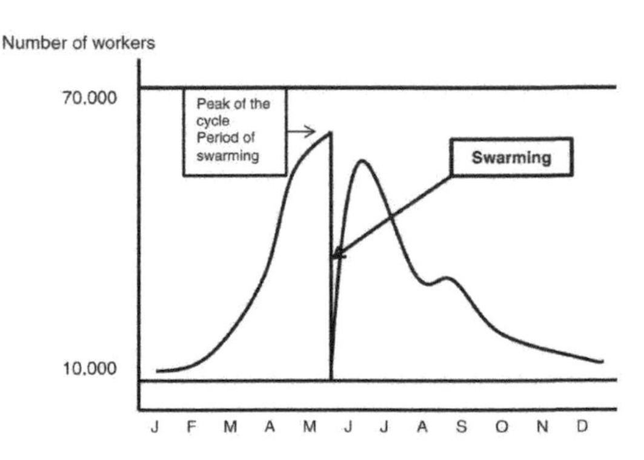

Figure 1.31 Life cycle of a swarming honeybee colony (temperate climate). Swarming occurs at the peak of the cycle. Secondary or even tertiary swarming can occur. Swarming allows the division of the colony and the perpetuation of the species. In apiculture, swarming poses a major risk to production. Swarming may be used by beekeepers in managed colonies to maintain or increase livestock. (Adapted from Le Conte, 2006.)

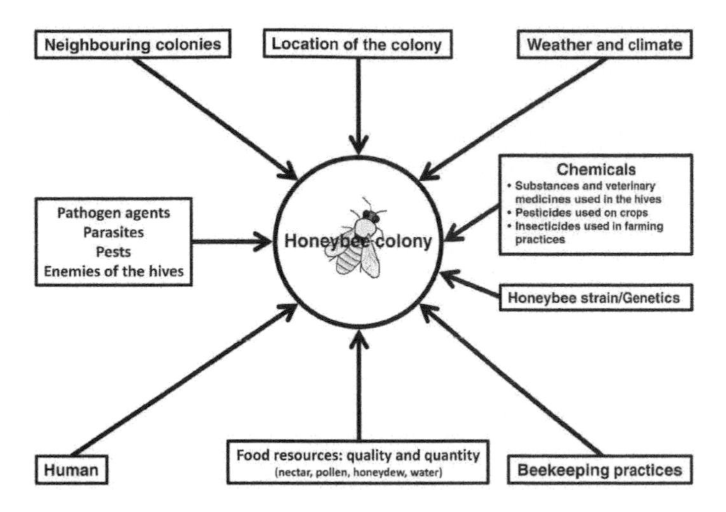

Figure 1.32 Factors acting as stressors on managed honeybee colonies.

allowing the colony to survive the winter. Their life span can last several months.

The peak of brood surface or number of workers within the colony occurs in mid–end spring when the maximal honey flow occurs.

This colony life cycle depends on subspecies, geographic situation, season, water resource, floral and agricultural environment, and consequently on the quality and quantity of honey plants. Feral and managed local honeybee strains are usually adapted to their own environment.

For example, in a northern hemisphere temperate climate zone, the colony cycle has one or two peaks (OIE, 2014a) (Figure 1.30).

This process can be described as follows:

- Development phase. After wintering, the colony develops when the queen resumes laying eggs in the cells.
- Peak period. The colony reaches a first brood peak in mid–end spring (the queen can lay up to 2,000 eggs a day). This is the time when swarming may occur, allowing the division of the colony and perpetuation of the species. In the case of swarming, the mother colony will lose many workers that depart with the old queen (Figure 1.31).
- At the end of July and into August, the queen's egg-laying activity decreases. The population decreases along with regional flowering.
- Preparation for the wintering phase (except in hot and tropical climates where there is no wintering period). At the end of August and in September, the queen continues to oviposit in order to allow the setting and rearing of the winter worker brood. The winter bees do not have to rear a brood or forage during overwintering. Their lifespan is longer. Their roles are to allow the colony to overwinter and to ensure the rearing of brood at the beginning of the new season (at the end of winter or in early spring according to the region). Thus, the ability of a colony to overwinter in good condition and start again in spring depends to a great extent on the winter bees' strength and lifespan (Noireterre, 2011).
- Overwintering phase. The population is reduced and lives around the queen in a cluster, feeding on stored honey (or carbohydrate feeding supplement in managed colonies). There is no brood in cold areas in winter. Overwintering is a risky period for the colonies. In managed colonies, mortality and dwindling mainly occur in this period.

Thus, there is a demographic explosion during spring, allowing pollination, pollen storage, and honey production. In autumn, the population declines and the emergence of winter bees, with specific physiological features (in particular well-developed fat bodies), allows the colony to survive the winter. In managed colonies, one of the main roles of the beekeeper is to ensure that both winter bees and colonies are strong enough for this critical period, especially if the climate and meteorological conditions are extreme.

As with any reared species, the life cycle and consequently the health (and thus productivity) of managed colonies depends on many factors (Figure 1.32). Impairment of one or several of these factors will affect the balance required for managed colonies:

- The geographical location, the climate, and the weather are some of the main factors influencing the life of honeybee colonies (Chapter 2).
- Food resources (nectar, pollen, honeydew, water) are crucial factors influencing the cycle and life of the colony. Both wild honey plants and crops around colonies are the only food resources. Monoculture and decreasing biodiversity pose the risk that bees will lack nutrients (Chapter 2).
- Phytosanitary products (pesticides) used on crops but also veterinary medicines and drugs used in hives (in particular in controlling the infestation by the mite *Varroa destructor*) may act as stressors on honeybees (Chapter 2). Pesticides used on crops are also stressors and chemical hazards for wild bees and bumblebees.
- Biological pathogens (viruses, bacteria, fungi, parasites) and pests and predators of the hives may seriously endanger colonies. The mite *V. destructor* (and bee mite parasitic syndrome) is one of the main biological hazards facing honeybees (Chapters 3–7).
- Human and beekeeping practices are also main 'factors' that may influence the life of managed colonies (Chapter 8).

The following chapters are dedicated to these stressors, their consequences, and how to manage and control them as far as possible.

The terms 'good health' and 'strong colonies', 'weakening', 'mortality', and 'collapse' are all used in the field of honeybee pathology to characterise the health status and strength of colonies. The definitions and features of these terms are developed in the Glossary and in Chapter 9 (section 1.4.5).

References

Agaisse H. and Perrimon N. (2004) The roles of JAK/STAT signaling in *Drosophila* immune responses. *Immunological Reviews*, 198: 72–82.

Allen, M.D. (1957) Observations on honeybees examining and licking their queen. *British Journal of Animal Behaviour*, 5: 81–84.

Amdam, G.V., Norberg, K., Hagen, A., and Omholt, S.W. (2003) Social exploitation of vitellogenin. *Proceedings of the National Academy of Sciences of the United States of America*, 100: 1799–1802.

Amdam, G.V., Hartfelder, K., Norberg, K., Hagen, A., and Omholt, S.W. (2004) Altered physiology in worker honey bees (Hymenoptera: Apidae) infested with the mite *Varroa destructor* (Acari: Varroidae): a factor in colony loss during overwintering? *Journal of Economic Entomology*, 97: 741–747.

Amdam, G.V., Fennern, E., and Havukainen, H. (2012) Vitellogenin in honey bee behavior and lifespan. In Galizia, C.G., Eisenhardt, D., and Giurfa, M. (eds), *Honeybee Neurobiology and Behavior*. Springer, Dordrecht, pp. 17–29.

Antúnez, K., Martín-Hernández, R., Prieto, L., Meana, A., Zunino, P., and Higes, M. (2009) Immune suppression in the honey bee (*Apis mellifera*) following infection by *Nosema ceranae* (*Microsporidia*). *Environmental Microbiology*, doi:10.1111/j.1462–2920.2009.01953.x

Arresse, E.L. and Soulages, J.L. (2010) Insect fat body: energy, metabolism, and regulation. *Annual Review of Entomology*, 55: 207–225.

Beesource (1978) *Overwintering of honey bee colonies*. Available at: http://www.beesource.com/resources/usda/overwintering-of-honey-bee-colonies/ (accessed 30 August 2014).

Beesource (2014) The different types of honey bees. Available at http://www.beesource.com/resources/usda/the-different-types-of-honey-bees/ (accessed 5 July 2014).

Blum, M.S. (1992) Honeybee pheromones. In *The Hive and the Honeybee*, rev. edn. Dadant & Sons, Hamilton, IL, pp. 385–389.

Bomtorin, A.D., Mackert, A., Rosa, G.C.C., Moda, L.M., Martins, J.R., *et al.* (2014) Juvenile hormone biosynthesis gene expression in the corpora allata of honey bee (*Apis mellifera* L.) female castes. *PLoS ONE*, 9(1): e86923. doi:10.1371/journal.pone.0086923

Bortolotti, L. and Costa, C. (2010) Chemical communication in honey bee society. In Mucignat-Caretta, C. (ed.), *Neurobiology and Chemical Communication*. Taylor & Francis, Boca Raton, FL, pp. 147–195.

Butler, C.G. (1957) The process of queen supersedure in colonies of honeybees (*Apis mellifera* L.). *Insectes Sociaux*, 4: 211–223.

Casteels, P., Ampe, C., van Damme, J., Elicone, C., Fleming, F., Jacobs, F., and Tempst, P. (1990) Isolation and characterization of abaecin, a major antibacterial response peptide in the honeybee (*Apis mellifera*). *European Journal of Biochemistry*, 187(2): 381–386.

Casteels, P., Ampe, C., Jacobs, F., and Tempst, P. (1993) Functional and chemical characterization of Hymenoptaecin, an antibacterial polypeptide that is infection-inducible in the honeybee (*Apis mellifera*). *Journal of Biological Chemistry*, 268(10): 7044–7054.

Chan, Q.W.T., Mutti, N.S., Foster, L.J., Kocher, S.D., Amdam, G.V., *et al.* (2011) The worker honeybee fat body proteome is extensively remodeled preceding a major life-history transition. *PLoS ONE*, 6(9): e24794. doi:10.1371/journal.pone.0024794

Claudianos, C., Ranson, H., Johnson, R.M., Biswas, S., Schuler, M.A., Berenbaum, M.R., Feyereisen, R., and Oakeshott J.G. (2006) A deficit of detoxification enzymes: pesticide sensitivity and environmental response in the honeybee. *Insect Molecular Biology*, 15(5): 615–636.

Cooper, P.D., William, M., Schaffer, W.M., and Buchmann, S.L. (1985) Temperature regulation of honeybees (*Apis Mellifera*) foraging in the Sonoran Desert. *Journal of Experimental Biology*, 114: 1–15.

Costa, J.T. and Fitzgerald, T.D. (2005) Social terminology revisited: where are we ten years later? *Annales Zoologici Fennici*, 42: 559–564.

Crespi, B.J. and Yanega, D. (1995) The definition of eusociality. *Behavioral Ecology*, 6(1): 109–115.

Dade, H.A. (2009) *Anatomy and Dissection of the Honeybee*, rev. edn. International Bee Research Association, London.

Dainat, B., Evans, J.D., Chen, Y.P., Gauthier, L., and Neumann, P. (2012) Predictive markers of honey bee colony collapse. *PLoS ONE*, 7(2): e32151. doi:10.1371/journal.pone.0032151

DeGrandi-Hoffman, G., Eckholm, B., and Anderson, K.E. (2012) Honey bee health: the potential role of microbes. In Sammatoro D. and Yolder J.A. (eds), *Honey Bee Colony Health Challenges and Sustainable Solutions*. CRC Press, Boca Raton, FL, pp. 1–12.

De Gregorio, E., Spellman, P.T., Tzou, P., Rubin, G.M., and Lemaitre, B. (2002) The Toll and Imd pathways are the major regulators of the immune response in *Drosophila*. *EMBO Journal*, 21(11): 2568–2579.

De La Rua, P., Jaffé, R., Dall'Olio, R., Munoz, I., and Serrano, J. (2009) Biodiversity, conservation and current threats to European Honeybees. *Apidologie*, 40, 263–284.

Donner, L.W. (1977) The sugars of honey – a review. *Journal of the Science of Food and Agriculture*, 28: 443–456.

Dor, R., Katzav-Gozansky, T., and Hefetz, A. (2005) Dufour's gland pheromone as a reliable fertility signal among honeybee (*Apis mellifera*) workers. *Behavioral Ecology and Sociobiology*, 58(3): 270–276.

El Hassani, A.K., Giurfa, M., Gauthier, M., and Armengaud, C. (2008) Inhibitory neurotransmission and olfactory memory in honeybees. *Neurobiology of Learning and Memory*, 90(4), 589–595. doi:10.1016/j.nlm.2008.07.018.

Engel, M.S. (1999a) The taxonomy of recent and fossil honeybees (Hymenoptera: Apidae; *Apis*). *Journal of Hymenoptera Research*, 8: 165–196.

Engel, M.S. (1999b) Augochlorini Beebe, 1925 (Insecta Hymenoptera): Corrected authorship and date (not Moure, 1943). *Bulletin of Zoological Nomenclature*, 56: 198.

Engels, W. (1987) Reproduction and caste development in social bees. In Eder, J. and Rembold, H. (eds), *Chemistry and Biology of Social Insects*. Verlag J. Peperny, Munchen, pp. 275–281.

Evans, J.D. and Spivak, M.L. (2010) Socialized medicine: individual and communal disease barriers in honey bees. *Journal of Invertebrate Pathology*, 103, S62-S72.

Fluri, P., Wille, H., Gerig, L., and Lüscher, M. (1977) Juvenile hormone, vitellogenin and haemocyte composition in winter worker honeybees (*Apis mellifera*). *Experientia*, 33: 1240–1241.

Free, J.B. (1987) *Pheromones of Social Bees*. Comstock, Ithaca, NY.

Free, J.B., Ferguson, A.W., and Simpkins, J.R. (1992) The behaviour of queen honeybees and their attendants. *Physiological Entomology*, 17: 43–55.

Garnery, L., Cornuet, J.-M., and Solignac, M. (1992) Evolutionary history of the honey *Apis mellifera* inferred from mitochondrial DNA analysis. *Molecular Ecology*, 1(3): 145–154.

Gliński, Z. and Buczek, K. (2003) Response of the Apoidea to fungal infections. *Apiacta*, 38 : 183–189.

Goodman, L. (2003) *Form and Function in the Honeybee*. IBRA, Cardiff.

Grimaldi, D.A. and Engel, M.S. (2005) *Evolution of the Insects*. Cambridge University Press, Cambridge.

Greenberg, J.K., Xia, J., Zhou, X., Thatcher, S.R., Gu, X., Ament, S.A., Newman, T.C., Green, P.J., Zhang, W., Robinson, G.E., and Ben-Shahar, Y. (2012) Behavioral plasticity in honey bees is associated with differences in brain microRNA transcriptome. *Genes, Brain and Behavior*, doi: 10.1111/j.1601-183X.2012.00782.x, available at: http://www.life.illinois.edu/robinson/Research/Pdf/GreenbergEtAl2012.pdf (accessed 19 September 2014).

Gregorc, A., Silva-Zacarin, M., and Nocelli R.C.F. (2012) Cellular response in honey bees to non-pathogenic effects of pesticides. In Sammatoro D. and Yolder J.A. (eds), *Honey Bee Colony Health Challenges and Sustainable Solutions*. CRC Press, Boca Raton, FL, pp. 161–180.

Guidugli, K.R., Nascimento, A.M., Amdam, G.V., Barchuk, A.R., Omholt, S., Simões, Z.L., and Hartfelder, K. (2005) Vitellogenin regulates hormonal dynamics in the worker caste of a eusocial insect. *FEBS Letters*, 579: 4961–4965.

Hammer, M. and Menzel, R. (1995) Learning and memory in the honeybee. *Journal of Neuroscience*, 15(3): 1617–1630.

Hatjina, F., Papaefthimiou, C., Charistos, L., Dogaroglu, T., Bouga, M., Emmanouil, C., and Arnold, G. (2013). Sublethal doses of imidacloprid decreased size of hypopharyngeal glands and respiratory rythm of honeybees in vivo. *Apidologie*, 44: 467–480, doi:10.1007/s13592-013-0199-4

Haydak, M.H. (1970) Honey bee nutrition. *Annual Review of Entomology*, 15: 143–156.

Hepburn, H.R. and Crewe, R.M. (1991) Portrait of the Cape honeybee, *Apis mellifera capensis*. *Apidologie*, 22: 567–580.

Heran, H. (1959). Wahrnehmung und Regelung der Flugeigengeschwindigkeit bei Apis mellifica. *Zeitschrift für vergleichende Physiologie*, 42: 103–163.

Heylen, K., Gobin, B., Arckens, L., Huybrechts, R., and Billen, J. (2011) The effects of four crop protection products on the morphology and ultrastructure of the hypopharyngeal gland of the European honeybee, *Apis mellifera*. *Apidologie*, 42: 103–116.

Hodges, D. (1952) *The Pollen Loads of the Honeybee*. Bee Research Association, London.

Imdorf, A., Ruoff, K., and Fluri, P. (2010) *Le développement des colonies chez l'abeille mellifère*. Station de recherche Agroscope Liebefeld-Posieux ALP, Berne.

Jung-Hoffmann, I. (1966) Die Determination von Königin und Arbeiterin der Honingbiene. *Z. Bienenforsch*, 8: 296–322.

Kamakura, M. (2011) Royalactin induces queen differentiation in honeybees. *Nature*, 473: 478–483.

Kirchner, W.H. (1993) Acoustical communication in honeybees. *Apidologie*, 24: 297–307.

Koschevnikov, G.A. (1899) Zur Kenntnis der Hautdrüsen der Apidae und Vespidae. *Anatomischer Anzeiger*, 15: 519–528.

Kovac, H., Stabentheiner, A., and Schmaranzer, S. (2010) Thermoregulation of water foraging honeybees – balancing of endothermic activity with radiative heat gain and functional requirements. *Journal of Insect Physiology*, 56(12): 1834–1845.

Le Conte, Y. (2006a) Les races d'abeilles. In *Traité Rustica de l'Apiculture*, 2nd edn. Rustica Editions, Paris, pp. 40–51.

Le Conte, Y. (2006b) La vie sociale de la colonie. In *Traité Rustica de l'Apiculture*, 2nd edn. Rustica Editions, Paris, pp. 54–83.

Lehane, M.J. (1997) Peritrophic matrix structure and function. *Annual Review of Entomology*, 43: 525–550.

Lindauer, M. (1952) Ein Beitrag zur Frage der Arbeitsteilung im Bienenstaat. *Zeitschrift für vergleichende Physiologie*, 34 : 299–345.

Lindauer, M. (1959) Angeborene und erlernte Komponenten in der Sonnenorientierung der Bienen. *Zeitschrift für vergleichende Physiologie*, 42: 43–62.

Maschwitz, U. (1964) Alarm substances and alarm behavior in social Hymenoptera. *Nature*, 204: 324–327.

Mitchell, A. (2006) Africanized killer bees: a case study. *Critical Care Nurse*, 26: 23–31.

Nelson, C.M., Ihle, K.E., Fondrk, M.K., Page, R.E., Jr, and Amdam, G.V. (2007) The gene *vitellogenin* has multiple coordinating effects on social organization. *PLoS Biol*, 5(3): e62. doi:10.1371/journal.pbio.0050062

Noireterre, P. (2011) Biologie et pathogénie de *Varroa destructor. Bulletin des GTV*, 62: 101–106.

Oldroyd, B.P., Ratnieks, F.L.W., and Wossler, T.C. (2002) Egg-marking pheromones in honeybees *Apis mellifera*. *Behavioral Ecology and Sociobiology*, 51(6): 590–591.

Otis, G.W., Wheeler, D.E., Buck, N., and Mattila, H.R. (2004) Storage proteins in winter honey bees. *Apiacta*, 38: 352–357.

Page, R.E., Jr (1980) The evolution of multiple mating behavior by honeybee queens (*Apis mellifera* L.). *Genetics*, 96: 263–273.

Pankiw, T. (1998) Queen mandibular gland pheromone influences worker honeybee (*Apis mellifera* L.) foraging ontogeny and juvenile hormone titers. *Journal of Insect Physiology*, 44: 685–692.

Philippe, J.M. (2007) *Le guide de l'apiculteur*. Edisud, Aix-en Provence.

Piulachs, M.D., Guidugli, K.R., Barchuk, A.R., Cruz, J., Simoes, Z.L.P., and Bellés, X. (2003) The vitellogenin of the honey bee, *Apis mellifera*: structural analysis of the cDNA and expression studies. *Insect Biochemistry and Molecular Biology*, 33: 459–465.

Plowes, N. (2010) An introduction to eusociality. *Nature Education Knowledge*, 3(10): 7.

Réaumur, R.A. (1734–1742) *Mémoires pour servir à l'Histoire des Insectes*. Vol 5. Imprimerie Royale, Paris.

Rembold, H., Lackner, B., and Geistbeck, I. (1974) The chemical basis of honeybee, *Apis mellifera*, caste formation. Partial purification of queen bee determinator from royal jelly. *Journal of Insect Physiology*, 20(2): 307–314.

Remolina, S.C. (2007) Senescence in the worker honeybee *Apis mellifera*. *Journal of Insect Physiology*, 53(10): 1027–1033.

Robinson, G.E., Underwood, B.A., and Henderson, C.E. (1984) A highly specialized water-collecting honey bee. *Apidologie*, 15 : 355–358.

Roma, G.C., Bueno, O.C., and Camargo-Mathias, M.I. (2010) Morpho-physiological analysis of the insect fat body: a review. *Micron*, 41: 395–401.

Rueppell, O., Bachelier, O., Fondrk, M.K., Robert, E., and Page, R.E., Jr (2007) Regulation of life history determines lifespan of worker honeybees (*Apis mellifera* L.). *Experimental Gerontology*, 42: 1020–1032.

Ruttner, F. (1988) *Biogeography and Taxonomy of Honeybees*. Springer Verlag, Berlin.

Ruttner, F. and Ruttner, H. (1966) Untersuchengen über die Flugaktivität und das Paarungs, verhalten der Drohnen. *Z. Bienenforsch.*, 8(9): 332–354.

Ruttner, F., Tassencourt, L., and Louveaux, J. (1978) Biometrical-statistical analysis of the geographic variability of *Apis mellifera* L. *Apidologie*, 9(4): 363–381.

Schmidt, J.O. (1999) Attractant or pheromone: the case of Nasonov secretion and honeybee swarms. *Journal of Chemical Ecology*, 25(9): 2051–2056.

Scientific Beekeeping (2014) The bee immune system. Available at: http://scientificbeekeeping.com/sick-bees-part-3-the-bee-immune-system/ (accessed 12 July 2014).

Scott, C.D. (1986) Biology and management of wild bee and domesticated honey bee pollinators for tree fruit pollination. Ph.D. thesis, Simon Fraser University, Burnaby, Canada.

Slessor, K.N., Kaminski, L-A., King, G.G.S., and Winston, M.L. (1990) Semiochemicals of the honeybee queen mandibular glands. *Journal of Chemical Ecology*, 16: 851–860.

Snodgrass, R.E. (1910) *The Anatomy of the Honeybee*. US Department of Agriculture.

Spitzner, M.J.E. (1788) *Ausführliche Beschreibung der Korbbienenzucht im sächsischen Churkreise, ihrer Dauer und ihres Nutzens, ohne künstliche Vermehrung nach den Gründen der Naturgeschichte und nach eigener langer Erfahrung*. Junius, Leipzig.

Spivak, M.S. (1996) Honeybee hygienic behavior and defense against *Varroa jacobsoni*. *Apidologie*, 7(4): 245–260.

Stabentheiner, A., Pressl, H., Papst, T., Hrassnigg, N., and Crailsheim, K. (2003) Endothermic heat production in honeybee winter clusters. *Journal of Experimental Biology* 206, 353–358.

Texas A&M University (2014) Honey Bee Biology. Available at: https://insects.tamu.edu/continuing_ed/bee_biology/ (accessed 12 July 2014).

Theopold, U. and Dushay, M.S. (2007) Mechanisms of *Drosophila* immunity – an immune system at work. *Current Immunology Reviews*, 3: 276–288.

Tofilski, A. (2012) Honey bee. Available at www.http://honeybee.drawwing.org (accessed 10 July 2014).

Towne, W.F. (1985) Acoustic and visual cues in the dances of four honeybee species. *Behavioral Ecology and Sociobiology*, 16(2): 185–187.

Unhoch, N. (1823) *Anleitung zur wahren Kenntnis und zweckmässigsten Behandlung der Bienen*. Munchen.

University of Illinois (2007) Bee Anatomy. Available at: http://www.uni.illinois.edu/~stone2/Bee_anatomy.html (accessed 12 July 2014).

Villa, J.D. (2004) Swarming behavior of honeybees (Hymenoptera: Apidae) in southeastern Louisiana. *Annals of the Entomological Society of America*, 97(1): 111–116.

Vidal-Naquet, N. (2009) L'abeille Apis mellifera: les castes et les cycles. *Bulletin des GTV*, 51: 86–90.

Vidal-Naquet, N. (2011) Honeybees. In Lewbart, G.L. (ed.), *Invertebrate Medicine*, 2nd edn. Wiley-Blackwell, Chichester, pp. 285–321.

von Frisch, K. (1953) *The Dancing Bees*. Harcourt, Brace & World, Inc., San Diego, CA.

von Frisch, K. (1967) *The Dance Language and Orientation of Bees*. Harvard University Press, Cambridge, MA.

von Frisch, K. (1969) *Vie et mœurs des abeilles (Aus dem Leben der Bienen)*. Albin Michel, Paris.

Watmouth, J. and Camazine S. (1995) Self-organized thermoregulation of honeybee clusters. *Journal of Theoretical Biology*, 176: 391–402.

Wendling, S. (2012) *Varroa destructor* (Anderson et Trueman, 2000), un acarien ectoparasite de l'abeille domestique *Apis mellifera* Linnaeus, 1758. Revue bibliographique et contribution à l'étude de sa reproduction. Thèse pour le Doctorat Vétérinaire, Ecole Nationale Vétérinaire d'Alfort, Créteil, France.

Weston, C.R. and Davis, R.J. (2007) The JNK signal transduction pathway. *Current Opinions in Cell Biology*, 19: 142–149.

Wheeler, D.E. and Kawooya J.K. (1990) Purification of honey bee vitellogenin. *Archives of Insect Biochemistry and Physiology*, 14: 253–267.

Williams, I.H., Pickett, J.A., and Martin, A.P. (1982) Nasonov pheromone of the honeybee *Apis mellifera* L. (Hymenoptera, Apidae). *Journal of Chemical Ecology*, 8(2): 567–574.

Winston, M.L. (1980) Swarming, after swarming, and reproductive rate of unmanaged honeybee colonies (*Apis mellifera*). *Insectes Sociaux*, 27(4): 391–398.

Winston, M.L. (1987) *The Biology of the Honeybee*. Harvard University Press, Cambridge, MA.

Winston, M.L. and Hugo, H.E. (1991) The role of queen mandibular pheromone and colony congestion in honeybee (*Apis mellifera* L.) reproductive swarming (Hymenoptera: Apidae). *Journal of Insect Behavior*, 4(5): 649–660.

Wirtz, P. and Beetsma, J. (1972) Induction of caste differentiation in the honeybee (*Apis mellifera*) by juvenile hormone. *Entomologia Experimentalis et Applicata*, 15(4): 517–520.

Woyke, J. and Jasinski, Z. (2008) Onset of oviposition by honeybee queens, mated either naturally or by various instrumental insemination methods, fits a lognormal distribution. *Journal of Apicultural Research*, 47(1): 1–9.

Yoder, J.A., Hedges, B.Z., Heydinger, D.J., Sammataro, D., and DeGrandi-Hoffman, G. (2012) Differences among fungicides targeting beneficial fungi associated with honey bee colonies. In Sammatoro D. and Yolder J.A. (eds), *Honey Bee Colony Health Challenges and Sustainable Solutions*. CRC Press, Boca Raton, FL, pp. 181–192.

2

Environmental problems and intoxication

Honeybee colonies are completely dependent on their surrounding environment. The honeybee is the only livestock species whose food supply cannot be controlled by its keeper. The beekeeper is often described as a landless farmer. The beekeeper has to 'provide' his or her managed colonies with a favourable environment featuring blossoming plants, aphid host plants (for honeydew production), and water. Supplementary feeding should only be necessary when the conditions are unfavourable.

Thus, all the factors influencing the environment of the colonies can affect their strength and health status. Changes in weather and climate, as well as the quality and quantity of food and water resources, may favour or impair the colony and the productivity of managed colonies. Some agricultural practices (monocultures, use of phytosanitary products and in particular insecticides such as neonicotinoids and phenylpyrazols) as well as inappropriate chemicals used within hives (e.g in attempts to control *Varroa destructor* infestation) may also endanger colony health by poisoning.

Because honeybee colonies entirely depend on their surrounding environment they are considered a primary indicator of the health of the environment (Lambert *et al.*, 2012).

1 Influence of meteorology and climate on colony welfare and health

1.1 Influence of meteorological factors

So-called 'good weather' is a necessity for colony welfare. In temperate countries, a colony needs water (but not too much rain), sun, and mild to hot temperatures. The weather is directly linked to the food resources of the colonies.

Meteorological factors such as sun, rain, temperature, wind, and humidity influence the life of the colony:

- High temperatures and sufficient precipitation are reported to be linked to increased nectar foraging and increased colony productivity (Shuel, 1992; Voorhies *et al.*, 1933).
- Unusually bad weather (long periods of rain, wind, and cold) that confines honeybees within the hive for long periods can weaken the colony. Such extended periods have been implicated in colony mortality (Kauffeld *et al.*, 1976; van Engelsdrop and Meixner 2010).

A recent study has shown that weather changes during flowering of highbush blueberry affect pollination and yield (Tuell and Isaacs, 2010). Comparing honeybees and bumblebees, it seems that honeybees are more likely to forage when the weather is fine and bumblebees when the weather is mild (Tuell and Isaacs, 2010).

A period of bad weather (rain, wind, cold), as soon as it begins, prevents foragers from flight and foraging activity. In such periods it has been shown that less trophallactic contact between honeybees occurs. Nurses seems to be 'highly sensitive' to alterations in the weather (Riessberger and Crailsheim, 1997). Brood nursing time is more than halved in bad weather conditions, and other nursing activities are also reduced. Thus, bad weather results in less activity with a reduced flow of stored food within the hive (Riessberger and Crailsheim, 1997).

Weather features may also directly or indirectly be a contributing factor to outbreaks of disease in colonies:

- In spring, if foragers have to remain confined in the hive because of cold or rain, the immediate and direct consequence is a lack of resources to feed larvae. If a long period of starvation occurs, the lack of pollen and proteins can rapidly affect brood rearing and weaken the colony. Confinement and food deficiency are predisposing factors to outbreaks of disease such as bacterial European foulbrood disease or viral sacbrood disease.
- Cold and humidity are unfavourable for colonies. They are in particular predisposing to the occurrence of fungal chalkbrood disease (*Ascosphaera apis*).
- Wind poses a hazard for colonies as it may be responsible for confinement, in particular if the entrance to the hive faces the direction of the wind, preventing foragers from seeking food resources.
- A long and cold winter may affect the health of colonies that have insufficient honey resources, resulting in weakening and collapse due to famine. It may also be favourable to the development of the fungus *Nosema apis*.

Electromagnetic changes are thought to have an influence on honeybees, in particular on foragers. A recent study in Germany has shown a lower returning percentage of foragers when they have been irradiated by standard commercial DECT telephones (Kimmel *et al.*, 2007). However, this fact is not well documented in the scientific literature.

Based on a personal observation by the author, hives moved to a location near a high-voltage power line in the south of France showed no change in almond tree pollination activity and colony strength at the beginning of a season.

1.2 Influence of climate change

As presented in Chapter 1, *Apis mellifera* is widely distributed and adapted to many climates around the world. By natural evolution and adaptation, their natural distribution ranges from northern Europe to southern Africa and from western Europe to the Middle East and eastern Europe, *A. mellifera* strains are adapted to many diverse climates and even microclimates. Moreover, managed colonies have been introduced in many territories because of their great pollination and honey-harvesting potential. Beekeeping activities (pollination, honey production, etc.) have led humans to import this species to the New World (South and North America) as well as to Asia and Oceania.

Thus, *A. mellifera* colonies are adapted to both a continental climate with a high annual temperature range (up to 40°C) as well as to the extreme heat of a Saharan climate. There are 25 sub-species or races of *A. mellifera* reported around the world, adapted to their own local climate and flora (Le Conte and Navajas, 2008).

Climate change has consequences on temperature and water flow in particular. Consequently, climate change influences the distribution of flower species and colony food resources (Thuiller *et al.*, 2005).

Thus, we can assume that the honeybee *A. mellifera*, by virtue of the diversity of its strains, sub-species, and races, is able to adapt to climate change as long as water resources and honey flowers are available.

The beekeeper will have to adapt his or her practices by choosing appropriate strains of honeybee and suitable apiary locations, and probably by migratory beekeeping.

1.3 Management

The management of meteorological factors and of the consequences of climate change involves applying good rules of husbandry. Prophylactic livestock, feeding supplementation, and material management must be applied not only during challenging periods or when faced by risk factors, but also during daily beekeeping.

Beekeepers and any stakeholders involved in apiculture must ensure that good sanitary beekeeping practices, as defined by the OIE and the FAO in the *Guide to Good Farming Practices for Animal Production Food Safety* (OIE and FAO, 2009; Vidal-Naquet, 2013), are applied in their apiaries and honey farms (cf. Chapter 8). The beekeeper can potentially control the honeybee strain and limit or avoid as far as possible the influence of bad weather and unfavourable environmental factors on honeybee colonies throughout the year – in early spring before the season, in autumn when the colony prepares to overwinter, and in the overwintering period.

In winter, the beekeeper must ensure that the colonies have enough honey or carbohydrate resources to go through the 'dangerous' overwintering period (Figure 2.1).

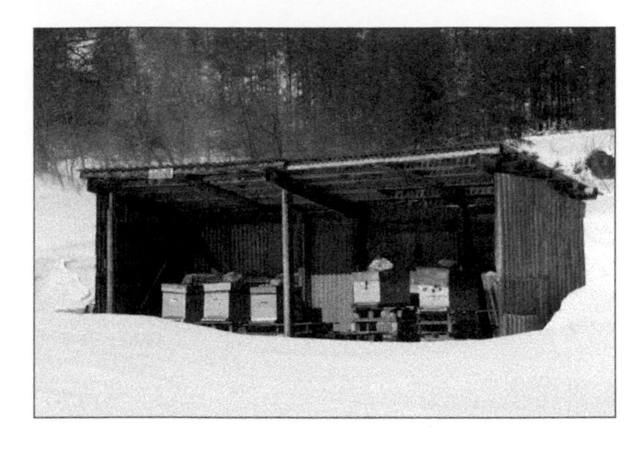

Figure 2.1 Overwintering colonies in the French Alps. Note the protection of the hives from wind and snow. The management of honey and/or carbohydrate resources is a crucial element for survival during this period in such regions (© Nicolas Vidal-Naquet).

2 Influence of food resources on colony welfare and health

Food resources are crucial for honeybees. The resources are mainly nectar, pollen, honeydew, and water. Pollen is the source of protein, and nectar and the honeydew provide the source of carbohydrates. Whereas pollen and honey are stored, water is not stored within the nest and must always be available for bees.

2.1 Pollen

Pollen is the only protein source for honeybee colonies. The crude protein content of pollen varies from 7 to 40% depending on the plant (Somerville, 2014). According to Somerville (2014), honeybees require pollens with minimum crude protein levels of between 20 and 25%. A diet containing high-protein pollen enhances the longevity of workers compared to pollen with a low protein level (Knox *et al.*, 1971; Somerville, 2014).

Pollen is also the colony's only natural source of lipids (pollen contains 0.8–19% lipids). These lipids are important, in particular as oils that are attractive to foragers.

Honeybee colonies are reported to collect and require 10–26 kg (sometimes up to 55 kg) of pollen per year (depending on certain factors such as the size and the strain of the colonies) (Winston, 1987; Brodschneider and Crailsheim, 2010). The pollen is stored as beebread in uncapped cells.

As well as the quantity, the quality of pollen is a crucial element of the food resources of honeybee colonies. Gathering diverse pollens from many flower species allows a balanced diet of amino acids (Brodschneider and Crailsheim, 2010). Recent publications suggest that both the quality and diversity of pollen may influence bee physiology (Di Pasquale *et al.*, 2013). Ten amino acids are considered as essential for a balanced honeybee diet (Somerville, 2014): threonine, valine, methionine, isoleucine, leucine, phenylalanine, histidine, lysine, arginine, and tryptophane. It has been shown that dietary deficiency in L-leucine, L-isoleucine, and/or L-valine alters the development of the colony (Brodschneider and Crailsheim, 2010).

Pollens have their own characteristic protein content, amino acid composition, lipid content, vitamins, and mineral elements. Few monopollen diets are considered a balanced diet for bees: according to Brodschneider and Crailsheim (2010), sweet clover and mustard provide a more balanced diet than some mixed-pollen diets. On the contrary, a monoflower (single-pollen) pollen diet of sunflower or sesame seems to act as a stressor for honeybees (and is reported to decrease their lifespan) compared with a mixed-pollen diet (Schmidt, 1984; Schmidt *et al.*, 1987).

Another study has shown that pollen quality influences nurse bee physiology. Pollen diversity seems to enhance the immune system of honeybees and their lifespan, in particular when the microsporidia *Nosema ceranae* is present (Di Pasquale *et al.*, 2013).

Hence, monocultures as single food resource pose a risk to honeybee health and can adversely affect metabolism, immunity, and lifespan (Figure 2.2). According to Alaux *et al.* (2010), 'malnutrition is probably one of the causes of immunodeficiency in honeybee colonies'.

An unbalanced protein diet may be a stressor at several levels (Brodschneider and Crailsheim, 2010):

- Protein deficiency or unbalanced diet and colonies. In the case of protein deficiency, brood rearing is quickly altered. Beebread is consumed and workers' body reserves are affected (Haydak, 1935). Workers can develop cannibalistic behaviour, feeding new larvae to older ones. If the deficiency level becomes too high, brood rearing will stop. Cannibalism on pupae has also been observed (after uncapping the cells) in cases of starvation.
- Protein deficiency or unbalanced diet and adult bees. Proteins are the major component of workers' bodies (on average 70% of the dry matter) (Hrassnigg and Crailsheim, 2005). A high-protein pollen diet is reported to enhance the lifespan of workers (Knox *et al.*, 1971; Somerville, 2014). Any deficiency may potentially alter maturation of muscles, storage of vitellogenin within fat bodies but also hypopharyngeal glands and ovaries in the queens. The immunocompetence of individual bees has been shown to depend on protein nutrition (Alaux *et al.*, 2010). According to Brodschneider and Crailsheim (2010), flight and foraging behaviour may be also affected.

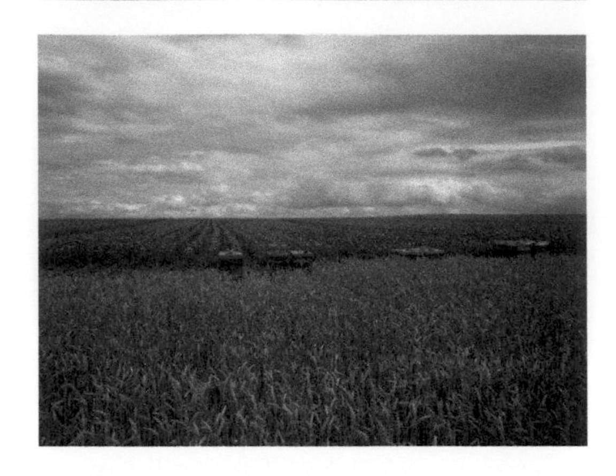

Figure 2.2 Monocultures cause amino acid deficiency. Here, a culture of seed-bearing onions (in the foreground is wheat, which not a bee plant). (© Claire Beauvais, DVM.)

- Protein deficiency or unbalanced diet and larvae. Malnutrition in the larval stage has consequences for the development of the bees. Protein deficiency causes honeybees to be smaller and weight, and ovaries of workers are reported to be less developed. In managed colonies, lifespan and brood rearing are reported to be better in colonies with a protein supplement diet. Particular attention must be given to pollen resources when the brood of winter bees is reared because of the importance of reserves within the fat bodies (which must be well developed in winter bees) to allow the colony to go through the winter (Imdorf *et al.*, 2010).

2.2 Nectar and honeydew

Nectar and honeydew, stored as honey in capped cells, are the colony's natural source of carbohydrates. Stored honey provides the carbohydrate reserve that allows the colony to meet the daily needs of the workers and also to survive long periods of starvation, e.g. winter. Honey is also the basic source of lipids synthesized by honeybee anabolism (e.g. wax).

Carbohydrate deficiency is a major risk for the colony during the active season and during overwintering. Adult bees are not able to survive long periods without carbohydrates because their bodies lack carbohydrate reserves. In winter, a lack of honey or carbohydrate supplement may cause weakening and collapse of the colony. In the active season, an absence of flowering, blooming, or honeydew resources may result in carbohydrate deficiency.

2.3 Water

Permanent access to water throughout the active season is essential for managed colonies. When the temperature increases there is a greater need for water to be used inside the hive for cooling; even when the risk of overheating has passed, the colony's need for water remains important (Kühnlolz and Seeley, 1997). Colonies adapt their water foraging activity to their needs.

Drought is a major risk for managed (and feral) colonies for two reasons: the lack of flowers due to the lack of water on crops and wild vegetation, and the lack of water for the colonies. A prolonged drought occurred in California in 2014, leading beekeepers to provide their colonies with feeding supplements (sugar and protein) and water to avoid or limit colony losses.

2.4 Plant toxicity

Some plants are toxic for honeybee colonies. Nectar and pollen of Tiliceae and Theaceae contain carbohydrates that are toxic for bees, namely mannose, galactose, arabinose, xylose, melibiose, raffinose, stachyose, and lactose (Brodschneider and Crailsheim, 2010).

According to Barker (1977), soybeans used in protein substitute contain toxic sugars (40%).

Other plants are poisonous to honeybee colonies due to the production of biotoxins, such as protoanemonin produced by Ranunculaceae and saponin produced by *Aesculus* species.

Asteraceae (Senecioneae and Eupatorieae), Borraginaceae, Orchidaceae (nine genera), and Fabaceae (genus *Crotolaria*) produce pyrrolizidine alkaloids and may be toxic for bees. Thus, in apiculture, it is necessary to prevent foragers from foraging species such as borage, groundsel, and viper's bugloss (Bruneau, 2014).

2.5 Management and supplement feeding

A balanced diet and access to water is fundamental for honeybee health, colony strength, and beekeeping productivity. Intensive cultures and monocultures may be a cause of colony weakening and a contributing factor to pathogen development. Access to a diversity of flowers and plants throughout the beekeeping season is important for the successful management of honeybee colonies. It may be necessary for the beekeeper to move his or her hives in order to provide the colonies with access to a more favourable environment. Permanent access to good-quality water is fundamental.

Feeding supplements containing carbohydrates and protein may be used if the colony is facing nutrient deficiency or malnourishment, or during high-risk periods (overwintering, beginning of the season, drought, etc.). The choice of feeding supplement must be adapted to the needs of the colony and will thus depend on many factors (the physiological status of the colony, time of year, hive products, floral and crop environment, etc.).

Syrup and fondant (also called bee candy or bee paste) are the main carbohydrate feeding supplements. They must contain carbohydrates assimilable by the bees (saccharose, fructose, glucose) and must not crystallize, which would render them unusable by bees. The hydroxymethylfurfural (HMF) content in sugar supplements must be less than 30 mg/kg (G. Therville-Tondreau, personal communication, 2013). HMF is an organic compound derived from the dehydration of certain carbohydrates found in honey (and other sugars), and is a toxic for honeybees (Rosatella *et al.*, 2011). The HMF content of the honey increases with time. Particular attention must be given to the use of honey as a feeding supplement because of the risk of introducing pathogenic agents such as *Paenibacillus larvae*, responsible for American foulbrood disease, and toxic compounds. Floral-origin (pollen) or non-floral (Torula or brewers yeast, soy flour) protein supplements may also be used when for whatever reason foragers bring back insufficient pollen to the colony. Protein supplements must be carefully chosen because of the risk of constipation. The use of frozen beebread is probably a good source of a protein supplement.

Feeding may be necessary in the event of starvation or risk of deficiency ('emergency' feeding), to stimulate colony activity ('speculative' or stimulating feeding), or to replace honey removed from the hive ('surrogate' feeding) (G. Therville-Tondreau, personal communication, 2013):

- Emergency feeding is used when famine threatens. Sugar candy is used in winter or early spring. Syrup is used in spring, summer, and autumn when the temperatures are not too cold.
- Speculative feeding can be used at the end of summer to stimulate the production of a larger winter population. Stimulating feeding may also be used in spring (at the beginning of the season). The principle is to feed honeybees little but regularly to stimulate the laying activity of the queen. Artificial swarming is used to divide the colony into two, by encouraging the natural process of swarming. Any artificial swarm thus produced will need feeding.
- Surrogate feeding can be given to substitute the honey removed, in particular at the end of summer and in autumn (syrup). It is also used to substitute the honey gathered for trade while overwintering (candy).

The management of feeding requires maintaining good sanitary beekeeping practices (Chapter 8).

3 Intoxication

The development of intensive agriculture, monocultures with the use of phytosanitary products on crops, as well as the use of miticides and other drugs in colonies, imply more and more potential contact between honeybees and chemicals.

Insecticides, herbicides, miticides, fungicides, molluscicides, bactericides, but also insect repellents and insect attractants, are some of the pesticides used on crops (Wood, 2012). Insecticides and miticides are also used in farm husbandry and by pet owners.

Insecticides are used in hives or in the apiary to control certain pests, such as small hive beetle *Aethina tumida* infestation or the damaging Asian hornet, *Vespa velutina*.

Miticides are used in colonies to control in particular the mite *V. destructor* (everywhere in the world), the tracheal mite *Acarapis woodi*, and also the mites *Tropilaelaps* spp. (in Asia).

Residues of pesticides used in crops and of miticides used in hives may be found in wax, honey, and pollen (Mullin *et al.*, 2010). They can be considered as environmental stressors for bee colonies.

Hence, honeybees may be sensitive to phytosanitary products used on crops and to miticides used in hives and to their post-therapeutic residues. Furthermore, there is a potential risk for honeybees and other crop pollinators not only because of just those phytosanitary products, and in particular insecticides, but also because of the synergy between insecticides and other pesticides or pathogenic agents.

The toxicity of pesticides may be acute, chronic, or sub-lethal. The clinical signs are various and often difficult to evaluate. The diagnosis of poisoning is not easy to perform, in particular at sub-lethal and chronic levels, often leading to controversial discussions between beekeepers, crop farmers, environmental associations, and chemical industries.

At this time, the use of phytosanitary products (mainly neonicotinoids and phenylpyrazols but also herbicides, fungicides ...) on crops and in particular as seed treatments are suspected by some authors and other stakeholders in the beekeeping sector to be heavily implicated in the health crisis affecting managed colonies (van Engelsdorp *et al.*, 2009; Mullin *et al.*, 2010; Henry *et al.*, 2012; Lu *et al.*, 2014). A few authors are more sceptical (Lawrence and Sheppard, 2013).

The role of pesticides, in particular neonicotinoids and phenylpyrazols, in colony weakening, disease, and collapse is a much-discussed subject in the present health crisis. Many studies, congresses, and national, regional and international meetings have focused on the role played by pesticides in colony losses, with the chemical industry facing opposition from environmental and bee-protection organizations. Many scientific studies on the toxicity of pesticides on honeybees have been and continue to be published.

The aim of this chapter is to present a veterinary approach if poisoning is suspected.

3.1 Insecticides and their targets (and other pesticides affecting honeybee health)

Insecticides (cf. Table 2.1) used on crops can be classified according to their chemical structure or their target tissue (or function): nervous activity, cell respiration activity, and insect growth and development (M.-E. Colin, personal communication, 2007; Vidal-Naquet, 2008; Wood, 2012).

Organochlorines, organophosphorus compounds (e.g. coumaphos), carbamates, pyrethroids (e.g. permethrin and deltamethrin), avermectins (e.g. ivermectin), formamidine (e.g. amitraz), phenylpyrazols (e.g. fipronil), neonicotinoids (e.g. imidacloprid and thiamethoxan) target the nervous system.

Amidinohydrazones, rotenone, and pyrazols all act on cellular respiration.

Benzoylurea and acylurea (e.g. lufenuron) compounds and benzhydrazides act on insect growth and metamorphosis. Brought back to the hive by foragers, they may affect the development of the brood and thus lead to a decrease of the population.

Genetically engineered plant varieties (GMOs, genetically modified organisms), due to their herbicide tolerance and/or insecticidal properties, can potentially be toxic for honeybees. For example, in some GMOs, the insecticide effect is the consequence of the introduction of a gene coding for an insecticidal protein from *Bacillus thuringensis* (Johnson *et al.*, 2012). These plants are used in USA and other countries. In the EU, GMOs are a controversial subject; although their use is legal in Spain, for example, their use is not permitted for crop production in France.

Since their appearance on the market in the beginning of the 1990s, neonicotinoid and phenylpyrazole insecticides have become widely and extensively used on crops in the USA and the EU. Because of their main use as seed treatments, they are systemic in plants and are found in the pollen and nectar of flowers during the blooming period, as well as in guttation drops (Tapparo *at al.*, 2011; Dively and Kamel, 2012). They are suspected by many stakeholders in the beekeeping sector to be one of the causes of the health crisis affecting honeybee colonies.

Ongoing research is considering the real, potential, or absence of toxicity of insecticides used on crops but also of the miticides used in hives to control *Varroa* infestation. In the EU, the USA and many other countries around the world, regulations concerning phytosanitary product use on crops demand in particular evaluation with respect to honeybee toxicity.

The insecticides shown in Table 2.1 include some compounds that are used in hives to control *Varroa* infestation. The level of insecticide toxicity of these miticides depends on the individual substance and their use in mite control must follow good veterinary practice.

Some other pesticides pose direct or indirect chemical hazards to honeybees. For example, fungicides used on crops have been reported to impair the presence of symbiotic fungi in beebread as well as to harm the beneficial mycoflora of honeybee colonies. Thus, exposure to fungicides used on crops and brought back to the hive by foragers may decrease the presence of this mycoflora (*Aspergillus* spp. and *Penicillium* spp.) and impair the resistance mechanisms of the honeybee colony (Yoder *et al.*, 2012, 2013). Some herbicides may alter the health of young bees, foragers, eggs and larvae (Morton and Moffett, 1972; Morton *et al.*, 1972). Herbicides may also impact on honeybee health by changing the attractiveness of plants by reducing resources for pollinators.

Table 2.1 Principal insecticides: target, classification, molecules and mode of action

Target	Classification		Insecticides (examples)	Mode of action
Nervous	organochlorine insecticides	diphenyl aliphaliques	DDT, DDD, Ethylan, Chlorobenzylate	blockage of axonal Na^+ channels
		cyclodiene	Aldrin, dieldrin, Chlordane, Chlordecone, endosulfan	blockage of the GABA-gated chloride channel
		hexachlorocyclohexane	Lindane	blockage of the GABA-gated chloride channel
		polychloroterpenes	Toxaphene	blockage of the GABA-gated chloride channel
	organophosphorus insecticides	organophosphates	Dichlorvos, phosphamidon	inactivate acetylcholinesterase
		organothiophosphates	Coumaphos, Endothion, Malathio, parathion	inactivate acetylcholinesterase
		phosphonates	Butonate, Trichlorfon	inactivate acetylcholinesterase
		phosphonothionates	Mecarphon, fonofos, cyanofenphos	inactivate acetylcholinesterase
		phosphoramidates	Crufomate, Fenamiphos, fosthietan, Pfosfolan, etc.	inactivate acetylcholinesterase
		phosphoramidothioates	Acephate, Chloramine Phosphorus, Isocarbophos	inactivate acetylcholinesterase
		phosphorodiamides	Dimefox, Mazidox	inactivate acetylcholinesterase
	carbamate insecticides		Carbaryl, benfuracarb, dimetan, dimetilan, pyramat, propoxur	inactivate acetylcholinesterase
	diamide insecticides		Chlorantraniliprole, flubediamid, anthranilamide	Ryanodine receptor modulator
	formamidine insecticides		amitraz, chlordimeform, formetanate, formparana, semiamitraz, medimeform	Inhibit monoamine oxidase – octopamine mimic
	macrocyclic lactone	Avermectin	Abamectin, doramectin, emamectin, eprinomectin, ivermectin, selamectin	blockage of GABA
		Milbemycin	lepimectin, milbemectin, milbemycin oxime, oxidectin	blockage of GABA
		Spinosym	spinetoram, spinosad	blockage of GABA
	neonicotinoids	nitroguanidine neonicotinoid	clothianidin, dinotefuran, imidacloprid, imidaclothiz, thiamethoxam	acetylcholine agonists

Target	Classification		Insecticides (examples)	Mode of action
		nitromethylene neonicotinoid	nitenpyram, nithiazine	acetylcholine agonists
		pyridylmethylamine neonicotinoid	acetamiprid, imidacloprid, nitenpyram, paichongding, thiacloprid	acetylcholine agonists
	pyrethrinoides	natural and synthesis	permethrine, deltamethrine, cypermethrine, etc.	maintain axonal Na^+ channels open
	Pyrazoles (and phenyl-)		Chlorantraniliprole, fipronil, flufiprole, etc.	inhibitor of GABA receptor
	Semicarbazone		Metaflumizone	blockage of Na^+ channels
Respiration	Amidinohydrazone		Hydramethylnon	cell respiration inhibition
	Rotenone		Rotenone	cell respiration inhibition
Growth	chitin synthesis inhibitors		buprofezin, cyromazine	chitin synthesis inhibition
		benzoylphenylurea	bistrifluron, chlorbenzuron, chlorfluazuron, dichlorbenzuron, diflubenzuron, flucycloxuron, flufenoxuron, hexaflumuron, lufenuron	juvenile hormone mimic
	juvenile hormones mimics		dayoutong, epofenonane, fenoxycarb, hydroprene, kinoprene, methoprene, pyriproxyfen, triprene	juvenile hormone
	juvenile hormone		Juvenile Hormone I,II,III	moulting hormone agonist
	moulting hormones agonists		Chromfenozide, furan tebufenozide, halofenozide, methoxyfenozide, tebufenozide, yishijing	moulting hormone agonist
	moultinghormones		α-ecdysone, ecdysterone	moulting hormone
	moulting inhibitors		Diofenolan	moulting inhibitor
	precocenes		Precocene I,II,III	
	unclassified insect growth regulators		dicyclanil	
	ketoenole	tetramic and tertronic acids	spirotetramat, spirodiclofen, spiroomesifen	lipid synthesis inhibition mainly in larvae and pupae
GMO	molecular biological origins		e.g. MON810 maize containing the gene *Cry1Ab* from *Bacillus thurigiensis*	insecticide action of the protein Cry1Ab

Source: Adapted from M.-E. Colin, personal communication, 2007; Vidal-Naquet, 2008; Wood, 2014.

Some chemicals have a synergistic effect with insecticides and may potentiate them (cf. section 3.6 below).

3.2 Factors affecting the severity of poisoning

Environmental factors (e.g. temperature, light, and humidity) may modify the toxicity of certain insecticides and pesticides. Chemical degradation of these molecules may also occur and produce metabolites that can be more toxic than the initial molecule (Barson, 1983; Colin, 1999).

The formulation of the pesticide for different applications, e.g. spraying, soil treatment, manure spreading, and seed treatment, may also modify the toxicity of such chemicals.

Neonicotinoids and phenylpyrazoles are used to treat seed crops. Seed treatment presents a double risk for honeybees (as well as for bumblebees and wild bees):

- Via drifted dust from seed treatment. Seed treatments (e.g. clothianidin) may be applied on the field in-furrow during sowing, which poses a risk of dust emission (EFSA Journal, 2013a). This dust may be deposited on neighbouring crops or plants attractive to bees. According to the EFSA, potential risks to 'non-target organisms' such as bees of dust formation due to seed coating arise with many crops: e.g spring cereals, winter cereals, maize, sweetcorn, sorghum, oilseed rape (canola), sunflower, beans, peas, cotton, flax, poppy, grasses, spinach, and beetroot (EFSA Journal, 2012, 2013b) (Figure 2.3).
- Via the systemic presence of insecticides within sap. Systemic insecticides can be found in pollen, nectar, and guttation drops, and therefore present a risk that foragers will be poisoned at the foraging site and/or bring the insecticide back to the hive (Dively and Kamel, 2012; Mullin *et al.*, 2010).

The toxicity of drugs used in hives to fight diseases and parasites may also be modified and may increase if incorrectly used or applied. For example, the use of pyrethroid on the soil and the in-hive use of coumaphos and fipronil (Schäfer and Ritter, 2014) to fight the small hive beetle, *A. tumida*, poses a major risk of poisoning for bees. Fipronil is also used in traps by some beekeepers to fight *V. velutina*, the Asian hornet, or *A. tumida*; this poses a high risk for bees.

Factors intrinisic to honeybees may also modify the toxicity: age, nutrition behaviour, sex, caste, as well as strain.

3.3 Modes of poisoning

Poisoning of honeybees may occur via several means and routes (cf. Figure 2.4). All stages and all castes may be affected by poisoning. The routes of exposures differ for nest bees, outside bees and immature forms. However, concerning brood and nest bees, toxic substances are mainly brought back by foragers in nectar, pollen, and water (EFSA Journal, 2012). The use of drugs and chemicals by beekeepers in order to control diseases, pests, and predators of the colonies (e.g. *V. destructor*, *A. woodi*, *A. tumida*) and to treat hive material (e.g. stored material) may be responsible of poisoning by ingestion, inhalation, and contact within the hive.

Several exposure routes may be involved in adult poisoning:

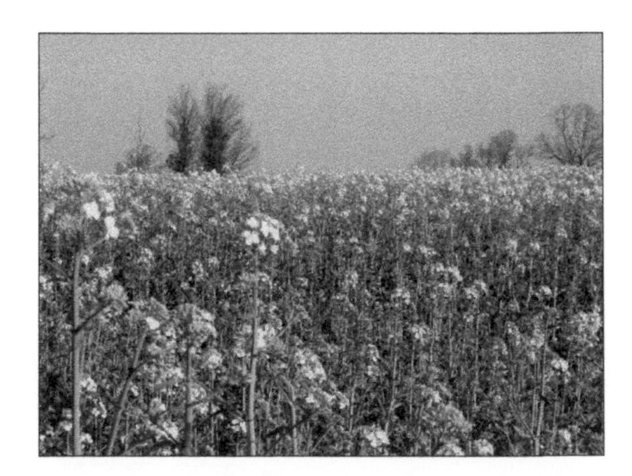

Figure 2.3 Canola crop. Coated canola seeds may present a chemical hazard to bees either systemically (i.e. due to the presence of insecticide in the sap and consequently in the nectar, pollen, and guttation drops) or via dust drift. (© Lydia Vilagines, DVM.)

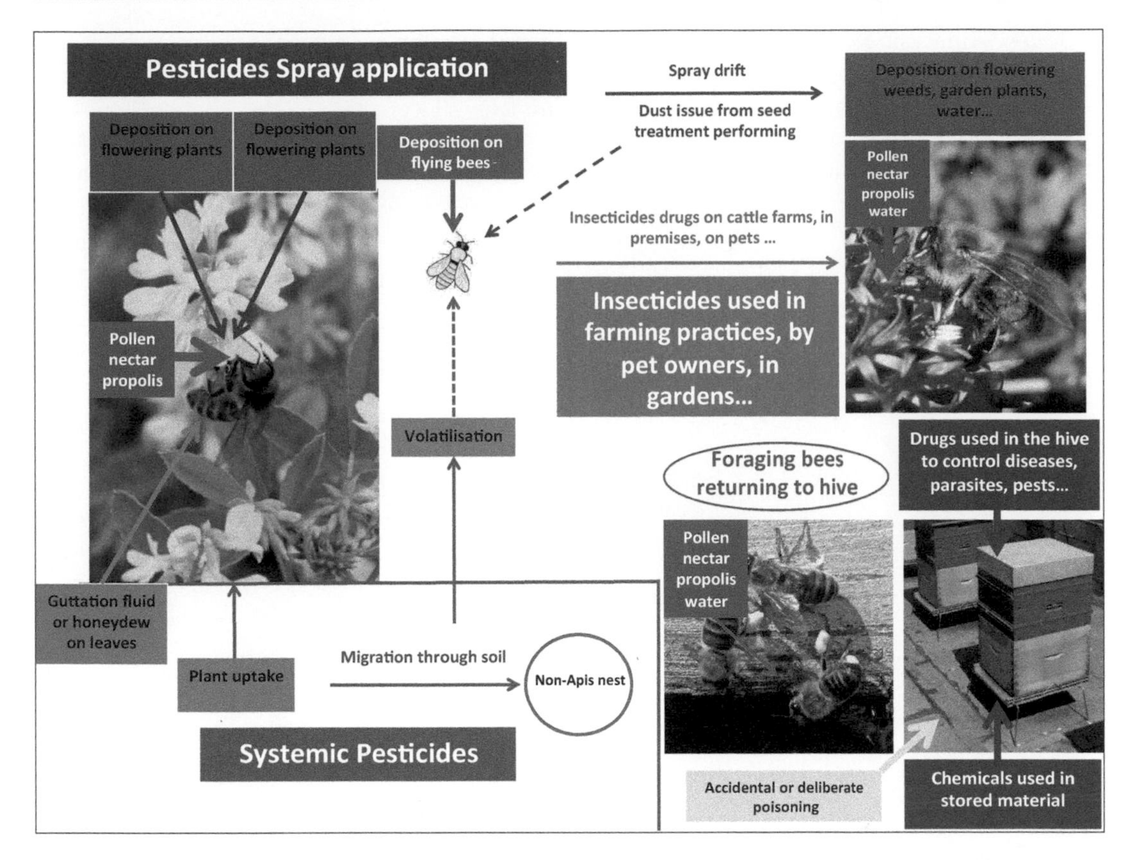

Figure 2.4 Major and potential exposure routes of honeybees to pesticides. (Adapted from EFSA Journal, 2012.)

- Ingestion of contaminated water or pollen, nectar, or guttation drops which may contain directly oversprayed or systemic residues (Thompson, 2012). This mainly occurs when foragers are out gathering pollen, nectar, and water. They may bring back the chemicals to the hive which will be stored within the honey, the beebread, and the wax:
  - Pollen is the main source of pesticides entering the hives. Bee-collected pollen has been shown in a study on managed colonies in the US to contain high levels of pesticides (miticides used for *Varroa* control, insecticides, fungicides, and herbicides) with on average seven different pesticides being found in pollen samples (Mullin *et al.*, 2010). According to Mullin *et al.* (2010), 'the potential for multiple pesticide interactions affecting bee health seems likely'.
  - Wax combs are 'uniformly contaminated with miticides' (Mullin *et al.*, 2010). The wax has been found to 'store' residues of miticides, including fluvalinate, amitraz, coumaphos, or bromopropylate used for *Varroa* control (Faucon *et al.*, 2002; Mullin *et al.*, 2010). Coumaphos can persist in wax for more than one year (Martel *et al.*, 2007). Fungicides have also been found in comb wax, and some of these may potentially have a synergistic effect with pyrethroids (Pilling *et al.*, 1995; Mullin *et al.*, 2010). Wax foundations used by beekeepers can contain residues of pesticides and veterinary medicines

depending on the origins of the wax used to make them (old combs, for example).
- In honey, various studies have shown the presence of residues of antibiotics, miticides, and neonicotinoids, often under the defined maximum residue limits (MRLs) (Martel *et al.*, 2007; Hammel *et al.*, 2008; Tanner and Czerwenka, 2011). An Austrian study found lower levels of neonicotinoids in forest honey samples than in flower honey samples (Tanner and Czerwenka, 2011).
- In water, contamination by pesticides may occur due to runoff of phytosanitary products used on crops. Seed treatments may result in the presence of insecticides and other pesticides in the guttation drops from the stomatal pores of plants that bees often forage for water intake. Insecticides used in animal management may potentially contaminate water; this has been suspected to have occurred in France in the fight against bluetongue disease transmitted by the midge *Culicoides* spp. (Vidal-Naquet, 2009).

• Inhalation occurs when the pesticide is volatile or/and applied by spraying.
• Contact: the bee interacts with the chemical and ingests the compound through normal grooming. This contact may occur with dust generated during drilling of treated seeds.

The main route by which larvae are poisoned is the brood-food (royal, worker, and drone jellies produced by the nurses). The brood may also be affected by chemical residues accumulated in the wax, e.g. certain miticides used in *Varroa* control and some fungicides (Faucon *et al.*, 2002; Mullin *et al.*, 2010).

3.4 Acute intoxication in the honeybee

Acute intoxication may be defined as the ability of a substance to cause severe damage or death after a single exposure. Specifically, the median lethal dose (LD_{50}) is the dose that kills 50% of the bees in a colony. Acute poisoning is a major problem for honeybees and for the colony. The clinical signs depend on the toxic substance(s) but also on the features of the honeybee colony. An acute intoxication of the whole colony will not have the same consequences as an acute poisoning of some specific forms (e.g. larvae, nurse bees, or foragers).

The clinical signs of insecticides in individuals depend on physiological system than is targeted. For example:

• Pyrethroids at or near LD_{50} rapidly induce neurotoxicity in adult bees. This results in loss of coordinated movements and flight, convulsive activity, and ultimately paralysis leading swiftly to death. This is termed the 'knock-down effect' (Moréteau, 1991).
• Organophosphorus compounds cause bees to become irritable and hyperexcitable.
• Imidacloprid and/or its metabolites are responsible for the rapid appearance of clinical signs of neurotoxicity, including hyporesponsiveness and hypoactivity following hyperresponsiveness, hyperactivity, and trembling (Suchail *et al.*, 2001).

At the colony level, acute poisoning may have direct or indirect consequences:

• Directly, via the death, following clinical signs, of bees inside the hive. Weakening and collapse may occur.
• Indirectly, by the loss of certain bees. For example, if foragers are compromised by acute poisoning at the foraging site, they may not be able to return to the hive because of death or disorientation, resulting in disorganization of the colony. If forager losses persist, the colony will initially react by accelerating its production of foragers thanks to the plasticity of the division of labour (see Chapter 1, section 12.1). The colony will then increase brood rearing, and there will be a high risk of an imbalance between the brood and the number of adult bees. Nurse and fanning workers will turn into foragers faster and will not be available to rear the brood as they should, potentially resulting in weakening of the colony and in brood diseases (Colin,

1999). Young bees and the queen may also abscond from the hive.

The global impact and the prognosis of acute poisoning will depend on the number and the category of the bees affected and on the ability of the colony to balance out the depopulation (Beauvais and Vidal-Naquet, 2014)

Thus, in the case of sudden colony mortality or weakening, but also when certain brood diseases occur, acute poisoning must be taken into account in the differential diagnosis.

3.5 Sub-lethal and chronic poisoning in the honeybee

3.5.1 Sub-lethal poisoning

A sub-lethal concentration is defined as one that induces no apparent mortality in the colony. Sub-lethal effects may be characterized by negative effects (either physiological or behavioural) on individuals that survive an exposure to a pesticide (Desneux *et al.*, 2007).

Clinical signs of sub-lethal poisoning vary depending on the toxic compound. Studies have often focused on the physiology, activity, abilities, and behaviour (e.g. olfaction and memory) of foraging honeybees. However, the workers affected are not only foragers, but also nurse bees that feed on pollen and honey stored in the cells. Larvae may be affected by the brood food produced by food-processing glands (from the metabolism of honey and pollen) and by lipophilic residues within the wax of the brood cell walls.

Sub-lethal poisoning by insecticides, e.g. neonicotinoides, in honeybees is reported to potentially impair the following functions:

- Cognitive functions (learning ability, memory, olfactory learning, gustation, navigation, and spatial orientation) (Decourtye *et al.*, 2005; Desneux *et al.*, 2007).
- Behaviour and in particular impairment of successful foraging. For example, as well as being potentially fatal, thiametoxam is reported to induce homing failure thereby impairing foraging (Henry *et al.*, 2012).
- Physiological functions such as thermoregulation and muscular activity (Belzunces *et al.*, 2012).
- Immunosuppression: sub-lethal neonicotinoid poisoning is reported to be responsible for suppression of the honeybee immune system (Desneux *et al.*, 2007; Mason *et al.*, 2013).

Furthermore, sub-lethal exposure of bees to thiametoxam 'causes high mortality due to homing failure at levels that could put a colony at risk of collapse' (Henry *et al.*, 2012). Colony weakening and/or mortality is a likely consequence of homing failure among foragers. Colony collapse can be the result of disorganization, starvation, and an imbalanced population.

3.5.2 Chronic poisoning

Honeybees may also be chronically exposed to chemicals and their residues. Pesticides used to treat crops, insecticide treatments used on domestic animals or their accommodation (and potentially on pets), and miticides used in hives to control *Varroa* infestation, all produce chemical residues and their metabolites that can contaminate honey, pollen, and wax. In the environment, there is 'widespread contamination of agricultural soils, freshwater resources, wetlands, non-target vegetation and estuarine and coastal marine systems', chronically exposing bees, pollinators, as well as other species to significant concentrations of neonicotinoids and fipronil (van der Sluijs *et al.*, 2014). These compounds may have a chronic poisoning effect on bees (Colin, 1999; Frazier *et al.*, 2008; van Engelsdorp *et al.*, 2009; Johnson *et al.*, 2012).

A review study published in 2010 in the US and Canada reported the presence of 121 pesticides and metabolite residues from 887 hive samples (wax, pollen, honey), i.e. an average of 6.2 detections per sample (Mullin *et al.*, 2010). Pyrethroids, organophosphates, carbamates, neonicotinoids, insect growth regulators, chlorinated cyclodienes, organochlorines, formamidine, miscellaneous miticides/insecticides, synergists, fungicides, and herbicides were found in those samples. Thus, honeybees, of all castes and stages, are chronically exposed to multiple chemicals with possible antagonistic or synergistic interactions. These multiple pesticides and metabolite residues are reported to be able to alter honeybee health and colony strength (at both the individual and colony level) (Johnson *et al.*, 2009; Gregorc *et al.*, 2012).

Chronic exposure to one or several of these residues (Johnson *et al.*, 2010) may have the following adverse effects:

- On larvae (Derecka *et al.*, 2013) and consequently on workers emerging therefrom. According to Wu *et al.* (2011), worker bee development is delayed in the early stages in combs containing pesticide residues. Furthermore, the lifespan of adults reared from such brood combs is shortened. Wu *et al.* (2011) also reported less impairment of brood development and lifespan with lower pesticide residue levels: 'Sub-lethal effects, including delayed larval development and adult emergence or shortened adult longevity, can have indirect effects on the colony such as premature shifts in hive roles and foraging activity' (Wu *et al.*, 2011).
- On queen reproduction (Thompson, 2003; Desneux *et al.*, 2007).
- On colony health, leading to weakening or even collapse (depending on the number of individuals affected and the brood-rearing ability of the colony).

Thus, sub-lethal effects and chronic poisoning caused by pesticides and their metabolite residues may alter colony strength and health and cause colony collapse too. Furthermore, they may cause nutritional deficiency and contribute to pathogen agent development and infectious diseases (Johnson *et al.*, 2009; Gregorc *et al.*, 2012).

3.6 Synergies and interactions

3.6.1 Between chemicals

The discovery of a number of pesticide residues in hive samples has led to the hypothesis that these may potentially have harmful synergistic effects on bees. In other words, 'the additive and synergistic effects of multiple pesticide exposures may contribute to declining honeybee health' (Johnson *et al.*, 2010). Chemicals found in beehives may act in synergy to 'create a toxic environment for the honeybee'. Thus, chronic exposure to neurotoxic insecticides associated with other pesticides, e.g. fungicides, is thought to be responsible for reducing 'honeybee fitness', and impairing honeybee health and colony strength (Belzunces *et al.*, 2012; Johnson *et al.*, 2012).

Some fungicides have been reported to have a synergistic or potentiating effect with pyrethoid on their toxicity to the honeybee. It has been shown that an ergosterol biosynthesis-inhibiting fungicide, prochloraz, increases the toxicity of a pyrethroid (γ-cyhalothrin) to honeybee colonies by affecting the metabolism and delaying in particular the mechanism of detoxification and excretion of this insecticide by the bees (Pilling *et al.*, 1995).

Furthermore, fungicides used on crops and found in pollens may adversely affect colony health because they impair the crucial 'mycoflora bees' involved in beebread processing (Yoder *et al.*, 2012).

A study has shown that oxytetracycline at a dose commonly used in hives to control American foulbrood disease (in the US, this antibiotic is approved for in-hive use) increases honeybee sensitivity to miticides (coumaphos, tau-fluvalinate) used to control *Varroa* infestation (and probably to other pesticide residues and their metabolites). Thus, 'seasonal co-application of these medicines to bee hives could increase the adverse effects of these and perhaps other pesticides' (Hawthorne and Dively, 2011).

3.6.2 Between chemicals and biological pathogenic agents

Interactions and/or synergy between biological stressors and chemicals have recently been highlighted.

Interactions between imidacloprid (neonicotinoid) and *Nosema* spp. (microsporidian parasite) cause increased mortality in honeybee colonies (Alaux *et al.*, 2009). Another study has shown a synergy between *N. ceranae* and fipronil (phenylpyrazole) on honeybees exposed to these biological and chemical stressors (exposure to fipronil has been performed both chronically and at a sub-lethal dose) (Aufauvre *et al.*, 2012).

Another example is a study showing that exposure to sub-lethal doses of fipronil and thiacloprid greatly increases the mortality of honeybees previously infected by *N. ceranae* (Vidau *et al.*, 2011).

The neonicotinoid clothianidin used on crops has been shown to alter honeybee immunity and to promote the replication of deformed wing virus (DWV) (Di Prisco *et al.*, 2013).

Thus, it is important to consider the possibility that sub-lethal poisoning of bees, or even their chronic exposure to pesticides and metabolites of pesticides within the hive, may favour outbreaks of infectious diseases (viral, bacterial, fungal) and may be a cause of weakening or collapse of colonies. Synergy between chemical and biological agents seems to have the potential to impair colony strength and health. In such cases, a colony might be compromised by a growing number of related and simultaneous problems.

3.7 Diagnosis

Diagnosis of poisoning is quite difficult and often a subject of discussion and debate between experts. A method based on veterinary practice is presented here.

3.7.1 Clinical diagnosis

Clinical diagnosis will usually be a diagnosis of suspicion and not a definitive diagnosis, at least in the field, before appropriate and thorough diagnostic tests are performed (Colin, 1999; M.-E. Colin, personal communication, 2007).

In the case of honeybee mortality or colony weakness, a diagnosis of poisoning will be based on consideration of the following factors:

- Absence of major infectious diseases (which by themselves could explain the symptoms observed).
- Colony history.
- Clinical signs: neurological issues, population decrease, lack of brood, mortality of bees and/or colonies, etc.
- Management of the livestock and analysis of beekeeping practices.
- The drugs used to control *Varroa* infestation or other pests and predators, and the chemicals used to treat stored material (hives, frames, supers, etc.).
- Knowledge, if possible, of crop management practices surrounding the apiary and the pesticides potentially used (as far as possible).
- Knowledge, if possible, of the anti-parasitic treatments used in nearby farms on livestock and their accommodation.
- Knowledge, if possible, of potential contacts between bees and chemicals (e.g. local industries).

3.7.2 Laboratory diagnosis

To confirm or refute the diagnosis of poisoning, residues should be identified and quantified in particular in dead honeybees sampled from within the hive. Although this is an essential step, it is not sufficient when honeybee poisoning is suspected: if only foragers are affected and die away from the hive, during their flight, sampling bees inside the hive will not yield any results. Crop samples, as well as honeybees, honey, wax, and pollen samples, must be analysed (Beauvais and Vidal-Naquet, 2014).

The diagnosis of pesticides and of their metabolites within those samples may give a positive diagnosis of poisoning. Nearby farmers and their pesticide usage and habits should be scrutinized (Colin, 1999).

The conditions under which sampling is performed may affect the diagnosis. The sampling method is crucial to the diagnosis. Sampling must be done carefully and immediately (or as soon as possible) after observing clinical signs (Appendix 3) (Franco *et al.*, 2012). Vigilance and routine inspections of colonies and apiaries are necessary, in particular for an early and optimum sampling if poisoning is suspected, but also to control any problem as soon as possible, regardless of its cause.

Sampling bees as soon as possible is crucial in terms of analysis and diagnosis because changes may occur quickly. Decomposition of dead honeybees and pesticide degradation occur due to the effects of rain, sun, and time. Well-preserved samples must be sent swiftly to the laboratory; samples can be frozen if necessary. However, the best way to respect good sampling practices is to contact the laboratory before or when performing sampling. When sampling for analysis, if the veterinarian suspects a particular pesticide, it is good practice to ask for investigation of this chemical in the sample sent.

Extraction of pesticide residues for laboratory tests is usually performed by the 'quick, easy, cheap, effective, rugged, and safe' (QuEChERS) method (EU Community Reference Laboratory for Residues of Pesticides, Fellbach, Germany) (Lehotay, 2006). Analyses are usually performed with liquid chromatography with tandem mass spectrometry (LC-MS/MS) and/or gas chromatography time-of-flight (GC-ToF) (Johnson, 2010; Wiest *et al.*, 2011). The analysis may provide only qualitative results, or both qualitative and quantitative ones.

Interpretation of results is a delicate process and must take into account several factors:

- The clinical signs observed in the apiary and/or in the neighbouring apiaries.
- Features of honeybee biology and physiology, such as the super-organism as a unit, bees as individuals, population renewal, labour task division, castes, and stages.
- The sampling conditions (time slot between first hypothetical signs observed and sampling; the meteorological impact – rain, sun, and/or heat – on samples from honeybees that died outside the hive; etc.)
- The results of the laboratory tests. The detection limits vary depending on the sample (bees, pollen, wax, honey, plants, water). If a residue is not found within a matrix, it does not mean that the bees have not been in contact with it or that it has caused poisoning. Indeed, it is necessary to take into account the kinetics of the molecule(s) degradation and the potential presence of toxic metabolites that may be unquantifiable, undetectable, undetected, or untested (Beauvais and Vidal-Naquet, 2014). For example, the metabolites of fipronil, i.e. desulfynil-fipronil and fipronil-sulfone, are more toxic than the parent molecule and should be tested for if there is a suspicion of fipronil poisoning (Hainzl *et al.*, 1998).
- The LD_{50} of the pesticide(s) found. LD_{50} is a delicate notion in honeybee poisoning compared to other species, as it is based not on the bee but on the colony as a super-organism. The LD_{50} must be used interpreted carefully (Beauvais and Vidal-Naquet, 2014).
- Field investigation findings, in particular search of potential/real use of pesticides on surrounding crops, insecticides on farm animals, etc.
- Beekeeping practices.

A veterinarian practitioner should contact the laboratory to define the samples needed and to interpret together the results according to the anamnesis (medical history) and the clinical examination performed.

3.7.3 Some basic keys for interpretation of laboratory tests results (Colin *et al.*, 2004; M.-E. Colin, personal communication, 2007; Beauvais and Vidal-Naquet, 2014)

The results of the chemical, pesticide and residue analysis when honeybee colony poisoning is suspected are frequently difficult to interpret, in particular in the case of sub-lethal and chronic poisoning, but sometimes also when acute poisoning is suspected.

Interpretation must be performed in coordination with the laboratory and taking into account the factors described in the previous section. Diagnosis of poisoning is often difficult and a source of misunderstanding and controversy. However, some basic keys are presented as follows to assist with interpretation.

If the result is negative (no residues found):

- It may not be a case of poisoning and other stressors must be sought.
- It may nevertheless be a case of poisoning for the following reasons:
  - The sampling method (sampling needs to be performed as carefully as possible; the quality and quantity of samples sent may alter the analysis): for example, if the dead bees were older bees (i.e. foragers) and only inside bees were sampled, the result may be negative; or if sampling is unduly delayed, changes in the dead bees may have occurred by decomposition/degradation.
  - The residue(s) is (are) under the detection limit of the laboratory.
  - The residue(s) has (have) been metabolized. It is advisable to search samples for metabolites and/or pesticide degradation products (this is in particular necessary for new insecticides used on crops).

If one or more residues are found in the analysis:

- If the laboratory test method allows only detection but not quantification of residue(s) and/or its metabolites and split products: this may provide a toxicological explanation for the problems observed in the colony. If possible, quantification of the residues or metabolites found should be performed if enough matrix samples have been sent to and kept by the laboratory.
- If the laboratory test method gives positive results with quantification of residues and metabolites and split products:
  - It is advisable to evaluate the part of the chemical(s) found which may have been naturally metabolized in the field, or during storage and transportation. This will give an idea of the initial level of residues within the sample sent.
  - It is necessary to interpret the answer to the following question: are the samples sent representative of the exposure risk for bees (in the case of analysis of plant samples, pollen and honey)?
    - ► Yes: it is a poisoning.
    - ► No: it may not be a poisoning.
  - It is also necessary to interpret the answer to the following question: can the chemical quantification found be linked to the level of dead or diseased bees observed in the field?

The diagnosis of poisoning is very difficult and often a controversial subject between stakeholders (beekeepers, farmers, health authorities, chemical industries, etc.). As with any disease, the diagnosis of poisoning requires taking the medical history, clinical examination of both individuals and colonies, analysis of beekeeping practices, and laboratory diagnosis. The conclusion will be the result of all these elements.

Sometimes, no definite conclusion can be reached. However, eliminating the diverse possible causes of the observed symptoms may give an accurate diagnosis in cases of suspected poisoning.

3.8 Management of poisoning

There is no treatment or antidote for bees in cases of poisoning. Strongly weakened colonies should be eliminated.

However, beekeeping techniques such as re-queening can assist the recovery of a colony after poisoning (Colin, 1999). Hives should eventually be moved to another location if the pesticide source remains in the surrounding environment of the affected apiary. Honey and pollen reserves must be removed. The colony must receive a feeding supplement and should be transferred onto new frames with new wax foundations (made with wax without residues, e.g. waxes from honey cells cappings) as soon as possible by the shaking bee method, also called the shock swarm method: see Chapter 4, section 1.8.3.

If chronic levels of pesticide are found in the surrounding environment, sedentary apiaries should be moved to another site.

Prophylactic measures are the best way to prevent poisoning as far as possible: in particular, beekeeping practices should be aimed at having strong colonies, and the beekeeper should know as far as possible the patterns of agriculture and pesticide use in the surrounding area. Control of *Varroa* infestation must follow good rules of veterinary medicine use and avoid any non-permitted chemicals. The fight against pests such as the small hive beetle or predators such as the Asian hornet must involve reasonable measures and avoid as far as possible the use of insecticides. It is sometimes necessary for beekeepers to practice migratory beekeeping to avoid certain poisoning risks.

In all cases, a beekeeper should get in touch with local crop, orchard and animal farmers to evaluate their use of pesticides and the risks these pose to his or her colonies. Sensible and proportionate application and good practice in the use of phytosanitary products on crops and orchards are necessary to at least limit the risk of poisoning honeybees as well as other wild or reared pollinators (bumblebees, solitary and wild bees).

References

Alaux, C., Brunet, J.L., Dussaubat, C., Mondet, F., Tchemitchen, S., Coucin, M., Brilard, J., Baldy, A., Belzunces, L., and Le Conte, Y. (2009) Interactions between *Nosema* microspores and a neonicotinoid weaken honey-bees (*Apis mellifera*). *Environmental Microbiology*, 3(3): 774–782.

Alaux, C., Ducloz, F., Crauser, D., and Le Conte, Y. (2010) Diet effects on honeybee immunocompetence. *Biology Letters*, doi:10.1098/rsbl.2009.0986. Available at : http://rsbl.royalsocietypublishing.org/content/early/2010/01/18/rsbl.2009.0986.full.html#cited-by (accessed 15 November 2014).

Aufauvre J., Biron D.G., Vidau C., Fontbonne R., Roudel M., Diogon M., Viguès B., Belzunces L.P., Delbac F., and Blot N. (2012) Parasite–insecticide interactions: a case study of *Nosema ceranae* and fipronil synergy on honeybee. *Scientific Reports*, 2: 326. doi:10.1038/srep00326(2012).

Barker, R.J. (1977) Some carbohydrates found in pollen and pollen substitutes are toxic to honey bees. *Journal of Nutrition*, 107: 1859–1862.

Barson, G. (1983) The effects of temperature and humidity on the toxicity of three organophosphorus insecticides to adult *Oryzaephilus surinamensis* (L.) *Pesticide Science*, 14: 142–152.

Beauvais, C. and Vidal-Naquet, N. (2014) Conduite à tenir face à une suspicion d'intoxication. In SNGTV (ed.), *Journées nationales des GTV. Les examens complémentaires: atouts du diagnostic et de la prescription raisonnée*. Reims, pp. 271–282.

Belzunces, L.P., Tchamitchian, S., and Brunet, J-L., (2012) Neural effects of insecticides in the honey bee. *Apidologie*, 43: 348–370.

Brodschneider, R. and Crailsheim, K. (2010) Nutrition and health in honey bees. *Apidologie*, 41: 278–294.

Bruneau, E. (2014) Risk management practices in beekeeping. In Ritter, W. (ed.), *Bee Health and Veterinarians* OIE, Paris, pp. 55–60.

Colin, M.E. (1999) Intoxications. In Colin, M.E., Ball, B.V., and Kilani, M. (eds), *Bee Disease Diagnosis, Options Méditerranéennes*, Series B: *Etudes et Recherches*, No. 25. CIHEAM Publications, Zaragoza, pp. 167–175.

Colin, M.E., Bonmatin, J.M., Moineau, I., Gaimon, C., Brun, S., and Vermandere, J.P. (2004) A method to quantify and analyze the foraging activity of honeybees: relevance to the sublethal effects induced by systemic insecticides. *Environmental Contamination and Toxicology*, 47(3) : 387–395.

Decourtye, A., Devillers, J., Genecque, E., Menach, K., Budzinski, H., Cluzeau, S., Pham-Delègue, M.H. (2005) Comparative sublethal toxicity of nine pesticides on olfactory learning performances of the honeybee *Apis mellifera*. *Archives of Environmental Contamination and Toxicology*, 48: 242–250.

Derecka, K., Blythe, M.J., Malla, S., Genereux, D.P., Guffanti, A., Pavan, P., Moles, A., Snart, C., Ryder, T., Ortori, C.A., Barreyy, D.A., Schuster, E., and Stöger, R. (2013) Transient exposure to low levels of insecticide affects metabolic networks of honeybee larvae. *PLoS ONE*, 8(7): e68191. doi:10.1371/journal.pone.0068191

Desneux, N., Decourtye, A., and Delpuech, J.M. (2007) The sublethal effects of pesticides on beneficial arthropods. *Annual Review of Entomology*, 52: 81–106.

Di Pasquale, G., Salignon, M., Le Conte, Y., Belzunces, L.P., Decourtye A, *et al.* (2013) Influence of pollen nutrition on honey bee health: do pollen quality and diversity matter? *PLoS ONE*, 8(8): e72016. doi:10.1371/journal.pone.0072016

Di Prisco G., Cavaliere V., Annoscia D., Varricchio P., Caprio E., Nazzi F., Gargiulo G., and Pennacchioa F. (2013) Neonicotinoid clothianidin adversely affects insect immunity and promotes replication of a viral pathogen in honey bees. *Proceedings of the National Academy of Sciences USA*, 110(46): 18466–18471.

Dively, G.P. and Kamel, A. (2012) Insecticide residues in pollen and nectar of a cucurbit crop and their potential exposure to pollinators. *Journal of Agricultural and Food Chemistry*, 60: 4449–4456.

EFSA Journal (2012) Scientific opinion on the science behind the development of a risk assessment of plant protection products on bees (*Apis mellifera*, *Bombus* spp. and solitary bees). Available at: http://www.efsa.europa.eu/fr/efsajournal/doc/2668.pdf (accessed 18 September 2014).

EFSA Journal (2013a) Conclusion on the peer review of the pesticide risk assessment for bees for the active substance clothianidin. Available at: http://www.efsa.europa.eu/en/efsajournal/doc/3066.pdf (accessed 5 November 2014).

EFSA Journal (2013b) EFSA Guidance Document on the risk assessment of plant protection products on bees (*Apis mellifera*, *Bombus* spp. and solitary bees). Available at: http://www.efsa.europa.eu/fr/efsajournal/doc/3295.pdf (accessed 30 October 2014).

Faucon, J.P., Mathieu, L., Ribière, M., Martel, A.C., Drajnudel, P., *et al.* (2002) Honey bee winter mortality in France in 1999 and 2000. *Bee World*, 83: 14–23.

Franco, S., Martel, A.C, Chauzat, M.P., Blanchard, P., and Thiéry, R. (2012) Les analyses de laboratoire en apiculture. In SNGTV (ed.), *Proceedings of the Journées nationales des GTV.* SNGTV, Nantes, pp. 859–867.

Frazier, M., Mullin, C., Frazier, J., and Ashcraft, S. (2008) What have pesticides got to do with it? *American Bee Journal*, 148: 521–523.

Gregorc A., Silva-Zacarin M., and Nocelli R.C.F. (2012) Cellular response in honey bees to non-pathogenic effects of pesticides. In Sammatoro D. and Yolder J.A. (ed.), *Honey Bee Colony Health Challenges and Sustainable Solutions*. CRC Press, Boca Raton, FL, pp. 161–180.

Hainzl, D., Cole, L.M., and Casida, J.E. (1998) Mechanisms for selective toxicity of fipronil insecticide and its sulfone metabolite and desulfinyl photoproduct. *Chemical Research in Toxicology*, 11: 1529–1535.

Hammel, Y.A., Mohammed, R., Gremaud, E., LeBreton, M.H, and Guy, P.A. (2008) Multiscreening approach to monitor and quantify 42 antibiotic residues in honey by liquid chromatography–tandem mass spectrometry. *Journal of Chromatography A*, 1177: 58–76.

Hawthorne D.J. and Dively G.P. (2011) Killing them with kindness? In-hive medications may inhibit xenobiotic efflux transporters and endanger honey bees. *PLoS ONE*, 6(11): e26796. doi:10.1371/journal.pone.0026796 (accessed 14 February 2014).

Haydak, M.H. (1935) Brood rearing by honeybees confined to a pure carbohydrate diet. *Journal of Economic Entomology*, 28: 657–660.

Henry, M., Béguin, M., Requier, F., Rollin, O., Odoux, J.F., Aurinel, P., Aptel, J., Tchamitchian, S., and Decourtye, A. (2012) A common pesticide decreases foraging success and survival in honey bees. *Science*, 336(6079): 348–350.

Hrassnigg N. and Crailsheim K. (2005) Differences in drone and worker physiology in honeybees (*Apis mellifera* L.). *Apidologie*, 36: 255–277.

Imdorf, A., Ruoff, K., and Fluri, P. (2010) *Le développement des colonies chez l'abeille mellifère.* Station de recherche Agroscope Liebefeld-Posieux ALP, Berne.

Johnson, R.M., Pollock H.S., and Berenbaum, M.R. (2009) Synergistic interactions between in-hive miticides in *Apis mellifera. Journal of Economic Entomology*, 99: 1046–1050.

Johnson, R. (2010) Honeybee Colony Collapse Disorder. Congressional Research Service. CRS Report for Congress. 7-5700. Available at: http://cursa.ihmc.us/rid=1JJM69DXL-27XB9CC-12CF/bees.pdf (accessed 31 August 2014).

Johnson, R.M., Ellis, M.D., Mullin, C.A., and Frazier, M. (2012) Pesticides and honey bee toxicity. In Sammatoro, D. and Yolder, J.A. (eds), *Honey Bee Colony Health Challenges and Sustainable Solutions.* CRC Press, Boca Raton, FL, pp. 145–160.

Kauffeld, N.M., Everitt, J.H., and Taylor, E.A. (1976) Honey bee problems in the Rio Grande Valley of Texas. *American Bee Journal*, 116: 220–222.

Kimmel, S., Kuhn, J., Harst, W., and Stever, H. (2007) Electromagnetic radiation: influences on honeybees (*Apis mellifera*). Available at: http://www.hese-project.org/hese-uk/en/papers/kimmel_iaas_2007.pdf (accessed 7 January, 2014).

Knox, D.A., Shimanuki, H., and Herbert, E.W. (1971) Diet and the longevity of adult honey bees. *Journal of Economical Entomology*, 64: 1415–1416.

Kühnholz, S. and Seeley, T.D. (1997) The control of water collection in honey bees colonies. *Behavioral Ecology and Sociobiology*, 41: 407–422.

Lambert, O., Piroux, M., Puyo, S., Thorin, C., Larhantec, M., Delbac, F., and Pouliquen, H. (2012) Bees, honey and pollen as sentinels for lead environmental contamination. *Environmental Pollution*, 170: 254–259.

Lawrence, T. and Sheppard, W.S. (2013) Neonicotinoid Pesticides and Honey Bees. Washington

State University Extension Fact Sheet. FS122E. Available at: http://cru.cahe.wsu.edu/CEPublications/FS122E/FS122E.pdf (accessed 21 September 2014).

Le Conte, Y. and Navajas, M. (2008) Climate change: impact on honey bee populations and diseases. *Scientific and Technical Review OIE*, 27(2): 499–510.

Lehotay, S.J. (2006) Quick, easy, cheap, effective, rugged, and safe approach for determining pesticide residues. *Pesticides Protocols Methods in Biotechnology*, 19: 239–261.

Lu, C., Warchol, K.M., and Callahan, R.A. (2014) Sub-lethal exposure to neonicotinoids impaired honey bees winterization before proceeding to colony collapse disorder. *Bulletin of Insectology*, 67: 125–130.

Martel, A.C., Zeggane, S., Aurières, C., Drajnudel, P., Faucon, J.P., and Aubert, M. (2007) Acaricide residues in honey and wax after treatment of honey bee colonies with Apivar® or Asuntol 50®. *Apidologie*, 38: 534–544.

Mason, R., Tennekes, H., Sanchez-Bayo, F., and Jepsen, P.U. (2013) Immune suppression by neonicotinoid insecticides at the root of global wildlife declines. *Journal of Environmental Immunology and Toxicology*, 1: 3–12.

Moréteau, B. (1991) Etude de certains aspects de la physiotoxicologie d'insecticides de synthèse chez le Criquet migrateur: *Locusta migratoria* R. & F. In Aupelf-uref (ed.), *La Lutte Anti-acridienne*. John Libbey Eurotext, Paris, pp. 167–178.

Morton, H.L., Moffet, J.O., and Macdonald, R.H. (1972) Toxicity of herbicides to newly emerged honey bees. *Environmental Entomology*, 1(1): 102–104.

Morton, H.L. and Moffet, J.O. (1972) Ovicidal and larvicidal effects of certain herbicides on honey bees. *Environmental Entomology*, 1(5): 611–614.

Mullin, C.A., Frazier, M., Frazier, J.L., Ashcraft, S., Simonds, R., van Engelsdorp, D., and Pettis, J.S. (2010) High levels of miticides and agrochemicals in North American apiaries: implications for honey bee health. *PLoS ONE*, 5(3): e9754. doi:10.1371/journal.pone.0009754

OIE and FAO (2009) *Guide to Good Farming Practices for Animal Production Food Safety*. FAO and OIE, Rome.

Pilling, E.D., Bromleychallenor, K.A.C., Walker, C.H., and Jepson, P.C. (1995) Mechanism of synergism between the pyrethroid insecticide λ-cyhalothrin and the imidazole fungicide prochloraz, in the honeybee (*Apis mellifera* L.). *Pesticide Biochemistry and Physiology*, 51: 1–11.

Riessberger, U. and Crailsheim, K. (1997) Short-term effect of different weather conditions upon the behaviour of forager and nurse honey bees (*Apis mellifera* carnica Pollmann). *Apidologie*, 28: 411–426.

Rosatella, A.A, Simeonov, S.P., Frade, R.F.M., and Afonso, C.A.M. (2011) 5-Hydroxymethylfurfural (HMF) as a building block platform: biological properties, synthesis and synthetic applications. *Green Chemistry*, 13: 754–793.

Schäfer, M.O. and Ritter, W. (2014) The small hive beetle (*Aethina tumida*). In Ritter, W. (ed.), *Bee Health and Veterinarians*. OIE, Paris, pp. 149–156.

Schmidt, J.O. (1984) Feeding preferences of *Apis mellifera* L. (Hymenoptera: Apidae): individual versus mixed pollen species. *Journal of the Kansas Entomological Society*, 57: 323–327

Schmidt, J.O., Thoenes, S.C., and Levin, M.D. (1987) Survival of honey bees, *Apis mellifera* (Hymenoptera: Apidae), fed various pollen sources. *Journal of Economic Entomology*, 80: 176–183.

Shuel, R.W. (1992) The production of nectar and pollen. In Graham, J.M. (ed.), *The Hive and the Honey Bee*, rev. edn. Bookcrafters, Hamilton, IL, pp. 401–433.

Somerville, D.C. (2014) Bee nutrition and plants visited. In Ritter, W. (ed.), *Bee Health and Veterinarians*. OIE, Paris, pp. 61–66.

Suchail, S., Guez, D., and Belzunces, L.P. (2001) Discrepancy between acute and chronic toxicity induced by imidacloprid and its metabolites in *Apis mellifera*. *Environmental Toxicology and Chemistry*, 20(11): 2482–2486.

Tanner, G. and Czerwenka, C. (2011) LC-MS/MS analysis of neonicotinoid insecticides in honey: methodology and residue findings in Austrian honeys. *Journal of Agricultural and Food Chemistry*, 59: 12271–12277.

Tapparo, A., Giorio, C., Marzaro, M., Marton, D., Soldà, L., and Girolami, V. (2011) Rapid analysis of neonicotinoid insecticides in guttation drops of corn seedlings obtained from coated seeds. *Journal of Environmental Monitoring*, 13(6): 1564–1568.

Thompson, H.M. (2003) Behavioral effects of pesticides in bees: their potential for use in risk assessment. *Exotoxicology*, 12: 317–330.

Thompson, H.M. (2012) Interaction between pesticides and other factors in effects on bees. Supporting Publications 2012:EN-340. Available online: www.efsa.europa.eu/publications (accessed 30 August 2014).

Thuiller, W., Lavorel, S., Araujo, M.B., Sykes, M.T., and Prentice, I.C. (2005) Climate change threats to plant diversity in Europe. *Proceedings of the*

National Academy of Sciences USA, 102(23): 8245–8250.

Tuell, J.K. and Isaacs, R. (2010) Weather during bloom affects pollination and yield of highbush blueberry. *Journal of Economic Entomology*, 103(3): 557–562.

van der Sluijs, J.P., Amaral-Rogers, V., Belzunces, L.P., Bijleveld van Lexmond, M.F.I.J., Bonmatin J-M., Chagon, M., Downs, C.A., Furlan, L., Gibbons, D.W., Giorio, C., Girolami, V., Goulson, D., Kreutzweiser, D.P., Krupke, C., Liess, M., Long, E., McField, M., Mineau, P., Mitchell, E.A.D., Morrissey, C.A., Noome, D.A., Pisa, L., Settele, J., Simon-Delso, N., Stark, J.D., Tapparo, A., Van Dyck, H., van Praagh, J., Whitehorn, P.R., and Wiemers, M. (2014) Conclusions of the worldwide integrated assessment on the risks of neonicotinoids and fipronil to biodiversity and ecosystem functioning. *Environmental Science and Pollution Research*, doi:10.1007/s11356-014-3229-5

van Engelsdorp, D., Evans, D.E., Saegerman, C., Mullin, C., Haubruge, E., Nguyen, B.K., Frazier, M., Frazier, J., Cox-Foster, D.L., Chen, Y., Underwood, R., Tarpy, D.R., and Pettis, J.S. (2009) Colony collapse disorder: a descriptive study. *PLoS ONE*, 4(8):e6481.

van Engelsdorp, D. and Meixner, M.D. (2010) A historical review of managed honey bee populations in Europe and the United States and the factors that may affect them. *Journal of Invertebrate Pathology*, 103, S80-S95.

Vidal-Naquet, N. (2008) Une classification des insecticides. Available at: http://www.apivet.eu/2008/03/une-classificat.html (accessed 11 October 2014).

Vidal-Naquet, N. (2009) Surmortalité d'abeilles en Ariège. Les antiparasitaires utilisés contre la FCO sont suspectés d'intoxiquer les abeilles. *La Semaine Vétérinaire*, 1349: 22.

Vidal-Naquet, N. (2013) Les bonnes pratiques apicoles. In SNGTV (ed.), *Proceedings of the Journées nationales des GTV.* Nantes, pp. 773–781.

Vidau C., Diogon M., Aufauvre J., Fontbonne R., Viguès B., Brunet J.L., Texier C., Biron D.G., Blot N., El Alaoui H., Belzunces L.P., and Delbac F. (2011) Exposure to sublethal doses of fipronil and thiacloprid highly increases mortality of honeybees previously infected by *Nosema ceranae. PLoS ONE,* 2011; 6(6):e21550. doi:10.1371/journal.pone.0021550.

Voorhies, E.C., Todd, F.E., and Galbraith, J.K., (1933) Economic aspects of the bee industry. *University of California College of Agriculture Bulletin*, 555: 1–117.

Wiest, L., Buleté, A., Giroud, B., Fratta, C., Amic, S., Lambert, O., Pouliquen, H., and Arnaudguilhem, C. (2011) Multi-residue analysis of 80 environmental contaminants in honeys, honeybees and pollens by one extraction procedure followed by liquid and gas chromatography coupled with mass spectrometric detection. *Journal of Chromatography A*, 1218(34): 5743–5756.

Winston, M.L. (1987) *The Biology of the Honeybee*. Harvard University Press, Cambridge, MA.

Wood, A. (2012) Compendium of Pesticide Common Names. Classified Lists of Pesticides. Available at: http://www.alanwood.net/pesticides/class_pesticides.html (accessed 10 October 2014).

Wu, J.Y., Anelli, C.M., and Sheppard, W.S. (2011) Sub-lethal effects of pesticide residues in brood comb on worker honey bee (*Apis mellifera*) development and longevity. *PLoS ONE*, 6(2): e14720. doi:10.1371/journal.pone.0014720

Yoder, J.A., Hedges, B.Z., Heydinger, D.J., Sammataro, D., and DeGrandi-Hoffman, G. (2012) Differences among fungicides targeting beneficial fungi associated with honey bee colonies. In Sammatoro D. and Yolder J.A. (eds), *Honey Bee Colony Health Challenges and Sustainable Solutions*. CRC Press, Boca Raton, FL, pp. 181–192.

Yoder, J.A., Jajack, A.J., Rosselot, A.E., Smith, T.J., Yerke, M.C., and Sammataro, D. (2013) Fungicide contamination reduces beneficial fungi in bee bread based on an area-wide field study in honey bee, *Apis mellifera*, colonies. *Journal of Toxicology and Environmental Health A*, 76(10): 587–600.

3

Honeybee viruses and viral diseases

As in other species and insects, the presence of viruses in honeybees is commonplace, and their effects have long been known. About 20 viruses have so far been identified in association with *Apis mellifera*; apart from two with DNA genomes, they are single-stranded RNA viruses approximately isometric in form (Culley *et al.*, 2003; de Miranda *et al.*, 2012).

As in other species, viruses may be diagnosed in apparently healthy colonies as asymptomatic, or as slight infections (Gauthier *et al.*, 2007). However, these viruses can be responsible for diseases in honeybees that can result in the weakening or death of colonies. If a virus becomes pathogenic and induces disease(s), the underlying cause(s), if they exist, are not always known, discovered, and/or reported.

1 Generalities on honeybee viruses

Among the approximately 18 honeybee-infecting known viruses, three are characterized by specific clinical signs: chronic bee paralysis virus (CBPV), deformed wing virus (DWV), and sacbrood virus (SBV) (de Miranda *et al.*, 2012).

After presenting the characteristics of these viruses, the diseases caused by CBPV, DWV, and SBV are discussed. Conditions caused by other viruses are also described. Table 3.1 presents some important features of the main honeybee viruses currently known.

1.1 Characteristics and elements of taxonomy

1.1.1 RNA viruses

Except for the unclassified CBPV and a heterogeneous group of other viruses (de Miranda *et al.*, 2012), most honeybee viruses are picorna-like viruses: iflaviruses and dicistroviruses. These are considered the most harmful viruses for bees.

Picorna-like viruses are single-stranded RNA viruses (Culley *et al.*, 2003; Ribière *et al.*, 2010; de Miranda et al., 2012). The capsid (protein shell) is isometric and exhibits icosahedral symmetry. Its role is to protect the RNA genome inside. Replication of these viruses occurs within the cellular cytoplasm. Iflaviruses and dicistroviruses are very similar insect-infecting viruses (the differences being the arrangement of genes in the genome).

The honeybee-infecting *Iflaviridae* are DWV, SBV, and slow bee paralysis virus (SBPV).

The honeybee-infecting *Dicistroviridae* are acute bee paralysis virus (ABPV), Kashmir bee virus (KBV), and Israeli acute paralysis virus (IAPV), forming the ABPV–KBV–IAPV complex (de Miranda *et al.*, 2012)

Other icosahedral RNA viruses are found in bees: cloudy wing virus (CWV), bee virus X (BVX), bee virus Y (BVY), and macula-like virus (MLV). These viruses are reported to be less damaging to honeybees and their colonies (de Miranda *et al.*, 2012).

Table 3.1 Honeybee viruses. (Adapted from Olivier and Ribière, 2006; Vidal-Naquet, 2011; de Miranda *et al.*, 2012.)

Virus	RNA/DNA	Taxonomy	Covert infection found	Clinical signs known (experimental observations)
Chronic bee paralysis virus (CBPV)	RNA	RNA virus unclassified	Y	Type-1 paralysis/Type-2: hairless, shorten abdomen, flightless
Acute bee paralysis virus (ABPV)	RNA	*Dicistroviridae*	Y	trailing bees, affected brood, etc.
Kashmir bee virus (KBV)	RNA	*Dicistroviridae*	Y	mortality without symptoms
Israeli acute paralysis virus (IAPV)	RNA	*Dicistroviridae*	Y	progressive paralysis and death
Black queen cell virus (BQCV)	RNA	*Dicistroviridae*	Y	queen pupa yellow with a tough sac-like skin/ black cell walls
Deformed wing virus (DWV)	RNA	*Iflaviridae*	Y	deformed wings and shortened abdomen/scattered brood
Sacbrood virus (SBV)	RNA	*Iflaviridae*	Y	larvae become a sac with an ecdysial fluid/scattered brood
Slow bee paralysis virus (SBPV)	RNA	*Iflaviridae*	Y	paralysis of the two first pairs of legs (exp.)
Cloudy wing virus (CWV)	RNA	miscellaneous virus	Y	clouding wings/not considered as highly pathologic
Bee virus X (BVX)	RNA	miscellaneous virus	Y	reduction of lifespan(with *Malpighamoeba mellifica*) infectious at 30°C or less
Bee virus Y (BVY)	RNA	miscellaneous virus	Y	found in young bees – infectious at 30°C or less
Arkansas bee virus (ABV)	RNA	miscellaneous virus	Y	no known symptoms
Berkeley bee virus (BBPV)	RNA	miscellaneous virus	Y	no known symptoms (associated with ABV)
Macula-like virus	RNA	miscellaneous virus	no data found	no known symptoms
Filamentous virus (AmFV)	DNA	baculo and asco-like virus	Y	no clinical signs, lifespan not affected significantly (clinical sign: whitish haemolymph)
Apis iridescent virus (AIV)	DNA	*Iridoviridae*	Y	adult flightless and inactive (*Apis cerana*)

Co, contact; O, oral; OF, oral–faecal; TO, transovarial; VB, vector-borne; Ve, vertical; Vn, venereal.

Effects on the colony	Main season occurence	Transmission (main routes)	*Varroa* role as vector	Association with another pathogen	Prevalence in the world
from mild to severe weakening	spring/summer	OF, Co	N	satellite virus: CBPSV	Worldwide distribution
weakening and mortality	summer/autumn	VB, Ve (Vn, TO)	Y	*Varroa destructor*	common in Europe
weakening and mortality	summer/autumn	VB, Ve (TO?)	Y	*Varroa destructor*	worldwide distribution
weakening and mortality	summer/autumn	VB, Ve (TO?)	Y	*Varroa destructor*	Europe, Asia, North America
weakening and mortality in association with *Nosema*	spring/summer	OF, VB?, Ve (TO)	Y (low)	*Varroa destructor/ Nosema*	worldwide distribution
colony weakening and even collapse	end of summer/ autumn	VB, Ve (Vn, TO)	Y	*Varroa destructor*	worldwide distribution
considered as not highly pathologic	spring/summer	O (jelly), Ve	Y	*Varroa destructor*	worldwide distribution
weakening and mortality	no evidence of seasonal occurrence	OF,VB	Y	*Varroa destructor* (?)	low prevalence in Europe
weakening and death exp.; not highly pathologic	no evidence of seasonal occurrence	unclear	no direct evidence	*Varroa destructor* (?)	Europe/ Worlwide?
weakening in association with *Malpighamoeba mellifica*	late winter/spring	OF	?	*Malpighamoeba mellificae*	low prevalence – seems on the decline
weakening in association with *Nosema apis*	late spring/early summer	OF	?	*Nosema apis*	First detected in Britain
no known symptoms	no data found	no data found	?	no data found	US
no known symptoms	no data found	no data found	?	found with ABV	US
no known symptoms	summer/autumn	VB	Y	*Varroa destructor*	common in France – virus of *Varroa*?
some cases of weakening suspected	spring	O	?	*Nosema apis*	worldwide?
weakening and mortality suspected	summer (*Apis cerana*)	no data found. VB?	?	*Nosema ceranae*	India, US?

1.1.2 DNA viruses

Apis mellifera filamentous virus (*Am*FV) and *Apis* iridescent virus (*A*IV) are the two DNA honeybee viruses currently known. *Am*FV seems to be related to both Baculoviruses and Ascoviruses. The structure of *Am*FV comprises a long filamentous nucleoprotein forming a figure of eight in order to fit in the envelope (Sitaropoulou *et al.*, 1989). *A*IV is an iridovirus (de Miranda *et al.*, 2012). Iridoviruses are large icosahedral viruses that infect insects and vertebrates.

1.2 Pathogenicity of viruses

The pathogenicity of viruses is the consequence of their replication within the cells of diverse organs of the honeybee. When pathogenic, some viruses have a tropism to specific organs, while others can replicate in many organs.

However, it seems that many honeybee-infecting viruses have a CNS tropism and are responsible for neurological problems. When pathogenic, viruses alter the lifespan of bees. If many bees are affected, the colony will suffer and weaken, and in some cases may die if the colony is not able to compensate for the lack of bees. If a few bees are affected, the colony will be only slightly affected, if at all, and able to compensate the population imbalance due to the ability of workers to adapt to different tasks.

Viruses are present in healthy colonies as asymptomatic or unapparent infections. It is generally considered that promoting factors are necessary to convert an asymptomatic infection into a symptomatic and overt infection. These factors are thought to be mainly environmental stressors: starvation; confinement; residues stored in wax, honey, or pollen (from pesticides used on crops, veterinary medicines used on cattle farms, or miticides used in hives); cold; humidity; other pathogens; and parasites, e.g. *Varroa destructor* (Genersch *et al.*, 2010; de Miranda *et al.*, 2012).

1.3 Transmission routes

Viral transmission may be horizontal between bees, vertical from queen to egg, venereal, and/or vector-borne, such as in the case of *V. destructor* or the mite *Tropilaelaps* spp. (Tentcheva *et al.*, 2004; Chen *et al.*, 2006).

- Horizontal transmission. Horizontal transmission can be oral or by contact. Feeding larvae and trophallaxis as well as oral communication are the main ways of oral transmission. Contact transmission seems to occur in the event of cuticle injuries or broken hairs allowing exposure of the epidermal cytoplasm (Chen *et al.*, 2006; de Miranda *et al.*, 2012). Confinement, wintering, and highly crowded colonies are conducive to contact transmission (Ball, 1999a).
- Vertical transmission. Viruses are frequently detected in queen ovaries, suggesting a vertical trans-ovarial transmission from queen to unfertilized male and fertilized female eggs. Vertical transmission may also be venereal during mating, from drone to queen, or trans-spermal (from the spermatozoa to the female egg).
- Vector-borne transmission. The acarian *V. destructor* is a vector of many honeybee viruses. The prevalence of the mite in managed colonies worldwide has probably increased virus transmission and outbreaks of viral disease. Thus, *V. destructor* infestations may transmit viruses and thus allow overt virus infections, impairing the health of colonies. The interaction between viruses and *V. destructor* has been termed 'bee parasitic mite syndrome' (Shimanuki *et al.*, 1994). The disease due to *Varroa*, varroosis, is not only caused by the infestation by the mite, but also incorporates the notion of virus transmission and overt virus infection (in particular DWV). The acarian *Tropilaelaps* spp. is also reported to be a vector of at least one virus, DWV. The acarian *Acarapis woodi*, a parasite of the tracheae, has been suspected to be related to paralysis syndrome (CBPV), though no evidence has been shown to confirm this suspicion (Ribière *et al.*, 2010; de Miranda, 2012).

1.4 Diagnosis of viral infection

As clinical signs are rarely pathognomonic, the diagnosis of viral diseases should rely on laboratory tests. Immunological methods can usually provide both qualitative and quantitative results and are generally affordable. However, these methods present a lack of sensitivity and adaptability (de Miranda *et al.*, 2012).

The most sensitive and reliable methods are the polymerase chain reaction (PCR) and the reverse-transcription polymerase chain reaction (RT-PCR) techniques. These methods give reliable quantitative and qualitative results, allowing virus identification and assessment of the viral load. Associated with the clinical examination, both identification and load are necessary for conclusive diagnosis of a viral disease.

Diagnostic test results should be interpreted in association with clinical signs, beekeeping techniques, blooming environment, *Varroa* infestation level, and other potential colony-weakening causes.

Unfortunately, because of their cost, PCR and RT-PCR are not yet routinely performed in honeybee veterinary medicine practice and have tended to remain a research technique.

2 Chronic bee paralysis virus (CBPV) disease: 'paralysis'

CBPV disease, also called paralysis, is a contagious disease.

The first bee virus isolated, CBPV has been recognized for decades (Ball, 1999a), though the disease itself has been known for much longer. CBPV is one of the most widely prevalent viruses, and found worldwide except for the Caribbean islands (Ribière *et al.*, 2010; de Miranda *et al.*, 2012). The disease pattern is usually characterized by two main syndromes: Type-1 CBPV disease (paralysis) and Type-2 CBPV disease ('black robbers' or 'little black' in the UK, 'hairless black' syndrome in the US, 'maladic noire', 'mal de mai' in France).

CBPV often persists as a covert infection in honeybee colonies throughout the year (Bailey and Ball, 1991; Ball, 1999a). The disease often presents in apparently strong colonies with thousands of dead bees being observed in front of the hives (Ribière *et al.*, 2010).

2.1 Characteristics of CBPV

CBPV is a positive-sense, single-stranded RNA virus, and is an unclassified virus (Ribière *et al.*, 2007). The particles of CBPV are anisometric (30–65 nm × 20 nm) (Bailey *et al.*, 1968). This virus has been reported to have an associated particle, the chronic bee paralysis satellite virus, CBPSV (previously called the CBPV associate). The role of CBPSV is not well known and understood at this time (de Miranda *et al.*, 2012), though it has been hypothesised to evoke an encoding role for either a capsid protein involved in CBPV replication or an abortive virus particle (Ribière *et al.*, 2010; de Miranda *et al.*, 2012).

2.2 Clinical signs

Two distinct syndromes characterize CBPV disease: Type-1 and Type-2 (Bailey and Ball, 1991; de Miranda *et al.*, 2012). In the case of overt CBPV infection, the two syndromes may occur simultaneously (de Miranda *et al.*, 2012).

In an apiary, when an outbreak of CBPV occurs within a colony, not all the colonies develop the disease. The affected colonies are usually strong and CBPV outbreaks do not usually cause 'massive colony losses' (Ribière *et al.*, 2010). However, CBPV disease may induce high-level losses of workers. A large carpet of dead or sick workers in front of the hives is frequently observed when outbreaks occur (Ribière *et al.*, 2010; de Miranda *et al.*, 2012).

2.2.1 Type-1 syndrome or 'paralysis'

Paralysis syndrome is the most serious consequence of CBPV. This syndrome is also called 'mal des forêts' ('sickness of the forest') because it is often observed in colonies gathering nectar or honeydew in forests. A large number of foraging bees can be affected. The deleterious effects are responsible for depopulation, disorganization, and even colony mortality.

Bees infected by CBPV present the following clinical signs during outbreaks (Ball, 1999a):

- Abnormal trembling wings and bodies.
- Ataxia.
- Circling.
- Inability to take off or fly, manifested by bees crawling on the ground and up grass stems.
- Bloated abdomens caused by distension of the honey sac with liquid.
- Mortality within a few days.

At the colony level, crawling bees, and a carpet of affected and dead bees with outspread wings, are seen on the floor of the hive and on the ground in front of or surrounding the hive (Figure 3.1).

A sudden collapse may occur in the terminal phase of this syndrome, leaving the queen and a few retinue workers within the hive (Bailey and Ball, 1991; Ribière *et al.*, 2010). Severely affected colonies may collapse in a week.

2.2.2 Type-2 syndrome

Bees affected by Type-2 syndrome are smaller, with a shortened abdomen. The honeybees become hairless and appear dark and shiny (Ball, 1999a) (Figure 3.2). At the beginning of the disease, bees are able to fly, but soon they begin crawling and trembling. They usually die soon after the onset of clinical signs.

In a colony, Type-2 syndrome usually appears in spring and summer and can sometimes significantly weaken colonies, although it is often considered only a minor problem. Indeed, frequently only a few Type-2 diseased bees are observed within a colony.

2.2.3 From two syndromes to one

According to Ribière *et al.* (2010), the question of whether there are two syndromes characterizing CBPV disease has to be challenged. Indeed, in some colonies affected by CBPV, both Type-2 and Type-1 syndromes have been described concurrently. In the same publication, Ribière *et al.* (2010) are clear that 'researchers have observed a general syndrome with clusters of trembling, flightless, crawling bees with some individual black, hairless bees standing at the hive entrance, sometimes rejected by bees of their colony'. These observations have also been made in the field by beekeepers and veterinarians. Moreover, the CBPV strains causing the two syndromes are serologically the same. This begs the questions: are these two

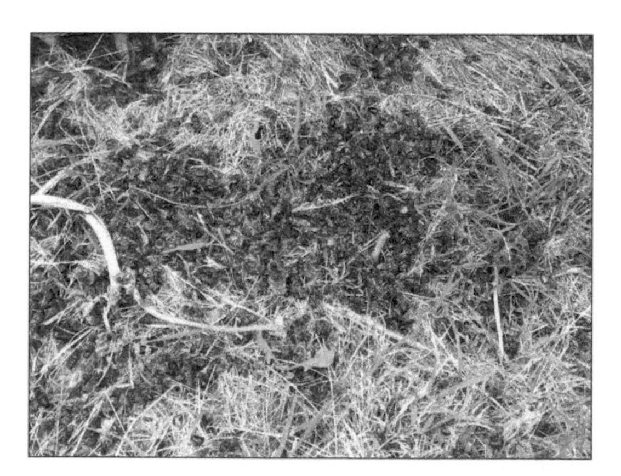

Figure 3.1 Typical carpet of diseased and dead bees observed in the front of a hive when a CBPV outbreak occurs within a colony. (Photo courtesy © Lydia Vilagines, DVM.)

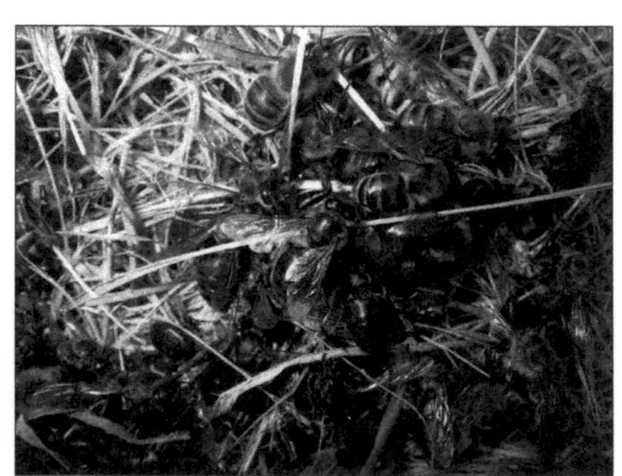

Figure 3.2 CBPV Type-1 syndrome (bee at the centre) and Type-2 syndrome with honeybees presenting as hairless and shiny with a shortened abdomen. (Photo courtesy © Lydia Vilagines, DVM.)

different stages of the CBPV viral disease and is there a particular sensitivity of bees' lineages within a colony?

The prognosis of CBPV infection is usually good with a spontaneous regression. However, if the disease persists in some colonies or occurs in autumn, the prognosis may become severe.

2.3 Epidemiological characteristics

Overt CBPV infection may occur throughout the year, even in winter. However, the prevalence of outbreaks is higher in the spring and summer beekeeping season.

In the case of overt infection, wound invasion is reported to be the main route of transmission via contaminated faeces (Bailey *et al.*, 1983; Ribière *et al.*, 2010). The mite *Varroa* probably plays a role in the transmission of CBPV. In strong and populous colonies, moving and contacts between bees assists the dissemination of the virus within the colony and explains the high number of bees affected and killed. The disease often regresses spontaneously in 3–4 weeks.

In asymptomatic colonies the persistence of the virus seems to be the consequence of oral exchange (trophallaxis), physical contact, and probably trans-ovarial transmission (Ribière *et al.*, 2010; de Miranda *et al.*, 2012).

Some studies reported by Ribière *et al.* (2010) show that CBPV particles have been found in other Hymenoptera species: the common and worldwide ant *Camponotus vagus* and the forest Northern European and Asian ant *Formica rufa*. In *C. vagus*, CBPV has been shown to replicate and it can be supposed that this species serves as a reservoir of infection and plays a role in the transmission of the virus. Within hives, ants are often found by beekeepers feeding on products of the hive and debris on the floor, the frames, the walls, and the feeders.

2.4 Pathogenesis

In asymptomatic colonies, bees are reported to present $\leq 10^4$ CBPV copies per bee (Ribière *et al.*, 2010). In symptomatic colonies, CBPV is more prevalent in older bees, with 10^{13} copies found in guards and symptomatic bees sampled at the front of the hive vs. 10^6 copies found in bees inside the nest (Ribière *et al.*, 2010). However, the causes inducing CBPV outbreaks within an asymptomatic colony (i.e. causing covert CBPV infection) remain mainly unknown.

CBPV may infect immature forms. Indeed, it has been found in all the stages of bees, from the egg to the adult (Blanchard *et al.*, 2007). In the eggs, larvae, and pupae, the viral load is low and is reported to remain mainly lower than in adult bees.

The tropism of CBPV is mainly the nervous system though other organs can also be affected (Ribière *et al.*, 2010). It has been shown that in an infected bee, half of the many million particles of CBPV found are located within the head (Blanchard *et al.*, 2007; Ribière *et al.*, 2010).

The higher-order integration centres of the brain are mainly infected by CBPV particles as shown by Olivier *et al.* (2008):

- The mushroom bodies involved in sensory, learning, memory and motor control.
- The central complex involved in locomotion control, orientation behaviour, and the regulation of insect arousal (the central complex is also a neurosecretory structure and a centre of sensory integration) (Olivier *et al.*, 2008; Ribière *et al.*, 2010).

CBPV has also been found in the optic and antennal lobes but also in structures in charge of antennae movement, the mouthparts, and olfaction.

This selected neurotropism is considered to be responsible for the neurological symptoms observed. The chronic bee paralysis satellite virus, CBPSV, have been found within the thoracic and abdominal nerve ganglia, but also in the mandibular and hypopharyngeal glands and in the brain (Ribière *et al.*, 2010).

The prognosis is usually good, with a spontaneous recovery; however, if the disease persists into autumn, the chances of recovery lessen.

2.5 Contributing factors

As noted previously, the mechanisms underlying the transformation of a covert CBPV infection into overt infection and activation of pathogenic virus are not fully understood. However, some factors seem to predispose to the occurrence of an outbreak.

Confinement (bad weather, failure of nectar flow, starvation, etc.) is reported to be a main cause of the occurrence of 'paralysis'. In this case, healthy honeybees are crowded with affected ones and their faeces, offering the potential for virus transmission and an outbreak of overt infection.

Bee concentration, inherited factors, environmental factors (e.g. consumption of honeydew by honeybees), protein deficiency, or even weakening factors (e.g. poisoning) may also play a part in CBPV disease outbreaks (Bailey and Ball, 1991; Ball, 1999a).

2.6 Diagnosis

2.6.1 Clinical diagnosis

The occurrence of two or more clinical signs is suggestive of CBPV disease.

At the level of the colony, the main symptoms are dead and trembling/crawling bees forming a carpet at the front of the hive. Affected colonies are usually the stronger ones within an apiary (not all the colonies in an apiary are affected, but all must nevertheless be examined).

At the level of bees, individuals with behavioural and neurological symptoms and/or presenting as smaller, shiny, and hairless with a broader abdomen favour a diagnosis of CBPV disease.

It has been observed that healthy worker bees attack affected bees to remove them from the colony, as they would do against robber bees.

2.6.2 Differential diagnosis

Other neurological diseases and poisoning by pesticides and/or chemicals should be ruled out. Many pathogens and chemicals can cause trembling and crawling. *Nosema apis*, *Malpighamoeba mellificae*, and *A. woodi* infestations (and/or the associated viruses BVX, BVY, *Am*FV) and the virus IAPV may be responsible for bees showing crawling symptoms (de Miranda *et al.*, 2012).

Clinical examination and the medical history (anamnesis) of the colony can give a presumptive diagnosis; however, laboratory analysis is usually necessary.

2.6.3 Laboratory diagnosis

Sampling bees for laboratory diagnosis must be performed according to certain rules. Usually, it is necessary to contact the laboratory who will assist in the choice of samples, and advise on performing the sampling and sending the samples. Tables of sampling management when poisoning or disease are suspected are given in Appendix 3. These sampling methods are those advised by the Sophia-Antipolis laboratory of ANSES which is the European Union Reference Laboratory for Bee Health (Franco *et al.*, 2012).

Identification and quantification of CBPV is necessary to diagnose the disease. Diverse techniques can be used, but RT-PCR (identification and viral load) is the most precise and selective diagnostic method (Blanchard *et al.*, 2007). Within an infected colony, the CBPV viral loads observed in symptomatic or dead bees (at the entrance of the hive) or guards are higher than in asymptomatic bees (foragers, nurses, drones).

According to Blanchard *et al.* (2007) and Ribière *et al.* (2010):

- CBPV levels of about 10^{12} copies per bee are found in symptomatic or dead bees.
- CBPV levels of 10^4–10^8 copies per bee are found in asymptomatic bees.
- CBPV can be found in all castes and all stages (egg, larva, pupa) in an infected colony.

The diagnosis will be the consequence of:

- Anamnesis.
- Clinical examination of the colony.
- Laboratory results.

- Analysis of various factors, e.g. beekeeping practices and the biological features of the bee colony.

In a suspected overt CBPV infection, it may be interesting to test for other viruses and perhaps pesticide residues as potential contributing factors, or as part of a differential diagnosis.

2.6.4 Management

Minimizing transmission and reducing viral loads within colonies are the two main pillars of the fight against viruses. As beekeeping practices may be a contributing factor to the development and transmission of viruses (and other pathogenic agents), good beekeeping practices are the best way to manage, prevent, and control viral diseases and in particular CBPV (cf. Chapter 8).

CBPV management involves in particular:

- Optimal *Varroa* control to avoid vector transmission of the virus.
- Overwintering without honeydew.
- Limiting risks of overcrowded colonies and confinement.
- Healthy and selected queens and colonies that exhibit good hygienic behaviour (see Chapter 4, section 1.9.3). Re-queening each year or every two years has become a necessity at the present time.

The management of diseased colonies affected by CBPV is described as follows:

- Clean the front and surrounding areas of the hive by removing dead bees (as they can be a source of contamination).
- Apply the shock swarm method to lower the viral load within the colony (cf. Chapter 4. section 1.8.3).
- Re-queen the colony.

3 Deformed wing virus (DWV) disease

Deformed wing disease is a contagious viral disease due to an *Iflaviridae*: DWV. The clinical signs mainly concern emerging bees (young bees) presenting deformities, and in particular wing deformities, and a reduction of their lifespan. The virus has also been identified in asymptomatic colonies.

Without *V. destructor* infestation, DWV infection remains a covert infection. Before the *Varroa* pandemic, DWV was unknown as

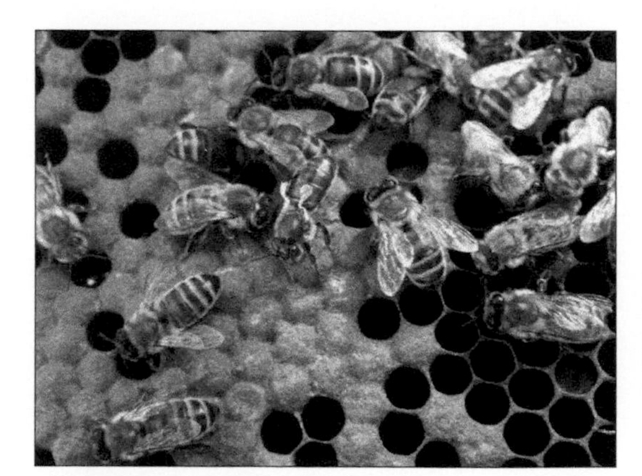

Figure 3.3 At the centre of the picture, a typical young bee symptomatically affected by DWV. Note the wing deformities. (Photo courtesy © Lydia Vilagines, DVM.)

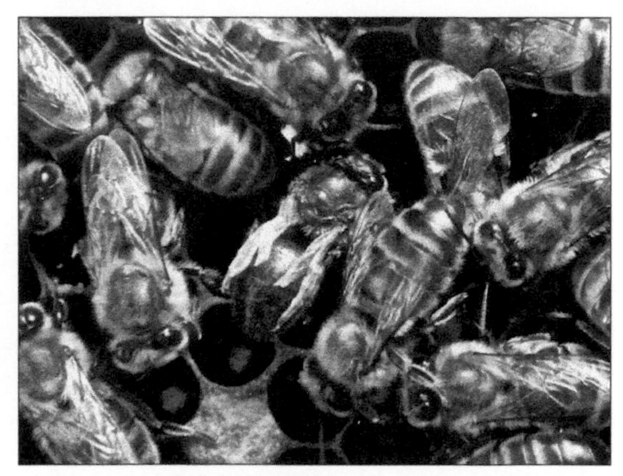

Figure 3.4 Emerging bee with wing and abdomen deformities due to DWV with a phoretic *Varroa* mite. (Photo courtesy © Lydia Vilagines, DVM.)

a pathogen. The occurrence of the disease is a consequence of the combination of DWV and *Varroa* infestation.

The virus was first isolated from Egyptian honeybee colonies in the 1970s, and hence first named Egypt bee virus (EBV). In 1982, a virus causing deformities in adult bees was described and found 'to be distantly related to EBV by serology' (Ribière *et al.*, 2008; de Miranda and Genersch, 2010; de Miranda *et al.*, 2012). With the *Varroa* pandemic, DWV has come to pose a serious threat to honeybee colonies.

To date, this virus has spread worldwide, except to Oceania where it has not yet been reported. It has been found in *A. mellifera* and *V. destructor* as well as in managed and wild bumblebees.

DWV is very similar to two other iflaviruses: Kakugo virus (KV) and *V. destructor* virus-1. KV is a considered as a close genetic variant of DWV, with mostly identical nucleotide sequences.

3.1 Clinical signs

Honeybee deformed wing disease usually occurs at the end of summer and in autumn.

This viral infection results in deformities of the body, and in particular of the wings, which occur during the metamorphosis of the pupae within the capped cell, where the *Varroa* reproductive cycle takes place. The clinical signs are then observed in emerging bees.

The wings are deformed, stubby, and useless (Figures 3.3 and 3.4) (Fievet *et al.*, 2006; Tentcheva *et al.*, 2006). The clinical signs also include rounded and shortened abdomens and miscolouring. The affected bees are, of course, unable to fly. Symptoms of paralysis may also be observed (Chen *et al.*, 2006). Infected bees, whose lifespan is severely reduced, are usually expelled from the hive by guards. DWV infection may also induce early death of pupae. The dead pupae are then removed from the brood cells and from the hive by cleaner workers.

After emergence, if bees do not present deformities, infection of adult bees is considered as asymptomatic (Ribière *et al.*, 2008). However, it seems that affected adult bees may present learning disabilities, in particular in foraging ability (Iqbal and Müller, 2007).

At the colony level, an irregular brood may be observed associated with pupae mortality, cannibalism, and a decrease in the bee population.

The occurrence of overt DWV infection is *always* linked to *Varroa* infestation (Figure 3.4). In cases of severe infection, with a high level of *Varroa* infestation, or if poor beekeeping practices have led to inadequate control of mite infestation, colony weakening and even collapse may occur, particularly during winter. A recent study has shown that the lifespan of overwintering workers without symptoms but with high levels of virus seems to be shortened (Dainat *et al.*, 2012a); hence DWV may play a role in winter colony mortality (cf. pathogenesis).

3.2 Epidemiological characteristics: spread and transmission

Adult honeybees are reservoirs of DWV and phoretic *V. destructor* are responsible of the spreading of the virus in a colony, between colonies, and between apiaries (Yue and Genersch, 2005). DWV may be found throughout the body, including queen ovaries, queen fat bodies, and drone seminal vesicles (Fievet *et al.*, 2006). All honeybee castes and stages may be DWV carriers, though pupae are most at risk of developing an overt infection.

Transmission may be vertical, venereal, and trans-ovarial (Yue *et al.*, 2007; de Miranda and Fries, 2008). It seems to present a low virulence level, remaining as a covert infection (asymptomatic) in the absence of *Varroa* infestation. Horizontal transmission (oral or contact) does not seem to play a significant role in DWV disease.

Vector-borne transmission by the mite *V. destructor* is the main route of DWV diffusion and is responsible of overt infection. The pathological effects of DWV are entirely linked to its association with *Varroa*. Not only does this mite carry the virus, but the virus can replicate within the organism. It has been reported that DWV is also transmitted by the mite *Tropilaelaps mercedesae* with the same consequences on bees (Dainat *et al.*, 2009). The small hive beetle, *Aethina tumida*, also seems to be a potential vector of DWV.

3.3 Contributing factors

Varroa destructor infestation is the main cause of overt DWV infection. The disease was unknown before adaptation of *Varroa* to *A. mellifera* (de Miranda *et al.*, 2012). The prevalence of DWV infection (and the viral load of DWV) within honeybees has followed *Varroa* infestation in colonies (Bowen-Walker *et al.*, 1999; Tentcheva *et al.*, 2006; de Miranda *et al.*, 2012). When the colony is free of mites, or nearly so, it has been shown by enzyme-linked immunosorbent assay (ELISA) that the DWV load is greatly reduced within the brood (even becoming undetectable in the capped brood) and within adult bees (Martin *et al.*, 2010).

Cold may also be a contributing factor. Winter colony weakening and mortality is associated with DWV infection in overwintering honeybees, irrespective of *Varroa* infestation (Martin *et al.*, 2010; de Miranda *et al.*, 2012).

The neonicotinoid crop pesticide clothianidin has been shown to alter honeybee immunity and to promote the replication of DWV (Di Prisco *et al.*, 2013).

3.4 Pathogenesis

In the absence of *V. destructor*, DWV virulence is minor and the development of the bee larvae is not affected. DWV is the main virus associated with *Varroa* and needs *Varroa* to become virulent (de Miranda and Genersch, 2010). It has been shown that optimal and efficient control of *Varroa* infestation drastically reduces viral load within the colonies (Dainat *et al.*, 2012b). DWV replication (and perhaps selection of variants) in mites is reported to be necessary for the virus to become pathogenic and to induce clinical signs in honeybees (Yue and Genersch, 2005; Gisder *et al.*, 2009; de Miranda *et al.*, 2012)

Due to their cuticle-piercing feeding habits, *Varroa* mites are responsible for DWV transmission and then replication in bees (de Miranda and Genersch, 2010; de Miranda *et al.*, 2012). The immunosuppression caused by *Varroa* probably stimulates both DWV replication and virulence (Yang and Cox-Foster, 2005). DWV replicates in various bee tissues, especially fat bodies, altering in particular immune defence and vitellogenin secretion (Dainat *et al.*, 2012b).

In cases of overt infection, the future health of the colony may be affected by both the outbreak of virus but also by mite infestation and varroosis (cf. Chapter 5). In summer, this infection can impair the production of strong winter bees and the prognosis for the strength of colony may be bleak during the overwintering period.

DWV and its vector *Varroa* play a major role in colony weakening and collapse by causing 'bee parasitic mite syndrome'. In summer and early autumn, when the brood decreases and is producing overwintering bees, uncontrolled *Varroa* infestation and DWV infection lead to massive losses of workers and then to the collapse of the colony.

In spring, if a DWV infection occurs, it is generally compensated by the development of the colony and massive brood rearing. However, the observation in spring of bees with deformed wings suggests poor control of *Varroa* infestation, endangering the colony and affecting the hive products.

Thus, it appears that colony collapse in association to DWV infection/*Varroa* infestation mainly occurs during wintering and is the consequence of interactions between *Varroa*, transmission and virulence of DWV, and the biology of the colony (in particular, population dynamics).

3.5 Diagnosis

3.5.1 Clinical diagnosis

A clinical picture presenting early death of pupae, deformed bees, bees without wings or with wing deformities, and bees with shortened abdomens is suggestive of DWV disease. These clinical signs are mainly observed at the end of the summer or in autumn.

In the case of winter colony weakening or mortality, the observation of workers with deformed wings strongly suggests overt DWV infection. If the sanitary management of *Varroa* is failing, the diagnosis is usually and undisputably in favour of DWV disease.

3.5.2 Laboratory diagnosis

Laboratory analysis (RT-PCR, PCR), associated with clinical examination, allows the diagnosis (Genersch, 2005). Analysis of a mite sample may prove interesting. A high viral load (10^{10}–10^{12} genome equivalent/mite) is correlated to DWV disease (de Miranda and Genersch, 2010).

DWV load within bees is one of the main tests to perform in cases of winter colony weakening or mortality associated with the evaluation of *Varroa* infestation. It may reveal a high *Varroa* infestation rate and/or a failure in *Varroa* control.

DWV is widely considered to be a predictive marker of colony collapse (Dainat *et al.*, 2012b). This property may prove of interest to the veterinary approach to infected colonies. Indeed, a laboratory test of DWV viral load within colonies in summer/autumn associated with a *Varroa* infestation evaluation, when the future winter bees are being reared, may be one interesting factor to evaluate the strength of the colony before wintering.

3.6 Management

Fighting DWV involves prophylactic methods against contributing factors, principally *V. destructor*: control of mite infestation is essential to limit or even avoid the risks of DWV outbreak and to prevent weakening and collapse, particularly in winter. Optimal and efficient control of *Varroa* infestation drastically reduces the viral load within colonies (Dainat *et al.*, 2012b).

Because DWV may be responsible for winter colony mortality, optimal control of mite infestation long before the colony starts to produce overwintering workers is essential. It has been shown (Martin *et al.*, 2010) that it takes at least 6 weeks after miticide treatment (at the end of July) to obtain undetectable DWV load in bees; this period extends to 23 weeks for an October treatment.

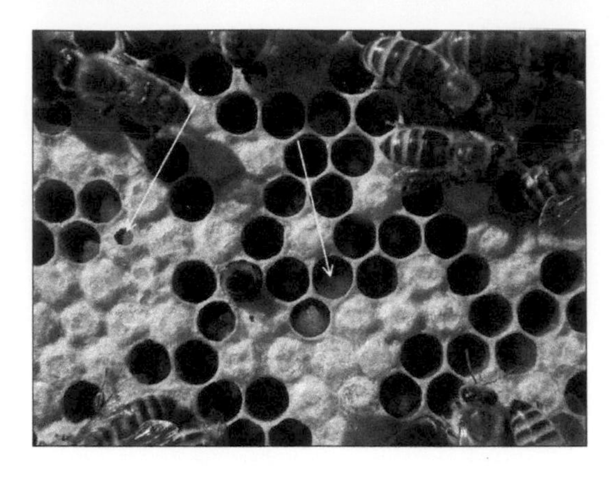

Figure 3.5 Scattered brood in a colony affected by sacbrood disease. The brood may appear irregular or scattered with punctured capped cells. In uncapped cells, diseased larvae can be observed (arrows). (Photo courtesy © Lydia Vilagines, DVM.)

As a result, the first prophylactic method is optimal control of *Varroa* infestation throughout the year and in particular at the end of the beekeeping season when the colony is about to rear overwintering bees.

Wintering demands healthy and strong colonies. Selection of strains that exhibit good hygiene, with cleaners able to detect and remove from the hive mite-infested and DWV-infected pupae, is an additional prophylactic method.

The process of RNA interference (RNAi) has been studied in bees to limit DWV load. Feeding both larvae and adult *A. mellifera* with a double-stranded (ds) RNA construct, DWV-dsRNA, has been reported to decrease viral load and the occurrence of symptoms (Desai *et al.*, 2012).

4 Sacbrood virus (SBV) disease

Sacbrood disease is a viral infectious disease of honeybee immature forms within the capped

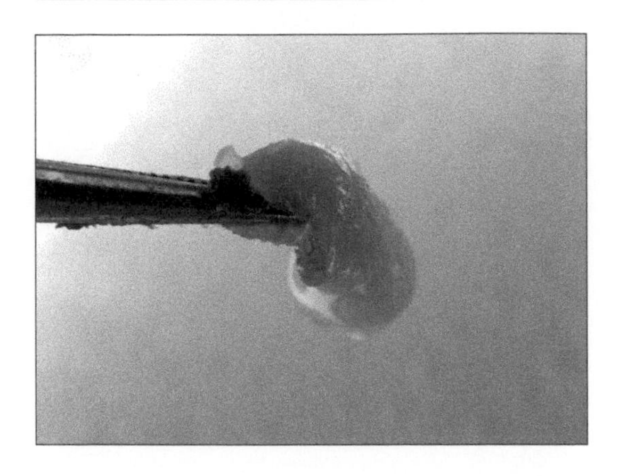

Figure 3.6 Sacbrood-diseased larva. Typical aspect of a sac containing ecdysial fluid. The sac is pale yellow and the cephalic part (on the left) is darker and drier. (Photo courtesy © Lydia Vilagines, DVM.)

brood (*A. mellifera* and *Apis cerana*) and adult bees due to an *Iflaviridae* (30 nm diameter): SBV (Ball, 1999b). SBV may remain as a covert infection in colonies. SBV may cause overt infection in the brood. The infection is mainly considered asymptomatic in adults but may be responsible for problems, in particular through the secretion of the brood-food. The disease is usually unimportant in *A. mellifera* (affecting some larvae, which are quickly removed from the cells and the hive by cleaners), but is highly lethal in *A. cerana*, easily killing colonies of this species (Ribière *et al.*, 2008; de Miranda *et al.*, 2012). Sacbrood disease was first described in 1917, but the virus was isolated much later (White, 1917; Bailey *et al.*, 1964). SBV is spread worldwide, is highly prevalent in apiaries, and is one of the commonest viral diseases of honeybees (Blanchard *et al.*, 2014a).

4.1 Clinical signs

There is a high prevalence of SBV in asymptomatic colonies. SBV causes a capped brood disease and may also asymptomatically infect adult bees. SBV disease usually occurs in spring or at the beginning of summer (when the brood is reared). In autumn, it may be observed concomitantly with varroosis. It may also occur if there is a food deficiency (Ball, 1999b; Tentcheva *et al.*, 2004). Clinical signs may not be observed due to the actions of cleaner bees. These workers detect the diseased larvae inside the capped cells and, after uncapping, remove them from the cells and the hive (Bailey and Fernando, 1972).

The brood may appear irregular or scattered with punctured capped cells. The cells with punctured cappings contain sacs (giving the name to the disease and the virus) or scales (Shimanuki and Knox, 2000).

Larvae infected by SBV fail to pupate after cell-capping and die. An ecdysial fluid, rich in SBV, accumulates under their unshed skin, forming a sac (Figures 3.5 and 3.6) (Bailey and Fernando, 1972; Ball, 1999b). The infectivity of this fluid decreases after a few days (Hitchcock, 1966).

The larval colour changes from pearly white to pale yellow.

The sacs are very fragile and odour-less. If cleaners do not operate:

- first, infected larvae become sticky and dark – a thread up to 1 cm long can be drawn from the dark larval remains (matchstick test)
- second, infected larvae become dry, non-adhesive, flattened, gondola-shaped scales (de Miranda *et al.*, 2012). The cephalic part of the infected larva is darker and drier than the body.

At the colony level, sacbrood is a perennial and common disease, though one that is generally not considered a serious threat to the strength of the colony. Indeed, usually only a few larvae are affected. However, it may sometimes cause colony weakening or impair the development of the colony and as such, is an important infection to identify.

In adult bees, the following clinical signs have been reported in experimental studies:

- Lifespan decrease and changes in behaviour are observed (Bailey and Fernando, 1972).
- Infected adults become foragers earlier in their life (Bailey and Ball, 1991); these bees

prefer to collect nectar and stop eating pollen (Bailey and Fernando; 1972).
- Secretion of royal jelly is impaired in infected *A. cerana* nurses compared to non-infected ones (Du and Zhang, 1985).

SBV disease occurs in spring and summer, and in some regions autumn when the brood is reared.

4.2 Spread and transmission

SBV infection begins with the excretion of the virus in the worker, drone, and royal jellies by the hypopharyngeal glands of nurses. In affected colonies, SBV may also be found in honey and stored pollen (Ribière *et al.*, 2008). Recent studies show that SBV is found in *Varroa*, which is believed to be a vector of this virus (Gauthier *et al.*, 2007). Oral and probably vector-borne transmission seem to be the main transmission routes of SBV.

4.3 Pathogenesis

The immature forms of the three castes can be infected. Two-day-old larvae are the most sensitive to the infection. After infection, a larva continues its development until the cell is capped. However, the infected larva fails to pupate and dies. The larva is unable to shed its skin during the final moult and the consequence is an accumulation of an ecdysial fluid under the unshed skin (Ball, 1999b). If overt infection occurs in a colony, cleaners quickly detect the affected larvae and remove these from the cells and hive (Ribière *et al.*, 2008). Infection of adult bees may only occur during the first days of emergence. The prognosis is usually good when an outbreak occurs. However, SBV disease often occurs in association with other brood disease(s). This may endanger the strength of the colony.

4.4 Contributing factors

If SBV is found in asymptomatic colonies, clinical signs usually arise when the brood reaches its peak size in spring/beginning of summer, when there may not be enough nurses to care for the brood (Ball, 1999b; Ribière *et al.*, 2008). Factors contributing to overt SBV infection are usually the consequence of nutritional deficiency:

- Lack of food.
- Confinement.
- Population unbalance.
- Poisoning is also supposed to be a predisposing factor.

The strain of the colony, the age of the queen, and other infections (e.g. European foulbrood disease) may favour the occurrence of sacbrood disease (Giraud, 2013). The mite *V. destructor* is considered to be a vector and a reservoir of SBV (Ribière *et al.*, 2008; Giraud, 2013).

4.5 Diagnosis

Diagnosis is primarily a clinical diagnosis in the field taking into account in particular the seasonal occurrence of the disease (spring, summer) associated with the finding of contributing factors. The clinical signs are quite specific to the disease and hence serve as reliable indicators.

A differential diagnosis should take into account other brood diseases, e.g. foulbrood diseases and brood mycosis. It should be considered that SBV disease is often associated with other brood diseases.

Laboratory testing with the RT-PCR method is possible but seldom performed in current veterinary practice because of the high cost. Laboratory examinations must take into account both identification and quantification of the viral load. It is possible to obtain a positive result in asymptomatic colonies (overt infection). Recent studies with a two-step real-time RT-PCR method suggest a threshold SBV load above which an overt SBV infection occurs. This threshold is set at 10^{10} SBV genome copies per individual irrespective of whether the sample comprises adult bees, larvae, or pupae (Blanchard *et al.*, 2014).

4.6 Management

The management of SBV disease involves good beekeeping sanitary practices, including optimal and measured control of *V. destructor* infestation.

Good practices usually allow clinical recovery (recovery is aimed at achieving covert status, rather than complete elimination), associated with a high-quality nectar flow and sufficient pollen. These practices are: removing infected brood, shaking bees (shock swarm) method with destruction and disinfection of contaminated equipment (cf. Chapter 4), re-queening the colony, and avoiding starvation and food deficiency (in particular by feeding them a protein supplement).

It is sometimes considered that if more than 20% of the brood is infected, then the colony should be eliminated because it is likely to be too weak to allow a sufficient renewal of its population.

5 Slow bee paralysis virus (SBPV) disease

SBPV, an Iflaviridus, was discovered in 1974. Two strains of SBPV have been described. SBPV may exist as covert infections. It has mainly been described in the UK in relation to mortality of colonies. However, its prevalence is considered as 'very low in Europe' (de Miranda *et al.*, 2012).

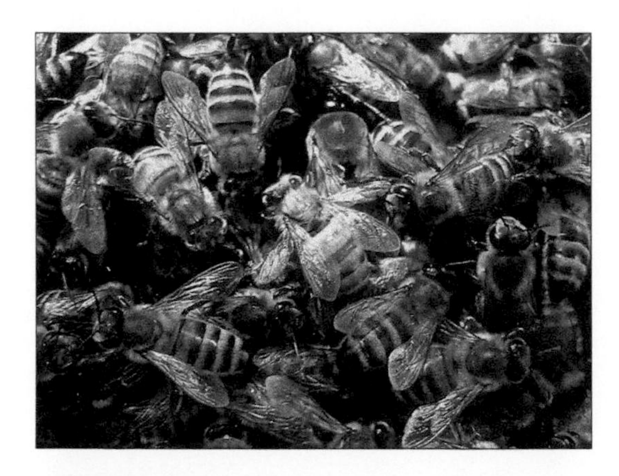

Figure 3.7 ABPV disease. Note, at the centre of the picture, a worker with an abnormal position of the wings. This picture was taken in a colony in which ABPV had been diagnosed by laboratory testing (Photo courtesy ©Lydia Vilagines, DVM)

Experimentally, injection of the virus is responsible for the occurrence of symptoms of paralysis affecting the two first pairs of legs on average 12 days after inoculation (Bailey and Woods, 1974). SBPV has a tropism for the CNS, the salivary glands, the fat bodies, and the forelegs. However, no tropism has been described for the hind legs and the honey stomach (Denholm, 1999).

Varroa is a vector of SBPV, allowing transmission to pupae and adult bees (Santillàn-Galicia *et al.*, 2010). SBPV has been linked to a high mortality of colonies infested by this mite (Carreck *et al.*, 2010a; Martin *et al.*, 1998). Management involves controlling *Varroa* infestation and also good sanitary beekeeping practices.

6 Dicistrovirus diseases

The three viruses ABPV, KV, and IAPV are very similar and, according to some searchers, must be considered as a complex, the so-called 'acute bee paralysis virus complex' (de Miranda *et al.*, 2010, 2012). These three viruses are genetically close but different. They are associated with colony mortality, in particular mortality linked to *Varroa* infestation, which is a vector of these viruses. Black queen cell virus is another Dicistrovirus affecting queen larvae and pre-pupae.

6.1 Acute bee paralysis virus (ABPV) disease

ABPV is a single-stranded RNA *Dicistroviridae* virus (Olivier and Ribière, 2006). This virus has been reported in several countries and is believed to have been a main cause of mortality of bees in France, the United States, and Germany. Before the *Varroa* pandemic, ABPV was rarely considered as responsible for disease and/or mortality of bees and colonies (Bailey, 1965a; Bailey *et al.*, 1981). ABPV may remain in colonies as a covert infection.

6.1.1 Clinical signs

ABPV virus is reported to become pathogenic following its direct injection into the haemolymph by *V. destructor* mites (Ball and Allen, 1988; Bakonyi *et al.*, 2002).

The clinical signs have been described as follows (Figure 3.7) (Békési *et al.*, 1999):

- Bees walking around, unable to fly, wandering more or less close to the hives before dying.
- The position of the wings is abnormal, asymmetric, and/or pointing straight out from the body.
- The brood cells can be punctured and mortality of immature forms can be observed.
- At the colony level, it may cause weakening and acute collapse.

6.1.2 Pathogenesis and diagnosis

ABPV is able to replicate and infect the brain and food-producing glands, allowing persistent infections in colonies (de Miranda *et al.*, 2012). Severely infected larvae may die. If they survive, asymptomatic bees will emerge (Bailey and Ball, 1991). Infected by *V. destructor*, adults and pupae die rapidly. Thus, at the colony level, ABPV infection associated with *Varroa* infestation may be lethal to the colony in one or two years if no control measures are performed.

It should be noted that ABPV infection associated with *Varroa* infestation is considered to be much more virulent than the association of mite infestation and DWV infection (Sumpter and Martin, 2004; de Miranda *et al.*, 2012).

The diagnostic method is to perform a RT-PCR test in the laboratory if ABPV infection is suspected. Identification and quantification of the virus load are necessary.

6.1.3 Management

The control of ABPV mainly involves sanitary and prophylactic methods, good husbandry practices, and in particular control of *Varroa* infestation within the colonies. As often evoked, control of any mite infestation must be measured and optimal to limit ABPV disease as for other infections linked to *Varroa* infestation.

6.2 Kashmir bee virus (KBV) disease

First described in *A. mellifera* experimentally infected with extracts from diseased Asiatic honeybees, *A. cerana*, in Kashmir, KBV is today found worldwide probably thanks to 'global apiculture' and the exchange and trade of bees (Allen and Ball, 1996; Ellis and Munn, 2005).

To date, KBV is considered experimentally as one of the most virulent honeybee-infecting viruses. When inoculated experimentally into the haemolymph of honeybees, it multiplies very rapidly and may induce bee mortality within three days (de Miranda *et al.*, 2012). When introduced via feeding it does not induce any clinical signs or mortality.

As with many honeybee viruses, KBV has been described in asymptomatic and healthy colonies, for example in France in 2012 (Evans, 2001; Blanchard *et al.*, 2014b). KBV can become virulent and lethal for honeybees due to the mite *V. destructor*, which inoculates the virus through the cuticle into the haemolymph while feeding. *Varroa* is a vector of the virus (Chen *et al.*, 2006).

KBV induces mortality without characteristic symptoms at all stages of honeybee life (de Miranda *et al.*, 2012). At the colony level, KBV may be responsible for sudden colony weakening and mortality in association with even moderate *Varroa* infestation (Todd *et al.*, 2007; de Miranda *et al.*, 2012).

Prophylactic and control management of KBV must mainly take into account optimal and measured *Varroa* infestation control.

6.3 Israeli acute paralysis virus (IAPV) disease

Discovered in 2004 in Israel, IAPV was prematurely and wrongly thought to be a major cause of colony collapse disorder (CCD) in the US (Cox-Foster *et al.*, 2007).

This virus may affect all stages and castes of *A. mellifera*. IAPV in experimental conditions is responsible for shivering wings, progressive paralysis, and death, while the body of the bee becomes darker and hairless (Maori *et al.*, 2007).

Varroa destructor is an active vector of this virus as well as ABPV and KBV, thus controlling mite infestation is necessary to prevent the associated IAPV infection.

6.4 Black queen cell virus (BQCV)

BQCV was first detected in affected queen larvae and pre-pupae (Bailey and Woods, 1977). It is today found worldwide and may persist as a covert infection in colonies.

Diseased drone pupae have been reported (Siede and Büchler, 2006). Worker bees can also be infected by BQCV but, in the field, they do not seem to develop clinical signs.

The cells with infected larvae develop dark brown or black cell walls. Within queen cells, the diseased pre-pupae or pupae cannot develop into adult queens, and die. The diseased larvae is a pale-yellow colour and forms a sac-like skin (a symptom somewhat similar to that induced by SBV). These pupae are full of virus particles.

The main transmission route is horizontal (oral transmission). BQCV is thought to be transmitted by brood-food through the glandular secretions of the nurse bees.

BQCV infection is closely associated with *Nosema* infestation and co-infection seems to be required to cause overt infection. BQCV outbreaks are reported to follow nosemosis. A peak of BQCV overt infection is mainly observed when the queens are reared in spring (after the nosemosis peak).

Two other honeybee-infecting viruses, filamentous virus and bee virus Y, are associated with *Nosema*. A *Nosema*–BQCV co-infection is believed to be necessary for BQCV overt infection to occur (Ribière *et al.*, 2008). Thus the prevalence of BQCV is parallel to *Nosema* infestation, with a peak when queens are reared (mainly in spring).

BQCV is also thought to be transmitted vertically because it has been found in queen ovaries (Chen *et al.*, 2006). BQCV has been also detected in *Varroa* but this parasite is not thought to be an important and active vector of this virus (Ribière *et al.*, 2008).

Controlling *Nosema* infestation is necessary to control as far as possible BQCV infection.

Diagnosis of BQCV infection must take into account clinical signs, seasonality, and *Nosema* infection. If suspected, laboratory tests should include analysis of the virus (identification and quantification) as well as *Nosema*.

7 Other viruses of honeybee colonies

7.1 Cloudy wing virus (CWV)

CWV is a small virus (17 nm diameter). It may remain as a covert infection and it is reported that 15% of managed colonies are naturally infected (de Miranda *et al.*, 2012).

This virus is not considered highly pathologic (Carreck *et al.*, 2010b). In a symptomatic infection, clouding wings, with a loss of transparency, is the main symptom.

The virus has a tropism for the head and the thorax, in which crystalline arrays of virus are found in the muscle fibres (Ribière *et al.*, 2008). In experimental conditions, CWV-infected adult bees present a decreased lifespan.

The transmission route of CWV is not well known; the hypothesis is mainly oral or vertical transmission. There is no evidence of vector-borne transmission (Carreck *et al.*, 2010b).

At the colony level, the virus has been experimentally associated with weakening and mortality (Carreck *et al.*, 2010b, de Miranda *et al.*, 2012).

Diagnosis of CWV infection requires identification and quantification of the virus by RT-PCR methods.

7.2 Bee X virus (BXV) and bee Y virus (BYV)

BXV and BYV are two genetically and pathologically similar viruses (35 nm diameter). Both these viruses are reported to be closely associated with an unicellular parasite.

BVX, first described in Arkansas (USA), is often associated with the protozoan *M. mellificae* in adult bees. However the virus and the parasite may be independently infectious. Co-infection reduces honeybee lifespan more than separate individual infections (Ribière *et al.*, 2008). The transmission route of BVX is oro-faecal. BVX becomes infectious when the temperature reaches 30°C or less. It is not infectious at 35°C. Thus, BVX disease is a winter disease. The infection is reported to develop slowly. If *M. mellificae* is usually a discrete spring infection, co-infection is more damaging for the winter survival of colonies (Bailey and Ball, 1991; de Miranda *et al.*, 2012). According to some researchers, BVX seems to be on the decline, *Varroa* and its vector-borne viruses being mainly responsible for winter weakening and mortality of colonies (Miranda *et al.*, 2012).

BVY, first described in Great Britain (Bailey *et al.* 1980), is more dependent on *N. apis* than BVX is on *M. mellificae*. Like BVX, BVY is infectious when the colony temperature decreases to 30°C. Therefore, the prevalence of overt infection is similar to *N. apis* infection and mainly occurs in spring (Ribière *et al.*, 2008).

The diagnosis of those two diseases needs laboratory tests to analyse both the virus and associated pathogens.

Controlling *M. mellificae* and *N. apis* infestations are the main ways to manage BVX and BVY infections.

7.3 Arkansas bee virus (ABV) and Berkeley bee picorna-like virus (BBPV)

ABV and BBPV are two RNA viruses (both icasohedral, 30 nm diameter) first identified in the US (Bailey and Woods, 1974; Lommel *et al.*, 1985; Bailey and Ball, 1991). To date, very little is known, other than that they are often found together naturally (even during transmission) (Bailey and Ball, 1991). At this time, no clinical signs have been described in colonies and at the level of adult bees and the brood.

Note that another virus, a macula-like virus, has been described in honeybee colonies in the US and France. It is thought to be very common, in particular in cases of significant *Varroa* infestation. It is thought to be primarily a virus of *V. destructor* (de Miranda *et al.*, 2012).

7.4 Honeybee-infecting DNA viruses

Apis mellifera filamentous virus (*Am*FV) is a baculovirus-like DNA virus (rod-shaped, 450 nm × 170 nm). Co-infection with *N. apis* has been reported (Bailey *et al.*, 1983).

The main clinical sign observed in *Am*FV infection is the appearance of the haemolymph in adult bees which becomes milky-white and in which are found viral particles (Clark, 1978; Bailey and Ball, 1991). However, *Am*FV infection is not related to significant adult bee symptoms or individual lifespan decrease and colony weakening. Rarely, *Am*FV has been suspected in some cases of bee mortality (presenting milky haemolymph at autopsy) and colony weakening.

Apis iridescent virus (*A*IV) is an Iridovirus (icasohedral, 140 nm diameter). It can be found in most tissues and organs of *A. mellifera*. It was originally described as a virus of *A. cerana* in India (de Miranda *et al.*, 2012). The symptoms of *A*IV overt infection are similar to the adult flightless clustering symptoms of CBPV (Bailey and Ball, 1978). The clinical signs of AIV disease have, to date, only been described in adult bees.

Iridoviruses associated with *Nosema ceranae* have recently been suggested to be associated with colony collapse disorder (Bromenshenk *et al.*, 2010), but there is no proof of their involvement at this time (de Miranda *et al.*, 2012).

References

Allen, M. and Ball, B. (1996) The incidence and world distribution of the honeybee viruses. *Bee World*, 77: 141–162.

Bailey, L. (1965) The occurrence of chronic and acute bee paralysis viruses in bees outside Britain. *Journal of Invertebrate Pathology*, 7: 167–169.

Bailey, L. and Ball, B.V. (1991) *Honey Bee Pathology*. Harcourt Brace Jovanovich, Sidcup.

Bailey, L. and Fernando, E.F.W. (1972) Effects of sacbrood virus on adult honey-bees. *Annals of Applied Biology*, 72: 27–35.

Bailey, L. and Woods, R.D. (1974) Three previously undescribed viruses from the honey bee. *Journal of General Virology*, 25: 175–186.

Bailey, L. and Woods, R.D. (1977). Two more small RNA viruses from honey bees and further observations on sacbrood and acute bee-paralysis viruses. *Journal of General Virology*, 37: 175–182.

Bailey, L., Gibbs, A.J., and Woods, R.D. (1964) Sacbrood virus of the larval honey bee (*Apis mellifera* Linnaeus). *Virology*, 23: 425–429.

Bailey, L., Gibbs, A.J., and Woods, R.D. (1968) The purification and properties of chronic bee paralysis virus. *Journal of General Virology*, 2: 25.

Bailey L., Carpenter J.M., Govier D.A., and Woods R.D. (1980) Bee virus Y. *Journal of General Virology*, 51: 405–407.

Bailey, L, Ball, B.V., and Perry, J.N. (1981) The prevalence of viruses of honeybees in Britain. *Annals of Applied Biology* 97: 109–118.

Bailey, L., Ball, B.V., and Perry, J.N. (1983) Association of viruses with two protozoal pathogens of the honeybee. *Annals of Applied Biology* 103: 13–20.

Bakonyi, T., Grabensteiner, E., Kolodziejek, J., Rusvai, M., Topolska, G., Ritter, W., and Nowotny, N. (2002) Phylogenetic analysis of acute bee paralysis virus strains. *Applied and Environmental Microbiology*, 68: 6446–6450.

Ball, B.V. (1999a) Paralysis. In Colin, M.E., Ball, B.V., and Kilani, M. (eds), *Bee Disease Diagnosis, Options Méditerranéennes*, Series B: *Etudes et Recherches*, No 25. CIHEAM Publications, Zaragoza, pp. 91–97.

Ball, B.V. (1999b) Sacbrood. In Colin, M.E., Ball, B.V., and Kilani, M. (eds), *Bee Disease Diagnosis, Options Méditerranéennes*, Series B: *Etudes et Recherches*, No 25. CIHEAM Publications, Zaragoza, pp. 81–89.

Ball, B.V. and Allen, M.F. (1988) The prevalence of pathogens in honeybee (*Apis mellifera*) colonies infested with the parasitic mite *Varroa jacobsoni*. *Annals of Applied Biology*, 113: 237–244.

Békési, L., Ball, B.V., Dobos-Kovács, M., Bakonyi, T., and Rusvai, M. (1999) Occurrence of acute paralysis virus of the honeybee (*Apis mellifera*) in a Hungarian apiary infested with the parasitic mite *Varroa jacobsoni*. *Acta Veterinaria Hungarica*, 47: 319–324.

Blanchard, P., Ribière, M., Celle, O., Lallemand, P., Schurr, F., Olivier, V., Iscache, A.L., and Faucon, J.P., (2007) Evaluation of a real-time two step RT-PCR assay for quantitation of Chronic bee paralysis virus (CBPV) genome in experimentally-infected bee tissues and in life stages of a symptomatic colony. *Journal of Virological Methods*, 141: 7–13.

Blanchard, P., Guillot, S., Antunez, K., Köglberger, E., Kryger, P., de Miranda, J.R., Franco, S., Chauzat, M.P., Thiéry, R., and Ribière, M. (2014a) Development and validation of a real-time two-step RT-qPCR TaqMan® assay for quantitation of sacbrood virus (SBV) and its application to a field survey of symptomatic honey bee colonies. *Journal of Virological Methods*, 197: 7–13.

Blanchard, P., Carletto, J., Siede, R., Schurr, F., Thiéry, R., and Ribière, M. (2014b) Identification of Kashmir bee virus in France using a new RT-PCR method which distinguishes closely related viruses. *Journal of Virological Methods*, 198: 82–85.

Bowen-Walker, P.L. Martin, S.J, and Gunn, A. (1999) The transmission of deformed wing virus between honey bees (*Apis mellifera* L.) by the ectoparasitic mite *Varroa jacobsoni* Oud. *Journal of Invertebrate Pathology*, 73: 101–106. http://dx.doi.org/10.1006/jipa.1998.4807

Bromenshenk, J.J., Henderson C.B., Wick C.H., Stanford M.F., Zulich A.W., *et al.* (2010) Iridovirus and microsporidian linked to honey bee colony decline. PLoS ONE 5(10): e13181. doi:10.1371/journal.pone.0013181

Carreck, N.L., Ball, B.V., and Martin, S.J. (2010a) Honey bee colony collapse and changes in viral prevalence associated with *Varroa destructor*. *Journal of Apicultural Research*, 49: 93–94.

Carreck N.L., Ball B.V., and Martin S.J. (2010b) The epidemiology of cloudy wing virus infections in honey bee colonies in the UK. *Journal of Apicultural Research*, 49(1): 66–71.

Chen, Y.P., Pettis, J.S., Collins, A., and Feldlaufer, M.F. (2006) Prevalence and transmission of honeybee viruses. *Applied and Environmental Microbiology*, 72(1): 606–611.

Clark, T.B. (1978) A filamentous virus of the honey bee. *Journal of Invertebrate Pathology*, 32: 332–340.

Cox-Foster, D.L., Conlan, S., Holmes, E.C., Palacios, G., Evans, J.D., Moran, N.A., Quan, P.L., Briese, T., Hornig, M., Geiser, D.M., Martinson, V., Van Engelsdorp, D., Kalkstein AL, Drysdale, A., Hui, J., Zhai, J., Cui, L., Hutchison, S.K., Simons, J.F., Egholm, M., Pettis, J.S., and Lipkin, W.I. (2007) A metagenomic survey of microbes in honeybee colony collapse disorder. *Science*, 318: 283–286.

Culley, A.I., Lang, S.L., and Suttle, C.A. (2003) High diversity of unknown picorna-like viruses in the sea. *Nature*, 424: 1054–1057.

Dainat, B., Ken, T., Berthoud, H., and Neumann, P. (2009) The ectoparasitic mite *Tropilaelaps mercedesae* (Acari, Laelapidae) as a vector of honeybee viruses. *Insectes Sociaux*, 56: 40–43.

Dainat, B., Evans, J.D., Chen, Y.P., Gauthier, L., and Neumann, P. (2012a) Predictive markers of honey bee colony collapse. *PLoS ONE*, 7(2): e32151. doi:10.1371/journal.pone.0032151

Dainat, B., Evans, J.D., Chen, Y.P., Gauthier, L., and Neumann, P. (2012b). Dead or alive: deformed wing virus and *Varroa destructor* reduce the life span of winter honeybees. *Applied and Environmental Microbiology*, 78: 981–987.

de Miranda, J.R. and Fries, I. (2008) Venereal and vertical transmission of deformed wing virus in honeybees (*Apis mellifera* L.). *Journal of Invertebrate Pathology*, 98(2): 184–189.

de Miranda J.R. and Genersch, E. (2010) Deformed wing virus. *Journal of Invertebrate Pathology*, 103: S48-S61

de Miranda, J.R, Gordoni, G., and Budge, G. (2010) The acute bee paralysis virus – Kashmir bee virus – Israeli acute paralysis virus complex. *Journal of Invertebrate Pathology*, 103: S30–S47.

de Miranda J., Gauthier L., Ribière M., and Chen Y.P. (2012). Honey bee viruses and their effect on bee and colony health. In Sanmarco, D. and Yoder J.A. (eds), *Honey Bee Colony Health Challenges and Sustainable Solutions.*CRC Press, Boca Raton, FL, pp. 71–102.

Denholm, C.H. (1999) Inducible honey bee viruses associated with *Varroa jacobsoni*. PhD thesis, Keele University.

Desai, S.D., Eu, Y.J., Whyard, S., and Currie, R.W. (2012) Reduction in deformed wing virus infection in larval and adult honey bees (*Apis mellifera* L.) by double-stranded RNA ingestion. *Insect Molecular Biology*, 21(4): 446–455.

Di Prisco, G., Cavaliere, V., Annoscia, D., Varricchio, P., Caprio, E., Nazzi, F., Gargiulo, G., and Pennacchioa, F. (2013) Neonicotinoid clothianidin adversely affects insect immunity and promotes replication of a viral pathogen in honey bees. *Proceedings of the National Academy of Sciences USA*, 110(46): 18466–18471.

Du, Z.L. and Zhang, Z.B. (1985) Ultrastructural change in the hypopharyngeal glands of worker honey bees (*Apis cerana*) infected with sacbrood virus. *Zoological Reseach*, 6: 155–162.

Evans, J.D. (2001) Genetic evidence for coinfection of honeybees by acute bee paralysis and Kashmir bee viruses. *Journal of Invertebrate Pathology*, 78(4): 189–193.

Ellis, J.D. and Munn, P.A. (2005) The worldwide health status of honey bees. *Bee World*, 86: 88–101.

Fievet, J., Tentcheva, D., Gauthier, L., De Miranda, J R., Cousserans, F.,Colin, M.E., and Bergoin, M. (2006) Localization of deformed wing virus infection in queen and drone *Apis mellifera* L. *Virology Journal*, 3: 16.

Franco, S., Martel, A.C, Chauzat, M.P., Blanchard, P., and Thiéry, R. (2012) Les analyses de laboratoire en apiculture. In SNGTV (ed.), *Proceedings of the Journées nationales des GTV.* SNGTV, Nantes, pp. 859–867.

Gauthier, L., Tentcheva, L., Tournaire, M., Dainat, B., Cousserans, F., Colin, M.E., and Bergoin, M. (2007) Viral load estimation in asymptomatic honeybee colonies using the quantitative RT-PCR technique. *Apidologie*, 38(5): 426–435.

Genersch, E. (2005) Development of a rapid and sensitive RT-PCR method for the detection of deformed wing virus, a pathogen of the honey bee (*Apis mellifera*). *Veterinary Journal*, 169(1): 121–123.

Genersch, E., von der Ohe, W., Kaatz, H., Schroeder, A., Otten, C., Büchler, R., Berg, S., Ritter, W., Mühlen, W., *et al.* (2010). The German bee monitoring project: a long term study to understand periodically high winter losses of honey bee colonies. *Apidologie*, 41: 332–352.

Giraud, F. (2013) Le couvain sacciforme (Sacbrood). *La santé de l'Abeille*, 254; 149–160.

Gisder, S., Aumeier, P., and Genersch, E. (2009) Deformed wing virus (DWV): viral load and replication in mite (*Varroa destructor*). *Journal of General Virology*, 90: 463–467.

Hitchcock, J.D. (1966) Transmission of sacbrood disease to individual honey bee larvae. *Journal of Economic Entomology*, 59: 1154–1156.

Iqbal, J. and Müller, U. (2007) Virus infection causes specific learning deficits in honeybee foragers. *Proceedings of the Royal Society B*, 106: 14790–14795.

Lommel, S.A., Morris, T.J., and Pinnock, D.E. (1985) Characterization of nucleic acids associated with Arkansas bee virus. *Intervirology*, 23: 199–207.

Maori, E., Lavi, S., Mozes-Koch, R., Gantman, Y., Peretz, Y., Edelbaum, O., Tanne, E., and Sela, I. (2007) Isolation and characterization of Israeli acute paralysis virus, a dicistrovirus affecting honey bees in Israel: evidence for diversity due to intra- and inter-species recombination. *Journal of General Virology*, 88: 3428–3438.

Martin, S.J., Hogarth, A., van Breda, J., and Perrett, J. (1998) A scientific note on *Varroa jacobsoni* Oudemans and the collapse of *Apis mellifera* colonies in the United Kingdom. *Apidologie*, 29: 369–370.

Martin, S.J., Ball, B.V., and Carreck, N.L. (2010) Prevalence and persistence of deformed wing virus (DWV) in untreated or acaricide-treated Varroa destructor infested honey bee (*Apis mellifera*) colonies. *Journal of Apicultural Research*, 49(1): 72–79.

Olivier, V. and Ribière, M. (2006) Les virus infectant l'abeille Apis *mellifera*: le point sur leur classification. *Virologie*, 10(4): 267–278.

Olivier, V., Massou I., Celle O., Blanchard P., Schurr, F., Ribière M., and Gauthier M. (2008) *In situ* hybridization assays for localization of the chronic bee paralysis virus in the honey bee (*Apis mellifera*) brain. *Journal of Virological Methods*, 153: 232–237.

Ribière, M., Lallemand, P., Iscache, A.-L., Schurr, F., Celle, O., Blanchard, P., Olivier, V., and Faucon, J.-P. (2007) Spread of infectious chronic bee paralysis virus by honeybee (*Apis mellifera* L.) feces. *Applied and Environmental Microbiology*, 73(23): 7711–7716

Ribière, M., Ball, B., and Aubert, M. (2008). Natural history and geographical distribution of honey bee viruses. In Aubert, M., Ball, B., Fries, I., Moritz, R., Milani, N., and Bernardinelli, I. (eds), *Virology and the Honey Bee*. EEC Publications, Brussels, pp. 15–84.

Ribière, M., Olivier, V., and Blanchard, P. (2010) Chronic paralysis virus. A disease and a virus like no other? *Journal of Invertebrate Pathology*, 103: S120–S131.

Santillàn-Galicia, M.T., Ball, B.V., Clark, S.J., and Alderson, P.G. (2010) Transmission of deformed wing virus and slow paralysis virus to adult bees (*Apis mellifera* L.) by *Varroa destructor*. *Journal of Apicultural Research*, 49: 141–148.

Shimanuki, H. and Knox, D.A. (2000) *Diagnosis of Honeybee Diseases*, Agriculture Handbook No. 690. United States Department of Agriculture.

Shimanuki, H., Calderone, N.W., and Knox, D.A. (1994) Parasitic mite syndrome: the symptoms. *American Bee Journal*, 134: 827–828.

Siede, R. and Büchler, R. (2006) Spatial distribution patterns of acute bee paralysis virus, black queen cell virus and sacbrood virus in Hesse, Germany. *Wiener Tierärztliche Monatsschrift*, 93: 90–93.

Sitaropoulou, N., Neophytou, E.P., and Thomopoulos, G.N. (1989) Structure of the nucleocapsid of a filamentous virus of the honey bee (*Apis mellifera*). *Journal of Invertebrate Pathology*, 53(3): 354–357.

Sumpter, D.J.T. and Martin, S.J. (2004) The dynamics of virus epidemics in *Varroa*-infested honey bee colonies. *Journal of Animal Ecology*, 73: 51–63.

Tentcheva, D., Gauthier, L., Zappulla, N., Dainat, B., Cousserans, F., Colin, M.-E., and Bergoin, M. (2004) Prevalence and seasonal variations of six bee viruses in *Apis mellifera* L. and *Varroa destructor* mite populations in France. *Applied and Environmental Microbiology*, 70(12): 7185–7191.

Tentcheva, D., Gauthier, L., Bagny, L., Fievet, J., Dainat, B., Cousserans, F., Colin, M.E., and Bergoin, M. (2006) Comparative analysis of deformed wing virus (DWV) RNA in *Apis mellifera* L. and *Varroa destructor*. *Apidologie*, 37: 41–50.

Todd, J.H., de Miranda, J.R., and Ball, B.V. (2007) Incidence and molecular characterization of viruses found in dying New Zealand honey bee (*Apis mellifera*) colonies infested with *Varroa destructor*. *Apidologie*, 38: 354–367.

Vidal-Naquet, N. (2011) Honeybees. In Lewbart, G.L. (ed.), *Invertebrate Medicine*, 2nd edn. Wiley-Blackwell, Chichester, pp. 285–321.

White, G.F. (1917) Sacbrood. US Department of Agriculture Bulletin, p. 431.

Yang, X. and Cox-Foster, D.L. (2005) Impact of an ectoparasite on the immunity and pathology of an invertebrate: evidence for host immunosuppression and viral amplification. *Proceedings of the National Academy of Sciences USA*, 102: 7470–7475

Yue, C. and Genersch, E. (2005) RT-PCR analysis of deformed wing virus in honey bees (*Apis mellifera*) and mites (*Varroa destructor*). *Journal of General Virology*, 86: 3419–3424.

Yue, C., Schröder, M., Gisder, S., and Genersch, E. (2007) Vertical-transmission routes for deformed wing virus of honeybees (*Apis mellifera*). *Journal of General Virology*, 88: 2329–2336.

4

Honeybee bacterial diseases

Bacterial diseases of the honeybee *Apis mellifera* mainly affect the brood, and are referred to collectively as foulbrood diseases: American foulbrood and European foulbrood disease are well known and may be harmful to both brood and colonies. The name 'foulbrood' comes from the foul smell emitted by an affected brood (Schirach, 1769). Foulbrood diseases seem to have been known since antiquity – Aristotle (384–322 BC) described a disease associated with a foul smell affecting hives in weakened colonies: 'Another diseased condition is indicated in a lassitude on the part of the bees and in malodorousness of the hive' (*The History of Animals*, IX, 40, trans. D'Arcy Wentworth Thompson, 1862).

1 American foulbrood disease (AFB)

AFB is an infectious and contagious disease of the capped brood of the honeybee *A. mellifera* and other *Apis* spp. It is caused by a Gram-positive spore-forming bacterium, *Paenibacillus larvae* (Genersch *et al.*, 2006; Genersch, 2010). AFB is a cosmopolitan disease occurring throughout the world where honeybees of the genus *Apis* are reared (OIE, 2014b).

AFB is a major threat to apiculture, since it is contagious and may be lethal for infected colonies. Therefore, AFB has the potential to cause beekeepers significant economic loss. Early detection is crucial because routine apiary management and practices, e.g. handling small hive tools, interchange of hive material (supers, frames, etc.), or even migratory beekeeping, can easily spread *P. larvae* to healthy honeybee colonies.

1.1 AFB disease sanitary status

AFB is a notifiable disease to sanitary authorities in many countries. AFB is a notifiable disease to the OIE (OIE, 2014b) (Appendix 2).

1.2 The pathogenic agent: *Paenibacillus larvae*

Paenibacillus larvae is a Gram-positive spore-forming bacterium (Heyndrickx *et al.*, 1996; Hansen and Brodsgaard, 1999; Genersch *et al.*, 2006). Four genotypes have been identified by repetitive-element PCR (Genersch *et al.*, 2006):

- The genotypes ERIC I and II correspond to the former subspecies *Paenibacillus larvae larvae*. Only these genotypes are isolated from AFB-affected colonies. These are the most prevalent genotypes with the following geographical distribution:
  - ERIC I and II are found in Europe.
  - ERIC I is the only one found in infected apiaries from the Americas (Genersch, 2010).
- The genotypes ERIC III and IV correspond to the former subspecies *Paenibacillus larvae pluvifaciens*. These strains have not been described in infected colonies in the field for years. At this time, ERIC III and IV considered to exist only in culture collections (Genersch, 2010).

The four genotypes ERIC I–IV are all pathogenic for honeybees (OIE, 2014a). However, each genotype has its own characteristic virulence (cf. section 1.5.1 below).

The bacterium is a slender, straight (though sometimes curved) rod with slightly rounded ends. The vegetative form has a tendency to grow in chains on culture medium (*in vitro* microscopic observations). The bacterium size varies greatly in length (2.5–5 µm × 0.5 µm). The spore is oval and about twice as long as it is wide, about 0.6 µm × 1.3 µm (Shimanuki and Knox, 2000).

The spores are the only infectious and contagious form of *P. larvae*. The spores may be found in wax, honey, pollen, on the hairs and the cuticle of honeybees, but also on the wood of the frames and the hive. They are very stable and resistant to chemical agents and to desiccation, heat, cold, freezing, draughts, and humidity (Hasemann, 1961). Spores can remain infectious for 3–10 years (some authors report a lifetime of more than 35 years in larval flakes) and purified spores even longer than 70 years (Rudenko, 1987; Genersch, 2010).

The spores can survive 8 hours at 100°C dry heat, 30 minutes in 20% formalin, solvents such as benzene, and UV. However, the spores are destroyed by 1.5% bleach, 1.5% caustic soda (in boiling water), by 30 minutes at 130°C dry heat, gamma rays, and finally by flames, though this last method is not 100% efficient.

The median infectious dose (ID_{50}) of *P. larvae* for a honeybee larva is between 8 and 9 spores per 24–48-hour-old larva. This infectious dose depends on a number of factors, including honeybee strain sensitivity and/or bacillus strain pathogenicity (Hansen and Brodsgaard, 1999; Genersch *et al.*, 2005; OIE, 2014a). The spores germinate into the vegetative form in the larval intestine. The vegetative form develops into spores when conditions are unfavourable (in particular exhaustion of nutritive elements and desiccation).

Paenibacillus larvae produces an antibacterial substance preventing the development of other bacterial pathogens (Fünfhaus *et al.*, 2009; Genersch, 2010). However, American and European foulbrood diseases have been described as occurring simultaneously in some colonies.

1.3 Clinical signs

The clinical signs of AFB are various and depend on the *P. larvae* genotype involved, the stage of the disease, and the strength of the colony (OIE, 2014a).

1.3.1 Clinical signs at the colony level

A colony affected by AFB is weakened through a decrease in honeybee population as well as impairment of population renewal of the infected brood. In severe cases, colonies may die following *P. larvae* infection.

At the beginning of the disease outbreak, the colony appears normal. At this time, only a few cells are affected (and it is sometimes difficult to observe these cells, hence the importance of routine inspections of colonies by beekeepers).

When the disease develops, the colony becomes more or less depopulated according to the infection level, *A. mellifera* strain (in particular according to the hygienic behaviour), and the bacillus strain involved. The activity level of the bees slows, and in some cases, dead bees are found on the hive floor or at the entrance of the hive. When the infection level is higher, the colony may become irritable and aggressive (Hansen and Brodsgaard, 1999; OIE, 2014a). When approaching and/or opening the hive, a slight to pronounced foul odour can be smelled if several larvae are affected (Shimanuki and Knox, 2000). When present, this odour is one clinical sign of AFB. When only few cells are affected, this odour is not present. In some cases, in particular in managed colonies without regular inspections, when the brood is severely infected, the colony may die.

1.3.2 Clinical signs at the brood level

The brood frame appears mottled and the cappings of affected cells become concave and punctured (Figures 4.1–4.3). Inside the affected cells, immature forms are dead and present the following main clinical signs:

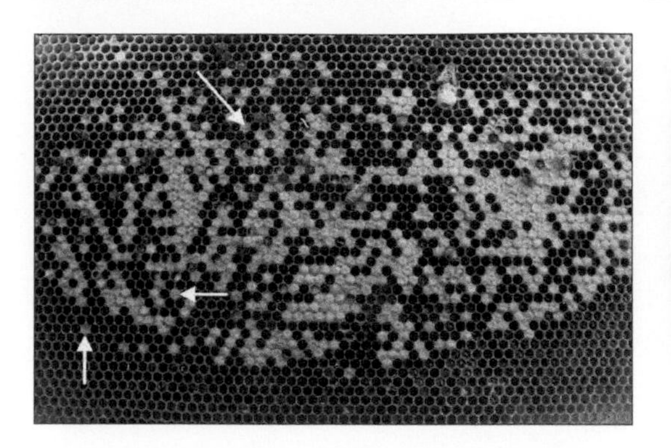

Figure 4.1 Brood comb affected by American foulbrood disease: mottled brood aspect of a brood comb with concave and punctured capped cells (arrows). (Photo © Nicolas Vidal-Naquet.)

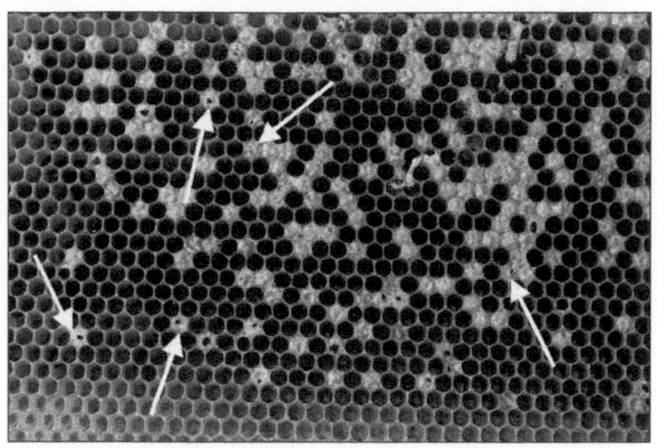

Figure 4.2 Brood comb of a colony killed by American foulbrood disease: note the presence of a mottled brood with numerous concave and punctured cells (arrows). (Photo © Nicolas Vidal-Naquet.)

- Larval colour turns progressively from creamy to dark brown.
- The larval remains become glutinous in consistency. On account of this viscosity, the larva 'can be drawn out as threads when a probe is inserted into the larval remains and removed from the cell (matchstick test)' (OIE, 2014a). Performing this test to evaluate the viscosity of the dead larvae represents the most obvious clinical symptom of AFB – the threads drawn out are usually ≥2 cm (De Graaf *et al.*, 2006) (Figure 4.4).

The remains of AFB-infected brood mainly arise from older larvae that die in the upright position immediately after the brood cell has been sealed. Rarely, larval remains can be found in uncapped cells.

As the infection progresses, inside cells with concave and punctured cappings, the dead brood specimens appear greasy and darkened. The remains of diseased larvae typically form dry, hard, and dark brittle scales sticking to the lower side of the cell (Figure 4.5).

When death occurs at the pupal stage, a characteristic pupal tongue protrudes from the pupal head, although this clinical sign is rarely observed (Figure 4.6).

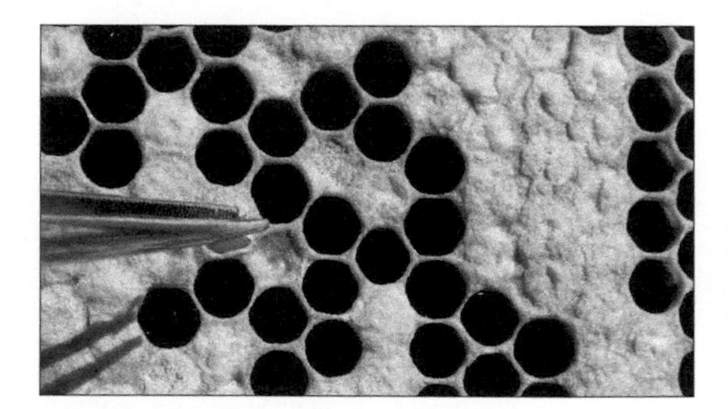

Figure 4.3 Brood comb of a colony affected by American foulbrood disease: concave capping. (Photo courtesy © Lydia Vilagines, DVM.)

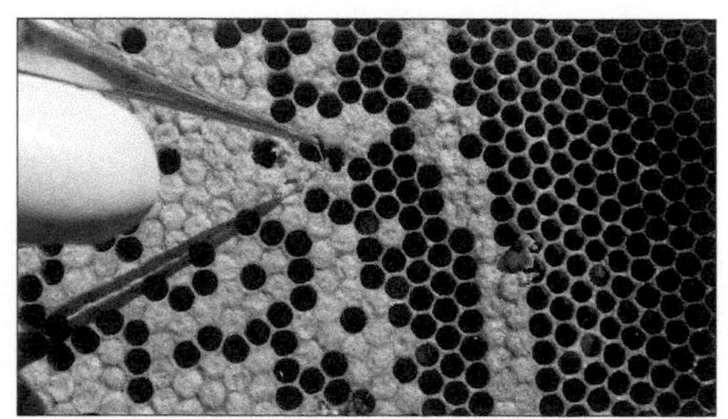

Figure 4.4 Brood comb of a colony affected by American foulbrood disease: performing a positive matchstick test on infected larval remains within a cell. (Photo courtesy © Lydia Vilagines, DVM.)

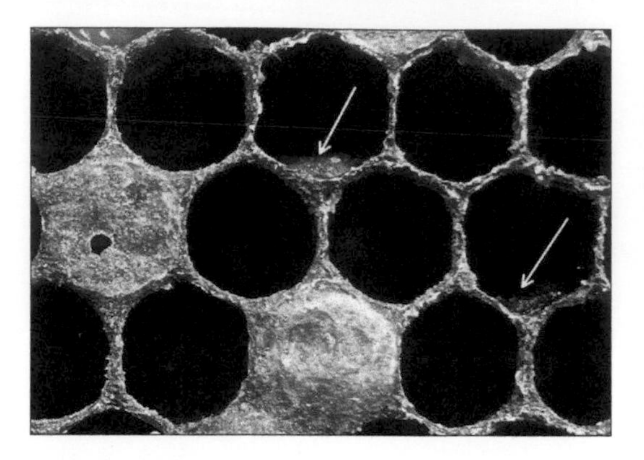

Figure 4.5 Brood comb of a colony affected by American foulbrood disease: dry, hard, and dark scales sticking to the lower side of the cell (arrows). (© Nicolas Vidal-Naquet.)

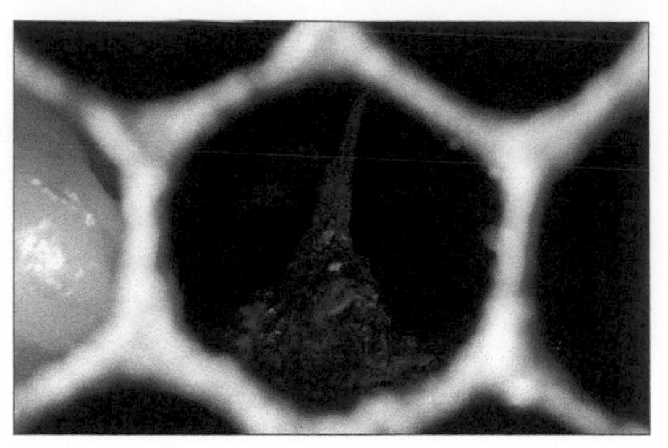

Figure 4.6 Characteristic pupal tongue stage in AFB disease. (© Courtesy The Animal and Plant Health Agency (APHA), Crown Copyright.)

1.4 Pathogenesis

AFB can affect the larvae of the three castes of honeybee (workers, drones, and queens) (Hansen and Brodsgaard, 1999). The spores are infectious only for larvae, and adult bees do not develop clinical signs after ingestion of *P. larvae* spores in the brood-food or honey (Wilson, 1971; Hitchcock *et al.*, 1979; Genersch, 2010).

Contamination usually occurs when the larvae are 12–48 hours old. Indeed, at this age in the early larval stages, they are especially sensitive to *P. larvae* infection. The ingestion of as few as 10 spores is considered sufficient to induce the clinical signs (Genersch, 2010).

After ingestion of contaminated brood-food, the spores germinate in the larval midgut on average 12 hours after ingestion (Yue *et al.*, 2008; Genersch, 2010).

The vegetative forms of *P. larvae* massively colonise the midgut:

- In the first stage, bacteria are contained in the midgut by the peritrophic membrane;
- In the second stage, the haemocel is contaminated through a breach made in the gut epithelium, probably due to proteases secreted by *Panibacillus larvae* (Genersch, 2010).

The infection thus turns into a septic stage and extends to all tissues, causing the death of the infected larvae (Figure 4.7). The larvae die when

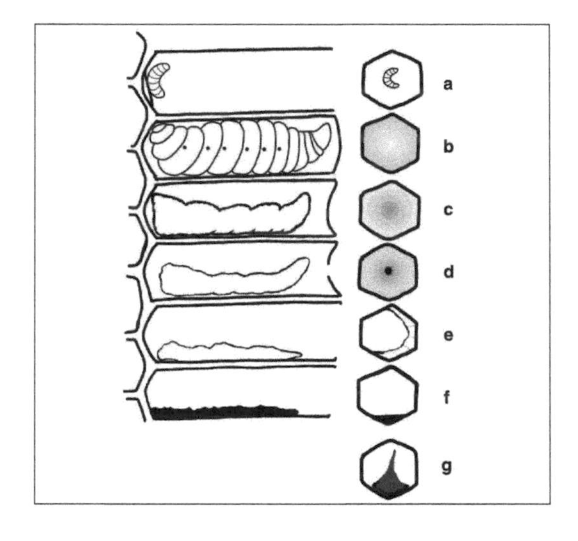

Figure 4.7 Progression of American foulbrood disease in a cell (front and profile view). (a) Point of infection. (b) Larval development to the prepupal stage within a capped cell. (c) Cell contents reduced and capping is drawn inwards or is punctured. (d) Cell contents reduced and capping is punctured. (e) Cell contents become glutinous. At this time, the matchstick test is positive. (f) At the end of the progression, residual scale containing millions of spores adheres tightly to the bottom of the cell. (g) If death occurs during the pupal stage, a characteristic tongue protrudes from the dead pupal head. (Redrawn by Nicolas Vidal-Naquet. Adapted from OIE, 2014a.)

the cell is capped. The dead larvae become viscous (ropey stage) and the developing infection results in gas release within the capped cell.

The viscous dead larvae gradually dry down to a hard brown scale, called foulbrood scale, sticking to the lower cell side (Genersch, 2010). These scales contain millions of spores and allow the transmission of *P. larvae* within and between colonies (Bailey and Ball, 1991; Genersch, 2010). Those spores are reported to remain infectious for at least 35 years and to be resistant to challenging weather conditions (in particular heat, cold, draughts, and humidity) (Hasemann, 1961).

1.5 Contributing factors

Several contributing factors may influence outbreaks of AFB. These factors concern mainly *P. larvae* and *A. mellifera* strains, and husbandry practices.

1.5.1 Virulence of *Paenibacillus larvae* strains

Four *P. larvae* genotypes have been described (Genersch *et al.*, 2006). They present differences in virulence level with different consequences for the larvae and colony (De Graaf *et al.*, 2006; Genersch 2010).

At the larval level, virulence can be evaluated by the 'time course of mortality' in experimentally infected hosts (Genersch *et al.*, 2005):

- The genotype ERIC I needs on average 12 days to kill an infected larva.
- The genotypes ERIC II–IV need on average 7 days to kill an infected larva.

Thus, at the larval stage, ERIC II–IV genotypes are more virulent than ERIC I.

However, at the colony level, ERIC I is the most virulent genotype because of the labour pattern of the nurse bees. Indeed, Genersh (2010) notes that 'removal of diseased larvae by nurse bees prior to the production of infectious spores efficiently disturbs disease transmission and disease development within an infected colony'.

The quicker the larvae die, the faster the nurse bees remove them from cells; as a result, less viscous remains and spore-containing foulbrood scale will be produced, and the less the disease will develop and spread within and between colonies (Genersch, 2010). On the contrary, the more slowly *P. larvae* develops (as in ERIC I infections), the more virulent it will be for the colony.

This is a prime example of immune defence at the colony level (Spivak and Reuter, 2001; Evans and Spivak, 2010; Genersch, 2010). This is also a major example of the particularity of honeybee pathology with certain features concerning the colony as a super-organism and others concerning the bees as individuals.

1.5.2 Other contributing factors

The development of AFB can be promoted by various factors:

- Robbing and drifting behaviours of bees.
- Insufficient hygienic behaviour by the bees.
- Inappropriate beekeeping practices, such as feeding colonies with unknown honey and beebread, artificial swarm forming, trading colonies, seasonal migrations (migratory beekeeping), lack of responsiveness of the beekeeper when confronted with affected hives, lack of routine inspection of the colonies, exchanges of material between hives and apiaries, lack or inadequate management of the material, etc.

1.6 Epidemiology

The epidemiological features of AFB are mainly the consequence of the sporulation of *P. larvae*. Spores may be found in the honey, the pollen, in the wax, on the wood hive material, and on adult honeybees (Vidal-Naquet and Boucher, 2013).

Within a colony and between colonies within an apiary or different apiaries, the disease can easily spread thanks to robbing or drifting behaviours of spore-vector adult bees but also thanks to beekeeping practices and migratory beekeeping.

An AFB transmission rate to neighbouring healthy colonies of 8% has been reported as being due to a low drifting level (i.e. when bees inadvertently enter hives other than their own) (Goodwin *et al.*, 1994). Robbing seems to pose a greater risk for local spreading between hives. It occurs when foraging bees enter the hives with weakened colonies affected by AFB and steal the honey stored (Mill *et al.*, 2013).

Beekeeping practices are likely to be responsible for the spread of AFB:

- Exchange of frames, supers, hive bodies, and other material between colonies.
- Use of external honey for feed; use of tools and contaminated materials.
- Inappropriate and flawed sanitary beekeeping practices (very risky for colonies).
- Abandoned hives and apiaries, but also empty hives left untouched after an infection, are a major risk of disease spreading and transmission.

The role of feral colonies in the spread of AFB remains unknown. However, we can suspect a potential role in transmission in the case of swarming or feral colony capture.

Global apiculture, with its trade in package bees, artificial swarms on frames, and queens, as well as migratory beekeeping (in particular, use of migratory sites, e.g. to produce local honey or to encourage pollination activity on large areas of crops or orchards), may also be involved in *P. larvae* transmission. Migratory beekeeping poses a major risk that strong colonies will rob honey from colonies weakened by AFB.

1.7 Diagnosis

Diagnosis must be performed as early as possible in order to limit or avoid the spread of the disease within the hive, between colonies within the apiary, and to neighbouring apiaries. This implies that the beekeeper must be able to monitor the health status of the colony and more particularly of the brood throughout the year during routine inspections.

The diagnosis of AFB is based the presence of clinical signs and on identification of the pathogenic agent (OIE, 2014a).

1.7.1 Clinical diagnosis

When it is suspected, and in order to take the necessary sanitary measures as soon as possible, all the brood frames have to be examined carefully. A routine inspection of the colonies is necessary throughout the season.

Opening and examination of the hives must be performed carefully and quickly, especially in autumn when the risk of robbing is more serious.

The following are the principal clinical signs of AFB:

- The colony may appear weakened, due to depopulation. Unusual aggressive behaviour of the bees can be observed.
- A mottled appearance of the brood combs.
- The presence of concave and punctured cell cappings.
- A foul smell from the brood combs may be detected.
- The presence of uncapped cells with larval remains.
- The larval remains are glutinous and can be drawn out like threads (usually >2 cm) with a probe (matchstick test). This is one of the main features of the clinical examination for AFB.
- The presence in the cells of dry dark scales in the lower sides of the cell may sometimes be noticed.
- The presence of protruding tongues in pupae remains one of the most characteristic but also one of the rarer clinical signs of AFB (OIE, 2014a).

1.7.2 Differential diagnosis

Differential diagnosis must take into account all the diseases of the brood, in particular European foulbrood disease (which in its most severe form affects capped brood) and sacbrood disease (which at a late stage may occasionally present black viscous larvae which can be drawn out like threads (<1 cm)). Differential diagnosis must also take into account a number of other possible problems:

- Chalkbrood disease caused by the fungus *Ascosphaera apis*.
- Baldbrood due to the small wax moth.
- Problems due to the laying activity of the queen or the presence of laying workers with multiple eggs oviposited within cells.
- Varroosis causing a mottled aspect of the brood.

1.7.3 Laboratory diagnosis

Identification of *P. larvae* is necessary to confirm the diagnosis in particular in the countries where AFB is a notifiable disease and sanitary measures must be taken by authorities.

Sampling

Sampling has to be done carefully, and shipping must be done according to regulations and to laboratory advice (Appendix 3) (Franco *et al.*, 2012).

According to where the samples are being sent, packaging is usually performed as follows:

- Brood-comb should be wrapped in a paper (*not* plastic) bag (or newspaper) and placed in a wooden or cardboard box for transportation.
- Larval remains, food stores (honey, pollen), and residues can be sent in tubes or plastic bags.
- Honeybee adults (at least 30) must be carefully stored before sending (freezing the honeybees is the best protocol).

In suspected overt infection, with clinical signs, affected brood sample must be collected. Usually, a 20 cm^2 comb piece containing as high a concentration of infected brood as possible is cut from the comb (OIE, 2014a). However, sampling neighbouring colonies is also necessary. Indeed, they have to be considered as suspect, and even without clinical signs, a laboratory test must be performed (OIE, 2014a). The following samples may be sent for analysis:

- Brood.
- Honey in cells close to the brood. Pollen, royal, and/or worker jelly may also be sent.
- Adult bees (the most reliable picture is obtained if these taken from the brood nest).
- Debris (wax).

Those samples can also be used to identify *P. larvae* in a monitoring or prevention programme (OIE, 2014a).

Laboratory analysis

- Microscopic examination can reveal the presence of spores (Figure 4.8) but also of the vegetative form, in infected larvae, either singly or in chains of Gram-positive rods.
- The detection and enumeration of spores in honey can be considered as indicative of the AFB infection status of a colony. It is also helpful to know if honey is unsafe for use as supplementary feed due to contamination, so that adequate prophylaxis and control measures can be taken.
- In honey above a threshold between 4,500 and 5,000 spores/g, the occurrence of an AFB outbreak is highly probable (Ritter, 2003; Otten and Otto, 2005). Thus, three categories of infection may be defined and determine the measures that must be implemented in the colony and the apiary (Ritter, 2003):
  - Category 0: 0 spores found in the honey.
  - Category I: <4,500–5,000 spores. Category I requires preventive management.
  - Category II: >4500–5000 spores. Category II needs control management.
- Sampling adult bees and determining the adult bee spore load may allow an early diagnosis of AFB even if the clinical signs are not observed. It may also give 'information on the actual health status of the colony' concerning *P. larvae* infection (Gende *et al.*, 2011). It is considered that a threshold of approximately 3,000 *P. larvae* spores per adult bee is needed experimentally for AFB overt infection in a colony (Gende *et al.*, 2011).
- Culture is possible on several media (*P. larvae* agar, MYPGP agar, etc.). This allows identification of *P. larvae*.
- Antibody-based techniques exist for the diagnosis of AFB. In the field, a veterinarian

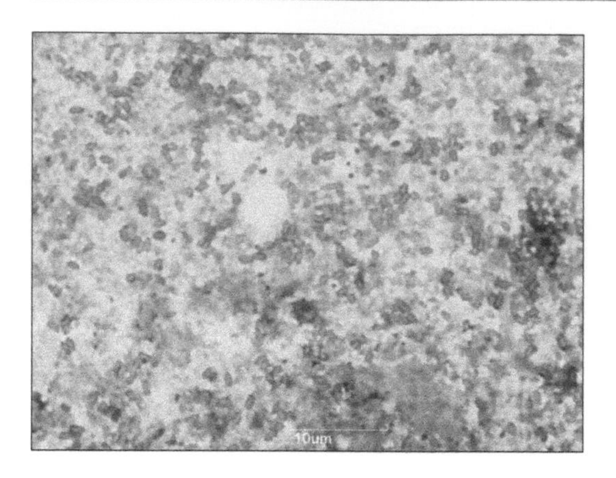

Figure 4.8 Spores of *Paenibacillus larvae*. Microscopic identification (×1,000). (Photo courtesy of © Anses Sophia-Antipolis.)

practitioner may perform on larvae samples a quick ELISA test for a diagnosis of AFB (VITA diagnostic kit: AFB Diagnostic Test Kit®). This allows an early detection of AFB (OIE, 2014a) and immediate management. Sanitary measures may be taken on the field when the diagnosis of AFB is positive. PCR is the most reliable method and allows identification of the genotype: usually ERIC I in Europe and the Americas and ERIC II in Europe only. ERIC III and IV have not been isolated in field samples for years (Genersch, 2010).

1.7.4 Prognosis

The prognosis for a colony infected by AFB must be considered from guarded to poor:

- The prognosis may be guarded if few larvae are affected and if control measures are quickly implemented after an early diagnosis.
- The prognosis is poor if a colony is highly infected.

However, within an apiary in which one or several colonies have been positively diagnosed with AFB, the prognosis must be considered as poor because of the high risk of spreading of spores by robbing, drifting, and beekeeping practices.

1.8 AFB control

AFB is a notifiable disease in many countries, and is on the list of the diseases notifiable to the OIE (OIE, 2014b). Thus, sanitary measures must be implemented in many countries according to the relevant legislation (destruction of colonies, shaking bees, regulation of local transportation, exchange and trade, etc.).

When one or more colonies within an apiary is affected by AFB, the beekeeper and all professionals operating there have an obligation to take sanitary measures with their equipment: hive tools, gloves, smokers, etc., have to be soaked in or scrubbed with a strong solution of washing soda between each hive inspection and of course between apiaries (FERA, 2013a). The veterinarian must also take sanitary protection measures when visiting a suspect or infected apiary.

1.8.1 Destruction of colonies, disinfection and sterilization of material

Destruction of infected colonies is a sanitary and reliable method to control AFB (Alippi, 1999). This is the best way to combat the spore resistance and long-lived viability of *P. larvae* in an apiary. The destruction of a colony is performed by asphyxiating the bees with a sulphur wick placed at the hive entrance and leaving the hive closed for about 15 minutes (Faucon, 2002).

The destruction of the colony must be combined with sanitary treatment of material: destruction of the brood frames and honey has to be performed by burning. The hive bodies and supers must be disinfected and sterilized (Alippi, 1999). Disinfection of bodies, supers, and feeders can be performed by scorching the wood with a blowtorch, then by applying or spraying bleach or caustic soda, and finally by immersion in hot microcrystalline wax or a mixture of paraffin and microcrystalline wax to achieve complete decontamination from spores (Dobbelaere *et al.*, 2001).

Gamma-rays may be used to sterilize beekeeping material. This method eliminates not only spores of *P. larvae*, but also *Melissococcus plutonius*, fungi such as *Nosema* spp., *A. apis*, and insects (e.g. moths) (Tremblay, 2010). This method is mainly used to treat all the frames of the hive body (where the brood is reared) (Tremblay, 2010). Gamma-ray sterilization is performed in specialized centres to which the beekeeper has to bring his/her material. Thus, irradiation is mainly of interest to professional beekeepers as a means of dealing with AFB.

1.8.2 Antibiotherapy

In the countries of the European Union, as well as in some other countries, the use of antibiotics as method of control or prevention of AFB, as well as other honeybee bacterial diseases, is banned.

In some countries, including the United States, the use of antibiotics is permitted for the control and prevention of foulbrood diseases and in particular AFB. However, antibiotics are only effective on the vegetative form of *P. larvae* (Alippi, 1999) and not on the infectious (and contagious) spores. Thus, the use of antibiotics will only deal with a covert (asymptomatic) infection of the colony and clinical signs may reappear at any time when the treatment ends.

On another hand, because of sporulation and the massive and inappropriate use of antibiotics (e.g. for prevention), there is a major risk that *P. larvae* will become resistant to antibiotics as occurred with oxytetracyclin (OTC) hydrochloride and sulfathiazole (Miyagi *et al.*, 2000; Kochansky *et al.*, 2001; Alippi *et al.*, 2007; Genersch, 2010). Resistance to OTC and sulfathiazole in *P. larvae* is widespread and has led to the use of new classes of antibiotics. Last but not least, antibiotherapy may affect the vitality of the brood and the lifespan of adult honeybees (Peng *et al.*, 1992; Genersch, 2010).

In the field of veterinary public health and of the 'One Health' principles (http://www.oie.int/doc/ged/d6296.pdf), the use of antibiotics can be responsible of the presence of residues in the products of the hive, e.g. honey. Consequently, for honeybee health, beekeeping management, and veterinary public health reasons, antibiotics are not the solution to controlling AFB.

Controlling AFB requires sanitary beekeeping management and furthermore implementation of good sanitary beekeeping practices throughout the year.

1.8.3 Shaking bee (or shock swarm) method

The shaking bee (or shock swarm) method is a husbandry technique to save strong colonies affected by AFB. This method must be implemented during the season and is usually effective if performed before August. In September it is too late because there are not enough wax-producing bees to build cells. The shaking method, a long-established approach to controlling honeybee disease, emulates the swarming behaviour of a colony to move to a new nest site when pressure from disease is high. Thus, changing the nest reduces the build-up of pathogenic agents (Howard, 1907; Budge *et al.*, 2010). New frames with pathogen-free (and residue-free) wax foundations in a new hive give a pathogen-free environment, inducing a break in the brood and disease cycles (Hansen and Brodsgaard, 2003).

In the case of AFB, the aim of this method is to help an affected colony eliminate spores. Studies have shown that in a swarm from asymptomatic infected colonies, spore load decreases within 2 months after swarming. After 13 months, the spore level was reported to be nearly undetectable (Fries *et al.*, 2006; Genersch, 2010). In swarms from symptomatic parent colonies, after an initial period of decrease, the spore load was increasing 3 months after swarming, and this load produced an overt infection when the new brood was reared. This is the basis of the shaking bees method used to control AFB (Pernal *et al.*, 2008; Genersch, 2010).

This beekeeping practice can be used on strong colonies with covert AFB or with poor clinical signs in order to save a colony deemed to be worth preserving. The implementation of the shaking bee method is not recommended for highly infected colonies, weakened colonies, or if a large part of the surface of the brood is affected.

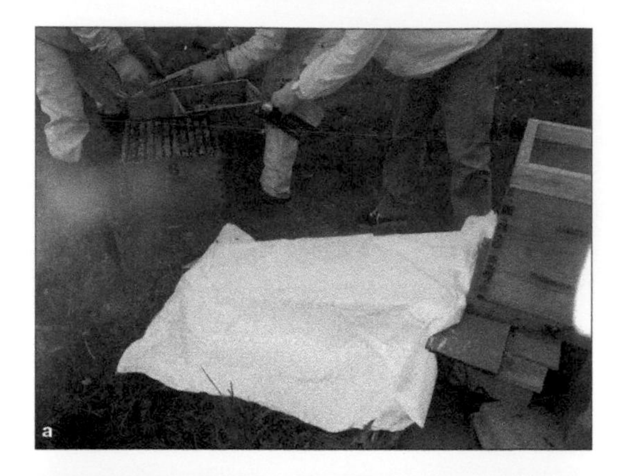

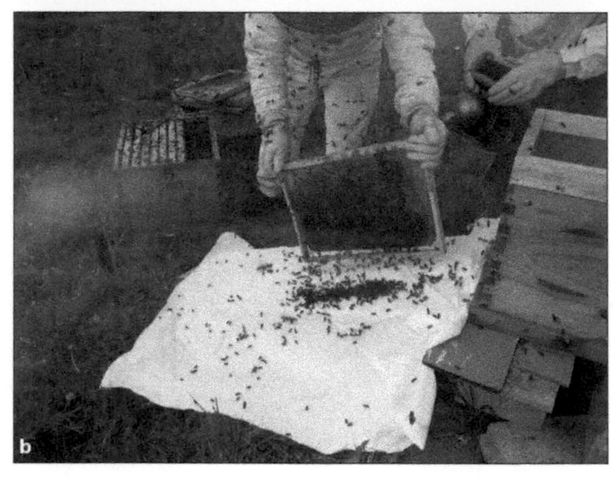

Figure 4.9a,b Transvasement: transferring method. The affected hive is removed from its site and replaced with a pathogen-free one with uncontaminated wax foundations. The bees are shaken onto a carpet in front of the new hive in order to enter the new hive. (Photo courtesy ©Lydia Vilagines.)

The method consists of shaking adult honeybees onto new frames with uncontaminated wax foundations, in a new hive. The shaken swarm method provides the colony with beehive material free of *P. larvae* spores. The removed infected combs and frames must be destroyed by burning. The body of the hive (and the super) must be disinfected and sterilized.

The shaking bees method reduces spore loads in colonies without the use of antibiotics and is a 'feasible option for managing AFB in commercial beekeeping operations' (Del Hoyo *et al.*, 2001; Pernal *et al.*, 2008). Another method, 'transvasement', consists of transferring bees from their hive to a new one with uncontaminated wax foundations. The new hive replaces the old one and the bees are shaken on a carpet (tissue, paper, cardboard) before entering the new hive, with the objective of them discarding some of the pathogens before entering. (Figure 4.9a,b). This method is reported by some beekeepers and veterinarians as presenting some risk for the queen.

This method involves significant labour and expense but seems to be effective at reducing spores load in colonies. However, controlling AFB also involved preventing the occurrence of overt infection by implementing good sanitary beekeeping practices.

1.9 Prophylaxis

Prophylactic measures are the best way to control AFB, as well as other infectious diseases, within an apiary. These measures concern beekeepers, bees, and apiaries, as well as management of beekeeping equipment (Matheson and Reid, 1992; Alippi, 1999; Vidal-Naquet, 2010; Vidal-Naquet and Boucher, 2013).

1.9.1 Beekeeper training

The beekeeper has to learn and know how to recognise bee diseases and AFB in particular. He or she must be able to detect the disease and intervene as soon as possible in order to prevent and limit the spread of AFB. Routine inspections of the colonies are a major pillar of prevention. Apiary inspections should begin with the strongest colonies.

1.9.2 Prophylaxis by honey and adult bee sampling and testing

The detection of *P. larvae* spores in honey produced in a colony, even without clinical signs, enables an early identification of the presence of AFB (Ritter and Kiefer, 1995; Ritter, 2003; Bassi *et al.*, 2010). In colonies neighbouring AFB-diseased colonies or apiaries, performing such a laboratory identification allows the early implementation of sanitary measures and prophylactic methods. Furthermore, honey sampling (to perform laboratory spore counting) allows the surveillance of sanitary measures taken in the event of an outbreak.

The detection of *P. larvae* spores in adult bees may allow prophylaxis and diagnosis. According to Gende *et al.* (2011), above a threshold of 3,000 spores per bee clinical signs of AFB will occur (experimental study). Thus performing laboratory spore counting on adult bees allows suitable prophylactic and sanitary measures to be taken.

1.9.3 Honeybees exhibiting hygienic behaviour

A high level of hygienic behaviour helps to control diseases (Spivak and Gilliam, 1998; Spivak and Reuter, 2001). This behaviour can be defined as the bee's ability in a colony to detect and remove diseased immature forms from the nest (in particular within the capped brood cells) (Rothenbuhler, 1964). Hygienic behaviour can be evaluated by a test described by Marla Spivak. The hygienic behaviour of honeybees involves all the challenges affecting the brood and in particular the capped brood. It is described here for AFB, but performing the test described by Spivak (Spivak and Reuter, 1998) is crucial in the context of a general prophylaxis against brood disease.

Performing the test to select bees that exhibit hygienic behaviour involves the following steps (Figure 4.10):

- Selection and removal of a piece of brood from a capped brood comb (usually a piece with an average area of 5 cm × 6 cm).
- Freezing this piece of brood for 24 hours (in order to kill immature forms within the cells).
- Replacing the piece at the same site.
- Recording the time taken for the colony to detect, uncap, and remove dead brood.

Colonies removing the freeze-killed brood from the comb section within 48 hours on two consecutive trials are considered to exhibit good hygienic behaviour (Spivak and Reuter, 1998). In colonies with good hygienic behaviour, the beginning of the detection and uncapping of the dead brood by bees may be observed 8 hours after the piece is replaced.

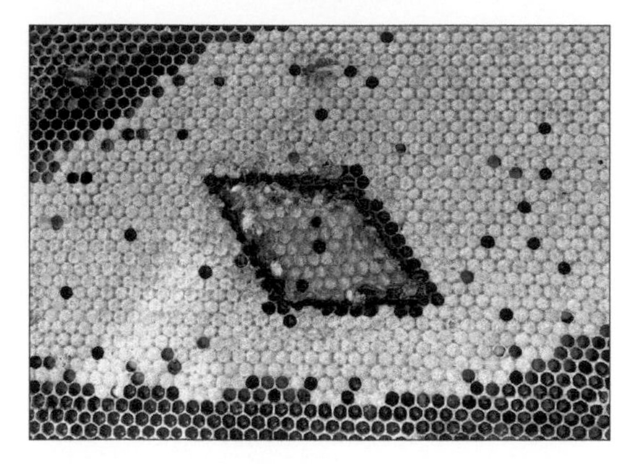

Figure 4.10 Performing a hygienic behaviour test. The piece of brood has been frozen for 24 hours and replaced; the honeybees have to remove the dead brood from the frozen cells within 48 hours (twice) to be considered as exhibiting hygienic behaviour. (© Nicolas Vidal-Naquet.)

Application of this test to managed colonies enables the selection of colonies with good hygienic behaviour. This behavioural feature is a crucial pillar of selection in apiculture but also of good sanitary beekeeping practices.

1.9.4 Apiary management

Visits and inspections of hives and combs allow for an early diagnosis (checking in particular the summer and winter bee broods).

Introducing and selecting honeybees with a high sanitary status in an apiary are necessary. A health certificate should certify any package bees, artificial swarms, or queens introduced into an apiary. Moving colonies, or grouping hives in close proximity, should only be done after evaluation of risk.

Limiting drifting and robbing is also important. Weakened colonies in an apiary will lead to robbing behaviour by other colonies. Weakened colonies should be destroyed as previously mentioned. According to the regulatory status of AFB, colonies should not be moved from the apiary.

Colonies should not be fed supplementarily with unknown honey or honey extracted from another apiary. These honeys may be the source of pathogens, such as *P. larvae* spores. In a German study performed in 1995 on 700 different honeys, 98% of the samples contained *P. larvae* spores (Ritter and Kiefer, 1995; Ritter, 2003). Moreover, in 200 different honeys from the EU, 62% of the samples contained spores (Ritter, 2003).

Quarantine before introducing colonies into an apiary is an interesting measure as illustrated by the successful no-drugs AFB programme implemented at country level in New Zealand (Von Eaton, 2000).

1.9.5 Material management

Good sanitary beekeeping practices in hives, supers, and frame management must be the rule. 'Ideal' management would involve associating combs to supers and those supers to hive bodies with no exchanges of material occurring between hives. However, though this is very feasible for small honey farms or hobby beekeeping, this management of hives, supers, and frames appears difficult to implement in professional beekeeping. In beekeeping management, it is usually considered that two or three frames in each hive must be replaced annually by new ones with wax foundations.

The use of a queen excluder between hive and super prevents the queen from laying in the frames of the supers and stops dissemination of the disease if supers are exchanged between hives.

Frames bearing honey and pollen from colonies that have died due to an unknown cause must not be used in other hives.

Material maintenance requires disinfection and sterilization (by scorching, washing soda (6% solution), bleach (2% solution), or gamma-radiation) (Alippi, 1999). Disinfection by heat may be performed using the following steps:

1. Scraping the wood and removing the remains of propolis, combs, etc.
2. Scorching of the wood with a blowtorch. The wood must become dark-brown in colour.
3. Dipping the material in hot molten microcrystalline wax (150°C for 10 minutes) to obtain 99.99% spore decontamination (Dobbelaere *et al.*, 2001).

Chemical disinfection and sterilization are not completely effective against *Panibacillus larvae* spores because of their strong resistance.

As previously noted, irradiation with gamma-rays provides effective sterilization.

2 European foulbrood disease (EFB)

EFB is an infectious and contagious disease affecting the uncapped brood of several honeybee species, namely *A. mellifera*, *Apis cerana* and *Apis laboriosa* (Alippi, 1999). It is caused by an anaerobic Gram-positive non-spore-forming bacterium: *Melissococcus plutonius* (Bailey and Collins, 1982). Several bacteria associated with *M. plutonius* develop secondarily. Infected larvae usually die rapidly when they are 4–5 days old. Overt EFB infection can cause significant weakening sometimes followed by collapse of colonies (Budge *et al.*, 2010). In many areas, the disease is endemic with occasional seasonal outbreaks (Forsgren *et al.*, 2013). In France, severe cases of EFB have occurred in recent

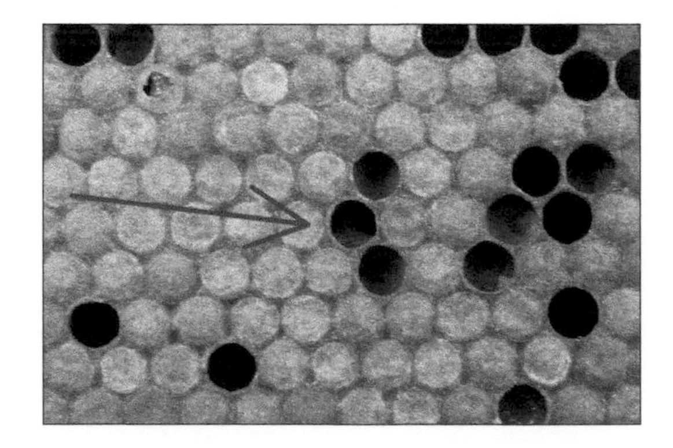

Figure 4.11 Dead larva in uncapped brood due to European foulbrood disease (arrow). Sometimes only a few larvae are affected. (Photo courtesy Lydia Vilagines, DVM.)

years, with colony mortality sometimes affecting all the colonies of an apiary.

EFB is found worldwide except in New Zealand (Forsgren, 2010). EFB is reported to be the most widespread bacterial bee disease in the UK, while in Switzerland severe outbreaks have increased each year since the late 1990s (Forsgren *et al.*, 2013).

2.1 Disease status

EFB is a notifiable disease to the OIE (2014b). In the EU, EFB is a notifiable disease in some countries (Appendix 2).

2.2 Pathogenic agent and associated bacteria

The causative agent of EFB is *M. plutonius*, a Gram-positive non-spore-forming microaerophilic to anaerobic bacterium. *M. plutonius* is phylogenetically close to the genus *Enterococcus*.

Several other bacteria are usually found associated with *M. plutonius* in affected larvae and have sometimes wrongly been considered to be the primary pathogenic agent. *Melissococcus plutonius* remains viable in brood cell walls and in larvae faeces, and may survive long periods of desiccation (Bailey, 1959a,b). *Achromobacter euridice*, *Enterococcus faecalis*, *Brevibacillus laterosporus*, and *Paenibacillus alvei* are the main secondary pathogens found with *M. plutonius.* Their roles in the pathogenesis of EFB remain unclear (Budge *et al.*, 2010).

2.3 Clinical signs

EFB affects the uncapped brood, killing larvae usually when they are 4–5 days old, 1–2 days before capping, sometimes just after in the most severe case, but always before pupation. The affected larvae move and die displaced in their cells. They may appear twisted within the cells around the walls, or stretched out lengthways (Forsgren, 2010).

Infected larvae become soft and their colour usually progresses from pearly white to yellow and then brown (Figure 4.11). Larvae may decay, forming dry and rubbery scales that can be easily removed. These dark scales are more malleable than those typically found in AFB (Forsgren *et al.*, 2013). In the more severe cases, the larvae may die within the cell after capping and symptoms may resemble those of AFB with sunken and punctured capping.

The brood pattern appears patchy and erratic (scattered or mottled brood) when a high proportion of larvae are affected (Figure 4.12).

The colony exudes a slightly sour to a foul and rotten smell when a high proportion of the larvae are affected (Shimanuki and Knox, 2000; Forsgren, 2010). This smell is due to the action of the associated secondary bacteria.

At the colony level, infection can develop over a long period (months, years). EFB outbreaks with spontaneous recovery a few weeks later have been reported (Bailey, 1961; Forsgren, 2010). EFB usually weakens but can on occasion kill the colony (FERA, 2013). Most larvae usually die within a brief period in late spring or mid-summer (Forsgren, 2010). Hence, there is a seasonal pattern, in late spring/mid-summer when the brood is well developed, with clinical signs increasing. If the disease occurs at the end of summer, or in some regions in autumn (when the winter worker brood is reared), a patchy brood is a sign that the disease must be considered as highly severe.

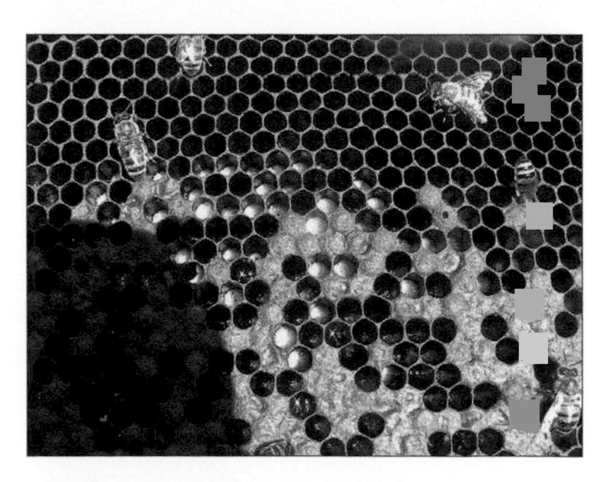

Figure 4.12 Scattered brood due to European foulbrood disease with dead larvae in uncapped cells. (Photo courtesy Lydia Vilagines, DVM.)

In some apiaries, EFB may remain as a covert infection, in particular because of mechanical contamination of the honeycombs. Thus, periodic outbreaks can occur in subsequent years (OIE, 2014a).

The prognosis of EFB may be:

- benign with spontaneous recovery if it occurs in strong colonies before the first honey flow;
- mild if the clinical signs persist after the honey flow;
- severe if the capped brood is affected (failing of detection of diseased larvae and super-infection) – the colony will probably die;
- severe in autumn if the brood presents a patchy pattern.

2.4 Epidemiology

EFB is endemic worldwide. In infected areas, outbreaks may occur in successive years, which can sometimes lead to massive colony weakening and even losses, as recently observed in Switzerland (Forsgren *et al.*, 2013). Frequently, colonies are debilitated. More often, only some cells are affected by EFB.

Melissococcus plutonius may be found in samples of worker bees from affected colonies. Hence, adult worker bees can spread the disease within the colony but also between colonies and apiaries by robbing and drifting behaviours (Belloy *et al.*, 2007; McKee *et al.*, 2004). *Melissococcus plutonius* has been found in a wide range of honey samples, suggesting that robbing is spreading the disease.

Furthermore, beekeeping practices are considered to be heavily implicated in the spread of EFB. Inadequate sanitary beekeeping practices, and exchanges of combs, honey, or hive equipment between EFB-free colonies and EFB-infected colonies are responsible for spreading the disease.

Swarm recovery is a potential danger for an apiary. Indeed, swarms from infected colonies are a potential carrier of *M. plutonius* and may become diseased after they are hived (FERA, 2013). Hence, symptomatic colonies from apiaries with EFB present an increased risk of carrying *M. plutonius* compared to asymptomatic colonies on apiaries free from EFB (Budge *et al.*, 2010)

Migratory beekeeping, trading in package bees, artificial swarms, and queens also pose a risk for colonies and can spread EFB.

2.5 Pathogenesis

EFB infection begins with the asymptomatic colonization of the gut of a larva after ingestion of contaminated brood-food. *M. plutonius* can only multiply within honeybee larval gut.

Usually, contamination occurs in larvae that are 1–2 days old. Older larvae may be infected but 'the older they are the less they are affected by the infection' (Bailey and Ball, 1991; Forsgren, 2010). *Melissococcus plutonius* then multiply strongly within the midgut.

A second phase of the infection leads to sepsis, tissue damage (after altering and entering the peritrophic membrane and the midgut epithelium), and death of the larvae (McKee *et al.*, 2004).

The infected larvae experience different fates (Bailey, 1959b, Forsgren, 2010):

- Some larvae die before capping and are removed from the colony by cleaners.
- Some larvae die after capping and defecate their infected and infective intestinal content within the cell.
- Some larvae do not die and succeed in pupating, forming undersized or normal adults.

The pathogenesis process but also the roles of secondary bacteria are not well understood and various hypotheses have been advanced. It has been suggested that competition between *M. plutonius* and the larvae for nutrients results in larval starvation (Bailey, 1983). However, in vitro studies did not confirm this hypothesis (McKee *et al.*, 2004).

Larval immunity, interaction between *M. plutonius* and secondary pathogens (and intestinal microflora), but also the hygienic behaviour of the colony, are also supposed to play a role in the pathogenesis process at the larval and colony stages (Forsgren, 2010).

2.6 Contributing factors

The main causes of EFB outbreaks are reported to be related to colony stress conditions and in particular to *protein deficiency*. EFB is most often seen at the brood spike in the late spring which is a critical time in the life cycle of the honeybee colony. At this time, there are large areas of brood to rear and to feed, and any stressor affecting feeding poses a major risk to the brood and the colony. Nursing the brood at this time can be disrupted by several factors:

- A deficiency in pollen, the bees' only protein source, is considered as one of the main predisposing factors (due to poor blossoming, inappropriate location of migratory beekeeping, etc.).
- Confinement due to bad weather conditions, preventing bees from foraging.
- An imbalance between the populations of nurses and larvae (i.e. an insufficient number of nurse bees to take care of the brood), resulting in a food shortage for the larvae. This may happen when performing artificial swarms.
- Infection of nurses by sacbrood bee virus. Nurses are young worker bees and SBV can affect their hypopharyngeal glands (cf. Chapter 3, section 4);
- Varroosis and a high level of *Varroa destructor* infestation.

Genetic factors and the geographic location of apiaries are also suspected to play a role in EFB outbreaks (Bailey, 1961).

2.7 Diagnosis

The clinical diagnosis of EFB first takes into account clinical signs observed on the brood comb and by the detection of diseased larvae. The main characteristic of the diagnosis is that EFB is the only disease of the uncapped brood.

A differential diagnosis must be developed with other brood diseases such as AFB and SBV in mind. Unlike AFB, the matchstick test is negative because the larval remains are not sticky and glutinous.

Analytical methods include microscopic examination, microbial cultivation, and immunological and PCR methods (PCR and real-time PCR) (Shimanuki and Knox, 2000; McKee *et al.*, 2003; OIE, 2014a; Budge *et al.*, 2010).

A field test kit (using a lateral flow device) allows the detection of *M. plutonius* in extracts of infected tissue with high specificity (Tomkies *et al.*, 2009). This kit uses an antibody test that reacts specifically to antibodies associated with *M. plutonius* (EFB Vita Diagnostic Test Kit®). The detection efficiency is reported to be high (96–100% of EFB-infected samples with no cross-reactivity with other bee brood pathogens) (Tomkies *et al.*, 2009). The use of such a test in the field is important and enables immediate sanitary control measures against EFB to be taken. Furthermore, a routine confirmation of covert *M. plutonius* infection in the field will allow much more efficient disease detection and control (Tomkies *et al.*, 2009).

The samples necessary for laboratory testing are mainly samples of brood and workers (cf. Appendix 3).

2.8 EFB control

Highly infected colonies should be destroyed (Wilkins *et al.*, 2007; Forsgren, 2010).

Antibiotic use in honeybee diseases is not permitted in the EU. Use of the antibiotic oxytetracycline (OTC) is authorized in the US and some other countries (Alippi, 1999; Waite *et al.*, 2003). In the US, OTC can be used for prevention and control according to state regulation. However, the use of antibiotics is not the solution, because of the risk of the occurrence of residues in the products of the hive and antibiotic resistance. Antibiotherapy (if allowed by regulation) should be performed only when combined with the shaking bee (shock swarm) method, which seems to lower the rate of recurrence of EFB in colonies (Waite *et al.*, 2003; Forsgren, 2010).

The shaking swarm method (shaking bees into a new hive with new combs and destroying the infected combs) is recommended for the control of EFB (Forsgren, 2010).

The shaking swarm method provides the colony with *M. plutonius*-free beehive material. It has been shown in the UK (England and Wales) that the shaking swarm method is more successful than OTC treatment at controlling EFB (Budge *et al.*, 2010).

Thus in an infected apiary, the following practice is recommended:

- Strongly infected colonies should be destroyed and the material disinfected.
- Covert infection or low-level overt infection should be managed by the shaking bee method, and by disinfection and sterilization of the material (managing disinfection and sterilization of material is described in section 1.9.5 above).
- If the EFB disease persists after the honeyflow, it is necessary to requeen (change the queen) in the colony,
- Feeding supplementary protein (pollen, etc.) is necessary to limit protein deficiency if the environmental conditions or the weather are bad.

The prophylaxis of EFB is achieved through the implementation of good sanitary beekeeping practices.

3 Other bacterial diseases

Some bacteria have been already described in adult diseased honeybees. However, they do not seem to endanger colonies significantly.

Septicaemia has been described in both brood and adults. The main causal agent is *Pseudomonas aeruginosa* and the clinical signs are dead or dying bees with a putrid odour. However, this bacterium, like some others found in dying bees or brood, is not specifically associated with honeybees, being common in water and soil. Infections are believed to occur, for example, after *V. destructor* feeds on the haemolymph through the cuticle (Ball, 1997).

Spiroplasmosis (*Spiroplasma apis* and *Spiroplasma melliferum*) has been described in honeybees (Mouches *et al.*, 1983; Evans and Schwartz, 2011). Spiroplasma can be found in the haemolymph of suspect infected bees and is thought to invade it through a breach in the gut epithelium. However, the scientific literature on spiroplasmosis is deficient and clinical cases have poorly been described.

References

Alippi, A.M. (1999) Bacterial diseases. In Colin, M.E., Ball, B.V., and Kilani, M. (eds), *Bee Disease Diagnosis, Options Méditerranéennes*, Serie B: *Etudes et Recherches*. No. 25. CIHEAM Publication, Zaragoza, pp. 31–55.

Alippi, A.M., Lopez, A.C., Reynaldi, F.J., Grasso, D.H., Aguilar, O.M. (2007) Evidence for plasmid-mediated tetracycline resistance in *Paenibacillus larvae*, the causal agent of American Foulbrood (AFB) disease in honeybees. *Veterinary Microbiology*, 125: 290–303.

Bailey, L. (1959a) An improved method for the isolation of *Streptococcus pluton*, and observations on its distribution and ecology. *Journal of Insect Pathology*, 1: 80–85.

Bailey, L. (1959b) Recent research on the natural history of European foulbrood. *Bee World*, 40: 66–70.

Bailey, L. (1961) European foulbrood. *American Bee Journal*, 101: 89–92.

Bailey, L. (1983) *Melissococcus pluton*, the cause of European foulbrood of honey bees (*Apis* spp.). *Journal of Applied Bacteriology*, 55: 65–69.

Bailey, L., and Ball, B.V. (1991) *Honey Bee Pathology*. Harcourt Brace Jovanovich, Sidcup.

Bailey, L. and Collins, M.D. (1982) Reclassification of *Streptococcus pluton* (White) in a new genus *Melissococcus*, as *Melissococcus pluton* nom. Rev; comb. Nov. *Journal of Applied Bacteriology*, 53: 215–217.

Ball, B.V. (1997) Varroa and viruses. In *Varroa! Fight the Mite*. IBRA, Cardiff, pp. 11–15.

Bassi, S., Carra, E., Carpana, E., Paganelli, G.L., and Pongolini, S. (2010) A scientific note on the detection of spores of *Paenibacillus larvae* in naturally and artificially contaminated honey: comparison of cultural and molecular methods. *Apidologie*, 41: 425–427.

Belloy, L., Imdorf, A., Fries, I., Forsgren, E., Berthoud, H., Kuhn, R., and Charriere, J.D. (2007) Spatial distribution of *Melissococcus plutonius* in adult honey bees collected from apiaries and colonies with and without symptoms of European foulbrood. *Apidologie*, 38: 136–140.

Budge, G.E., Barrett, B., Jones, B., Pietravalle, S., Marris, G., Chantawannakul, P., Thwaites, R., Hall, J., Cuthbertson, A.G.S., and Brown, M.A. (2010) The occurrence of *Melissococcus plutonius* in healthy colonies of *Apis mellifera* and the efficacy of European foulbrood control measures. *Journal of Invertebrate Pathology*, 105: 164–170.

De Graaf, D.C., Alippi, A.M., Brown, M., Evans, J.D., Feldlaufer M., Gregorc, A., Hornitzky, M., Pernal, S.F., Schuch, D.M.T., Titěra, D., Tomkies, V., and Ritter, W. (2006) Diagnosis of American foulbrood in honey bees: a synthesis and proposed analytical protocols. *Letters in Applied Microbiology*, 43(6): 583–590.

Del Hoyo, M.L., Basualdo, M., Lorenzo, A., Palacio, M.A., Rodriguez, E.M., and Bedascarrasbure, E. (2001) Effect of shaking honey bee colonies affected by American foulbrood on *Paenibacillus larvae larvae* spore loads. *Journal of Apicultural Research*, 40: 65–69.

Dobbelaere, W., de Graaf, D.C., Reybroeck, W., Desmedt, E., Peeters, J.E., and Jacobs, F.J. (2001) Disinfection of wooden structures contaminated with *Paenibacillus larvae* subsP. larvae spores. *Journal of Applied Microbiology*, 91: 212–216.

Evans, J.D. and Schwartz, R.S. (2012) Bees brought to their knees: microbes affecting honey bee health. *Trends in Microbiology*, 19(12): 614–620.

Evans J.D. and Spivak M.L. (2010) Socialized medicine: individual and communal disease barriers in honey bees. *Journal of Invertebrate Pathology*, 103: S62-S72.

Faucon, J.P. (2002) Conduite à tenir en cas de loque américaine. Available at: http://www.apiculture.com/sante-de-labeille/articles/conduite_loque_americaine.htm (accessed 19 August 2014)

FERA: Food & Environment Research Agency (2013) *Foulbrood Disease of Honey Bees and other Common Brood Disorders*. Food and Environment Research Agency, York.

Forsgren, E. (2010) European foulbrood in honeybees. *Journal of Invertebrate Pathology*, 103(1): S5-S9.

Forsgren E., Budge G.E., Charrière J-D., and Hornitzky, A.Z., (2013) Standard methods for European foulbrood research. *Journal of Apicultural Research*, 52(1): doi:10.3896/IBRA.1.52.1.12

Franco, S., Martel, A.C, Chauzat, M.P., Blanchard, P., and Thiéry, R. (2012) Les analyses de laboratoire en apiculture. In SNGTV (ed.), *Proceedings of the Journées nationales des GTV.* SNGTV, Nantes, pp. 859–867.

Fries, I., Lindström, A., and Korpela, S. (2006) Vertical transmission of American foulbrood (*Paenibacillus larvae*) in honey bees (*Apis mellifera*). *Veterinarian Microbiology*, 114: 269–274.

Fünfhaus, A., Ashiralieva, A., Borriss, R., and Genersch, E. (2009). Use of suppression subtractive hybridization to identify genetic differences between differentially virulent genotypes of *Paenibacillus larvae*, the etiological agent of American foulbrood of honeybees. *Environmental Microbiology Reports*, 1: 240–250.

Gende, L., Satta, A., Ligios, L., Ruiu, L., Buffa, F., Fernandez, N., Churio, S., Eguaras, M., Fiori, M., and Floris, I. (2011) Searching for an American foulbrood early detection threshold by the determination of *Paenibacillus larvae* spore load in worker honey bees. *Bulletin of Insectology*, 64(2) : 229–233.

Genersch, E. (2010) American foulbrood in honeybees and its causative agent, *Paenibacillus larvae. Journal of Invertebrate Pathology*, 103: S10-S19.

Genersch, E., Ashiralieva, A., and Fries, I. (2005) Strain- and genotype-specific differences in virulence of *Paenibacillus larvae* subsP. larvae, a bacterial pathogen causing American foulbrood disease in honeybees. *Applied and Environmental Microbiology*, 71(11): 7551–7555.

Genersch, E., Forsgren, E., Pentikåinen, J., Ashiralieva, A., Rauch, S., Kilwinski, J., and Fries, I. (2006) Reclassification of *Paenibacillus larvae* subsp. *pulvifaciens* and *Paenibacillus larvae* subsP. larvae as *Paenibacillus larvae* without subspecies differentiation. *International Journal of Systematic and Evolutionary Microbiology*, 56: 501–511.

Goodwin, R.M., Perry, J.H., and Tenhouten, A. (1994) The effect of drifting honey-bees on the spread of American foulbrood infections. *Journal of Apicultural Research*, 33: 209–212.

Hansen, H. and Brodsgaard, C.J. (1999) American foulbrood: a review of its biology, diagnosis and control. *Bee World*, 80(1): 5–23.

Hansen, H. and Brodsgaard, C.J. (2003) Control of American foulbrood by the shaking method. *Apiacta*, 38: 140–145.

Hasemann, L. (1961) How long can spores of American foulbrood live? *American Bee Journal*, 101: 298–299.

Heyndrickx, M., Vandemeulebroecke, K., Hoste, B., Janssen, P., Kersters, K., de Vos, P., Logan, N.A., Ali, N., and Berkeley, R.C.W., (1996) Reclassification of *Paenibacillus* (formerly *Bacillus*) *pulvifaciens* (Nakamura 1984) Ash et al. 1994, a later synonym of *Paenibacillus* (formerly *Bacillus*) *larvae* (White, 1906) Ash et al. 1994, as a subspecies of *P. larvae*, with emended descriptions of *P. larvae* as *P. larvae* subsP. larvae and *P. larvae* subsp. *pulvifaciens*. *International Journal of Systematic and Evolutionary Microbiology*, 46: 270–279.

Hitchcock, J.D., Stoner, A., Wilson, W.T., and Menapace, D.M., (1979) Pathogenicity of Bacillus pulvifaciens to honeybee larvae of various ages (Hymenoptera: Apidae). *Journal of the Kansas Entomological Society*, 52: 238–246.

Howard, L.O. (1907) Report of the meeting of inspectors of apiaries. *USDA, Bureau of Entomology, Bulletin 70*. USDA, San Antonio, TX.

Kochansky, J., Knox, D.A., Feldlaufer, M., and Pettis, J.S. (2001) Screening alternative antibiotics against oxytetracycline-susceptible and -resistant *Paenibacillus larvae*. *Apidologie*, 32: 215–222.

Matheson, A. and Reid, M. (1992) Strategies for prevention and control of American foulbrood. *American Bee Journal*, 132: 399–402.

McKee, B.A., Djordjevic, S.P., Goodman, R.D., and Hornitzky, M.A.Z. (2003) The detection of *Melissococcus* pluton in honey bees (*Apis mellifera*) and their products using a hemi-nested PCR. *Apidologie*, 34: 19–27.

McKee, B.A., Goodman, R.D., and Hornitzky, M.A.Z. (2004) The transmission of European foulbrood (*Melissococcus plutonius*) to artificially reared honey bee larvae (*Apis mellifera*). *Journal of Apicultural Research*, 43: 93–100.

Mill, A.C., Rushton, S.P., Shirley, M.D.F., Smith, G.C., Mason, P., Brown, M.A., and Budge, G.E. (2013) Clustering, persistence and control of a pollinator brood disease: epidemiology of American foulbrood. *Environmental Microbiology*, doi:10.1111/1462-2920.12292.

Miyagi, T., Peng, C.Y.S., Chuang, R.Y., Mussen, E.C., Spivak, M.S., and Doi R.H. (2000) Verification of oxytetracycline-resistant American foulbrood pathogen *Paenibacillus larvae* in the United States. *Journal of Invertebrate Pathology*, 75: 95–96.

Mouches, C., Bové, J.M., Tully, J.G., Rose, D.L., McCoy, R.E., Carle-Junca, P., Garnier, M., and Saillard, C. (1983) *Spiroplasma apis*, a new species from the honey-bee *Apis mellifera*. *Annals of Microbiology (Paris)*, 134A(3): 383–397.

OIE (2014a) Manual of Diagnostic Tests and Vaccines for Terrestrial Animals 2014. Apinae. Section 2.2, available at: http://www.oie.int/en/international-standard-setting/terrestrial-manual/access-online/ (accessed 24 August 2014).

OIE (2014b) OIE Listed Diseases, available at http://www.oie.int/en/animal-health-in-the-world/oie-listed-diseases-2014/ (accessed 29 April 2014).

Otten, C. and Otto, A. (2005) Epidemiology and control of the American Foulbrood in Germany, *Apiacta*, 40: 16–22.

Peng, C.Y.S., Mussen, E.C., Fong, A., Montague, M.A., and Tyler, T. (1992) Effects of chlortetracycline of honey bee worker larvae reared in vitro. *Journal of Invertebrate Pathology*, 60: 127–133.

Pernal, S.F., Albright, R.L., and Melathopoulos, A.P., (2008) Evaluation of the shaking technique for the economic management of American foulbrood disease of honey bees (Hymenoptera: Apidae). *Journal of Economic Entomology*, 101: 1095–1104.

Ritter, W. (2003) Early detection of American foulbrood by honey and wax analysis. *Apiacta*, 38: 125–130

Ritter, W. and Kiefer, M.B. (1995) A method for diagnosing *Bacillus larvae* in honey samples. *Animal Research and Development*, 42: 7–13.

Rothenbuhler, W.C. (1964) Behaviour genetics of nest cleaning in honey bees. IV. Responses of F1 and backcross generations to disease-killed brood. *American Zoologist*, 4(2): 111–123. http://dx.doi.org/10.1016/0003-3472(64)90082-X.

Rudenko, E.V. (1987) American foulbrood of honey bees and its vaccine prophylaxis. Dissertation for Doctorate of Veterinary Science, Minsk (in Russian).

Schirach, G.A. (1769) *Histoire des Abeilles*, Chapter 3, p. 56.

Shimanuki, H. and Knox, D.A. (2000) *Diagnosis of Honeybee Diseases*. United States Department of Agriculture (USDA), Agriculture Handbook No. 690.

Spivak, M. and Gilliam, M. (1998) Hygienic behaviour of honeybees and its application for control of brood diseases and varroa. Part 1. Hygienic behaviour and resistance to American foulbrood. *Bee World*, 79: 169–186.

Spivak, M.S. and Reuter, G.S., (1998) Performance of hygienic honey bee colonies in a commercial apiary. *Apidologie*, 29: 291–302.

Spivak, M.S. and Reuter, G.S. (2001) Resistance to American foulbrood disease by honeybee colonies *Apis mellifera* bred for hygienic behavior. *Apidologie*, 32: 555–565.

Tomkies, V., Flint, J., Johnson, G., Waite, R., Wilkins, S., Danks, C., Watkins, M., Cuthbertson, A.G.S., Carpana, E., Marris, G., Budge, G., and Brown, M.A. (2009) Development and validation of a novel field test kit for European foulbrood. *Apidologie*, 40: 63–72.

Tremblay, N. (2010) L'utilisation d'une chambre d'irradiation pour la désinfection du matériel apicole. Available at: http://www.agrireseau.qc.ca/

apiculture/documents/Irradiation_%20désinfection%20%20matériel%20apicole_NT%202010.pdf (accessed 24 November 2014).

Vidal-Naquet, N. and Boucher, S. (2013) La loque américaine: épidémiologie et méthodes de lute. *Bulletin des GTV*, 68: 101–107.

Von Eaton, C. (2000) Controlling AFB without drugs. New Zealand's approach. *Bee Cult*, 128: 36–40.

Waite, R., Brown, M., Thompson, H., and Bew, M. (2003) Controlling European foulbrood with the shock swarm method and oxytetracycline in the UK. *Apidologie*, 34: 569–575.

Wilkins, S., Brown, M., Andrew, A., and Cuthbertson, G.S. (2007) The incidence of honey bee pests and diseases in England and Wales. *Pest Management Science*, 63: 1062–1068.

Wilson, W.T. (1971) Resistance to American foulbrood in honey bees XI. Fate of Bacillus larvae spores ingested by adults. *Journal of Invertebrate Pathology*, 17: 247–255.

Yue, D., Nordhoff, M., Wieler, L.H., and Genersch, E. (2008) Fluorescence in situ-hybridization (FISH) analysis of the interactions between honeybee larvae and *Paenibacillus larvae*, the causative agent of American foulbrood of honeybees (*Apis mellifera*). *Environmental Microbiology*, 10: 1612–1620.

5

Parasitic diseases

Of all the stressors that can affect honeybee colonies, the mite *Varroa destructor* probably poses the greatest threat.

Numerous parasitic agents may endanger honeybee colonies:

- Mites (super-order Acari), principally *V. destructor*, *Acarapis woodi*, and *Tropilaelaps* spp. – the most significant parasites of bees.
- Insects, such as Diptera (*Braula caeca*).
- Members of the Fungi kingdom, notably the microsporidia *Nosema apis* and *Nosema cerana* and the fungus *Ascosphaera apis*.
- The amoeba *Malpighamoeba mellificae*, which is a parasite of the Malpighian tubes.

This chapter is dedicated to mites and mainly to varroosis caused by *V. destructor*; Chapter 6 will deal with fungi and amoebae; and Chapter 7 will focus on pests and predators of the hives and the colonies.

1 Varroosis: infestation by the mite *Varroa destructor*

Varroosis is a parasite of the adult and brood of the honeybee *Apis mellifera* due to a haematophagous ectoparasite Acari, *V. destructor* (Anderson and Trueman, 2000). Originally, the natural host of this mite was the Asian honeybee *Apis cerana*, and the mite is endemic in Asia. A stable mite–*A. cerana* relationship developed over a long period of co-evolution (Rosenkranz *et al.*, 2010). Sometime around the middle of the 20th century, *V. destructor* transferred to a new host, the honeybee *A. mellifera* (Oldroyd, 1999).

Today, *V. destructor* poses a major health problem as it has spread worldwide, in particular via honeybee trade and exchange practised as part of global apiculture.

Australia and some isolated locations, such as the Finnish Åland Islands and the Isle of Man (self-governing dependency of the British Crown) are *Varroa*-free areas (Official Journal of the EU, 2013, 2015; OIE, 2014a).

Varroosis, often referred to as a plague, is widely considered to be the most destructive disease of *A. mellifera*, and causes great economic loss (Boecking and Genersch, 2008). Fighting the mite in apiaries is both a necessity and a duty for beekeepers. Hence, knowledge of *V. destructor* and its biology is necessary and crucial to controlling infestation of honeybee colonies.

1.1 Regulatory status

Varroosis is a notifiable disease to the OIE (2014b). In some European countries, it is a regulated disease (Appendix 2)

1.2 History of the *Varroa destructor* global pandemic

The history of the *Varroa* pandemic begins in 1904 when an entomologist, Edward Jacobson, discovered and collected a mite present on *A. cerana* on the island of Java. This mite was named *Varroa jacobsoni* in his honour by an acarologist, Antoon Cornelis Oudemans (Oudemans, 1904).

At the beginning of the 20th century, there was no connection between the ranges of *A. cerana* and *A. mellifera*: *A. cerana* was distributed mainly in Asia, and was separated from the range of *A. mellifera* by Siberia to the north and by the desert areas of Iran and Afghanistan to the west.

In 1918 the stages of development of the mite were described in Sumatra (Lux, 1987). Between 1939 and 1953, *Varroa jacobsoni* was observed in *A. cerana* colonies in French Indochina (Toumanoff, 1939), in Singapore (Gunther, 1951), and in the far-eastern Soviet territory of Ussouriysk (Breguetova, 1953).

In the 1930s, *A. mellifera* colonies were imported into Asia to exploit their beekeeping features (in particular, their larger colonies compared to those of *A. cerana*) (Donzé, 1995). The transfer and adaptation of *Varroa* from *A. cerana* to its new host, *A. mellifera*, is supposed to have occurred between 1940 and 1960 (Grobov, 1976; Colin, 1982). However, the presence of *V. destructor* within the brood of *Apis mellifera* seems to have been first reported in Korea in 1950 (Topolska, 2001). Further observations were reported in Japan and on the north bank of the Amur River in China in 1958, and in 1963 in Hong Kong and in the Philippines (Wendling, 2012). *Varroa* expanded westward across the Soviet Union between 1953 and 1964; by the end of the 1960s it was found in Bulgarian apiaries. *Varroa* gradually spread to colonies of *A. mellifera* worldwide, due to the international trade in honeybees (package bees, artificial swarms, queens).

In 1966, the pathogenic effect and damage the mite caused to *A. mellifera* colonies was first highlighted. In 1971, during the Apimondia World Congress in Moscow, an official alert was raised. Varroa was first described in European apiaries in 1976 in Bulgaria (Grobov, 1976). *Varroa* was reported in Germany in 1981, in France in 1982, and in the US in 1987. In 1992, its arrival in England was reported (FERA, 2013a).

Today, *Varroa* is spread worldwide. Australia and the Åland Islands in Finland are the only officially *Varroa*-free zones thanks to quarantine measures by the authorities.

1.3 *Varroa destructor*: taxonomy

Varroa destructor belongs to the class Arachnida, subclass Acari, order Mesostigmata, and family Varroidae. Until recently, *Varroa* on *A. mellifera* was identified as *Varroa jacobsoni*. However, in 2000, Anderson and Trueman identified 18 haplotypes of the mite and proposed classing these into two species (Anderson and Trueman, 2000; Wendling, 2012):

- *Varroa jacobsoni* (9 haplotypes) infests only *A. cerana*.
- *Varroa destructor* (6 haplotypes) infests *A. cerana*, though two of these haplotypes may also parasitize *A. mellifera*.
- Three haplotypes could not be classified as belonging to either of these two species.

Thus, the mite causing varroosis in *A. mellifera* is *V. destructor*.

1.4 *Varroa destructor*: morphology and anatomic details

A distinct sexual dimorphism characterizes *V. destructor* adults. The immature stages are: egg, protonymph, and deutonymph.

1.4.1 The female adult

The mites observed on adult honeybees are exclusively adult females: they are in the phoretic phase of their life cycle and called phoretic *Varroa* (Figures 5.1 and 5.2).

Female adults of *V. destructor* have an oval-shaped and dorsoventrally flattened body, approximately 1.2 mm × 1.7 mm (Anderson and Trueman, 2000). The colour of the body changes from light brown after the last moult to dark reddish in 24–48 hours (Donzé, 1995).

The weight of this mite is on average 325 μg when phoretic and may reach approximately 480 μg when breeding within the capped brood cell (Garrido *et al.*, 2000). *Varroa* mites are eyeless and blind.

The body is composed of two well-defined parts: the idiosoma and the gnathosoma (Figures 5.3 and 5.4) (Rosenkrantz *et al.*, 2010, Wendling, 2012):

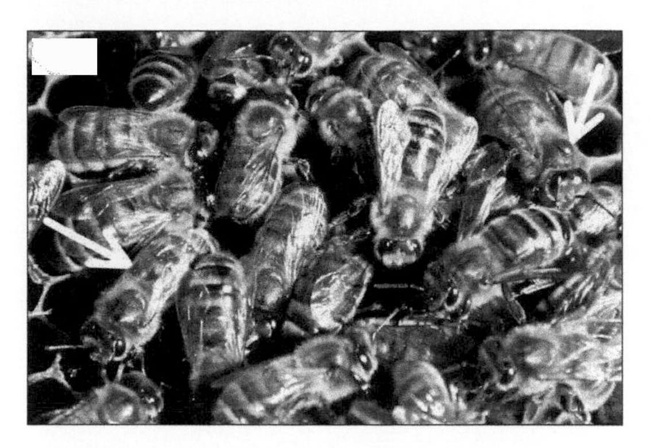

Figure 5.1 Phoretic *Varroa destructor* on adult worker honeybees (see white arrows). (© Nicolas Vidal-Naquet.)

- The idiosoma is composed of one dorsal sclerotized shield also called the scutum and several ventral sclerotized scuta. The shields are bound together with thin and flexible membranes, allowing dilatation of the body during periods of feeding and breeding. On the ventral side and between the shields open the genital and anal orifices. The four pairs of legs are short and strong. They are attached to the ventral shields. The first pair of legs is believed to play a sensory role with an olfactory pit organ, and gustatory and thermosensitive chemoreceptors located on the tarsis. The three other pairs of legs are involved in locomotion and terminate in the apoteles, specialized structures for adherence to the host (De Ruijter and Kaas, 1983).
- The gnathosoma forms the mouthparts and is situated cranially on the ventral side. It is composed of the oral cavity opening at the basis of the hypostoma, two sensory pedipalps, and two chelicerae. The two chelicerae are formed by three segments: the basal, middle, and distal digits (Rosenkranz *et al.*, 2010). The distal one is movable and has two teeth forming a blade able to pierce the cuticle of the host for feeding. The tritosternum is a Y-shaped sensory structure caudally located to the gnathosoma.

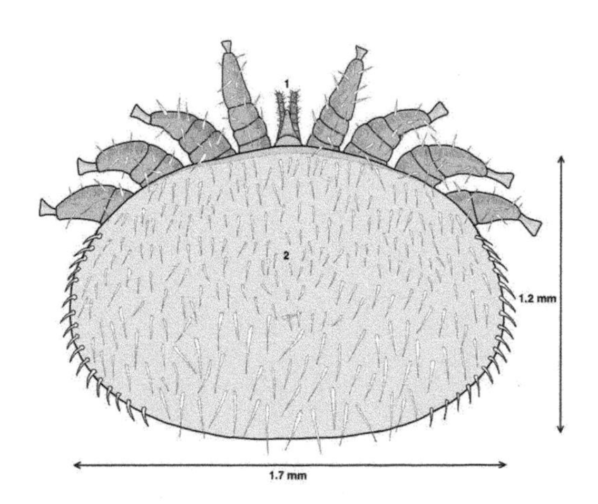

Figure 5.3 Dorsal morphology of *Varroa destructor* mature female: (1) gnathosoma; (2) dorsal scutum. (Nicolas Vidal-Naquet adapted from Langhé *et al.*, 1976.)

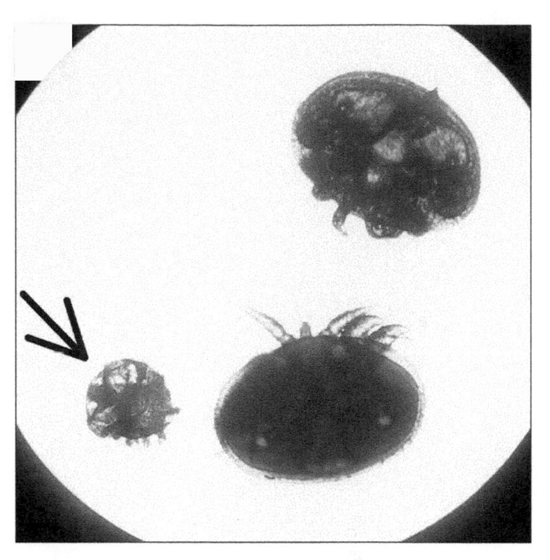

Figure 5.2 Microscopic examination of two adult females and one male (arrow) *Varroa destructor*. (Photo courtesy © Lydia Vilagines, DMV.)

The whole body is covered with different types of hairs. Some of these have sensory functions, in particular as mechano- and chemoreceptors.

The female genitalia is composed of two systems:

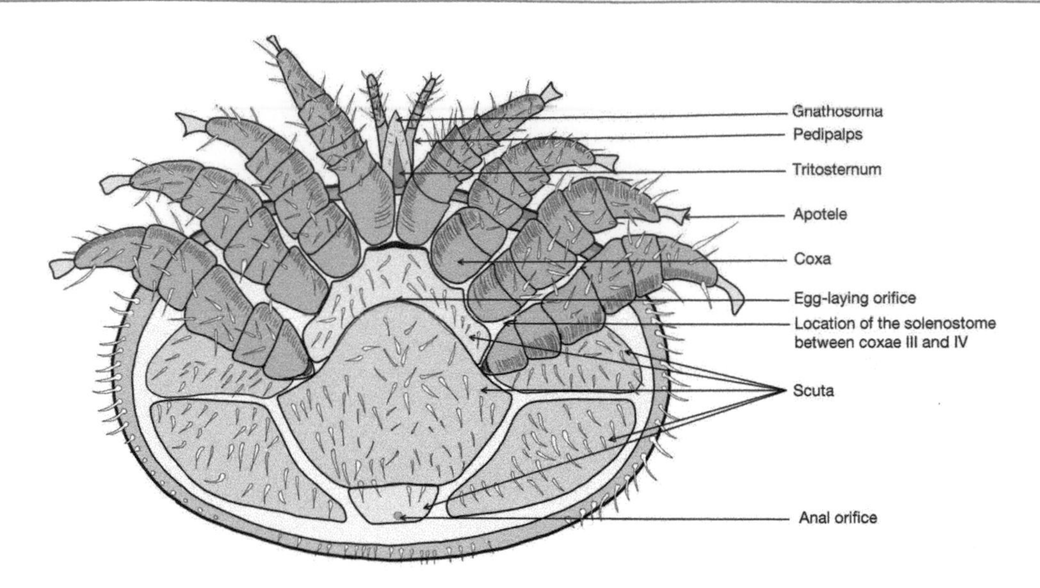

Figure 5.4 Ventral morphology of *Varroa destructor* mature female (Nicolas Vidal-Naquet adapted from Wendling, 2012; Tofilski, 2012; The World's Best Photos of *Varroa*, 2014.)

- One ovary, a uterus, and a vagina releasing the eggs via a genital (egg-laying) orifice situated between the second pair of legs.
- The second part is dedicated to the reception and maturing of the spermatozoa. Two pores, the solenostomes, situated between coxae III and IV, allow copulation. Each one opens up into a tubulus followed by a ramus. The two rami coalesce to form the sperm duct, which leads to the spermatheca (which serves as a reservoir for the spermatozoa).

The spermatheca, the ovary, and the uterus are connected to form a structure called the camera spermatica. The ovary with two lyrate organs (which have a nutritional function during oogenesis) is located ventrally to the spermatheca (De Ruijter and Kaas, 1983; Alberti and Zeck-Kapp, 1986).

1.4.2 The male adult

The *Varroa* male lives inside the capped brood cell. It is reported to be unable to feed by itself and is very sensitive to dehydration and dies quickly after the emergence of the parasitized young honeybee (Moritz and Jordan, 1992).

The male body is smaller than the female's (on average 0.75 mm × 0.70 mm), and is almost spherical (pear-shaped) with a light yellow colour (Colin *et al.*, 1999; Rosenkranz *et al.*, 2010). The body is weakly sclerotized except at the level of the legs (Figure 5.2).

The male genital system is composed in a single testis in the rear of the body. Two vasa deferens emerge from the testis and coalesce into an ejaculatory duct opening at the edge of the sternogenital scutum between the long second pair of legs. Spermatozoa are transferred into the female genital tract at the level of the solenostomes by means of the spermatodactyl (Alberti and Hänel, 1986). This tubular structure is an adaptation of the distal digit of the chelicera to fertilization. This mode of fertilization is called podospermy (Wendling, 2012).

1.4.3 The life cycle

The life cycle of *V. destructor* has two distinct phases:

- A phoretic phase when the female mites stay on the adult honeybees.
- A reproductive phase which occurs inside the capped drone and worker brood cells.

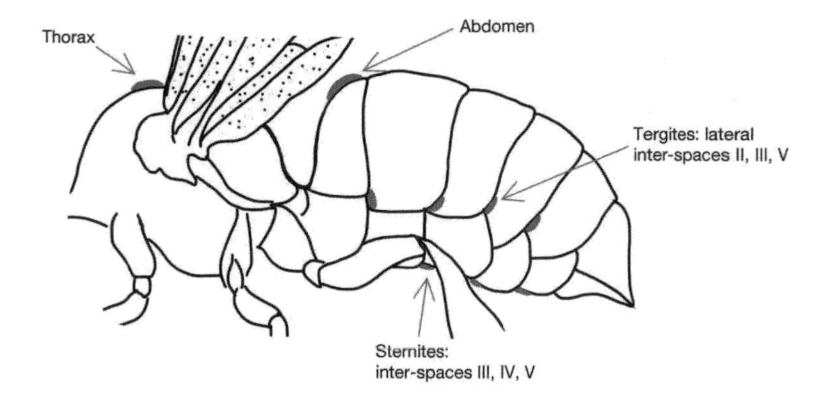

Figure 5.5 Prime positions of *Varroa destructor* in the phoretic stage to escape the grooming behaviour of bees. (Adapted from Delfinado-Baker *et al.*, 1992; Wendling, 2012.)

The phoretic phase

The phoretic phase allows mites to be transported by adult bees to brood cells for reproduction but also to spread by foraging, robbing, drifting, and swarming. The mites feed on honeybee haemolymph, withdrawing substantial amounts from adults and pupae (Rosenkranz *et al.*, 2010). On adult honeybees, the mites usually stay and hide in the inter-sternite and inter-tergite spaces but also on the thorax and the abdomen in order to protect themselves from the grooming behaviour of the host (Figure 5.5) (Delfinado-Baker *et al.*, 1992). In the wintering period when the colony is broodless, *Varroa* females may survive the overwintering period and continue their life cycle when the brood is reared again in spring.

After emerging on young bees, the mites infest older workers, aged on average 12–14 days. These middle-aged workers are mainly nurse bees. This strategy is believed to be an adaptation *Varroa* has made to achieve successful reproduction.

Another crucial point is the role of the fifth instar larvae of the honeybee just before cell capping. The fifth instar larvae secrete volatile organic compounds that have an attractive effect on the phoretic mite (Pernal *et al.*, 2005). Attractive chemicals, and in particular aliphatic esters secreted by the honeybee larvae, play a crucial role throughout the *Varroa* life cycle (Le Conte *et al.*, 1989).

The reproductive phase

After entering the cell, the reproductive phase of the mites begins (Figure 5.6). The mite entering the cell is called the founder mother mite.

The reproductive cycle of *V. destructor* occurs more often in drone brood than in worker brood. The mite tends to reproduce in drone brood for several reasons: the uncapped brood period in drones' cells is longer than in workers, drone larvae are visited more frequently by nurses and receive more food than worker larvae, and the cells of drone brood are larger than those of workers (Wendling, 2012). This tendency is important to consider in the management of *Varroa* infestation.

The founder mother mite passes between the cell wall and the larva and then stays in the larval jelly. This may be an adaptation to hide from cleaning workers (Rosenkranz *et al.*, 2010). Immediately before capping, the mite feeds on the haemolymph after piercing the larval cuticle. Several mites may enter a brood cell before capping in order to reproduce (Martin, 1995).

The mite weight increases and its morphology changes with the ventral part becoming convex. Oogenesis followed by vitellogenesis allows the laying of a first egg on average 70 hours after cell capping (Rosenkranz *et al.*, 2010). The sex determination of *V. destructor* is a haplodiploid system. The first egg laid is unfertilized and develops into a haploid male. Subsequent eggs

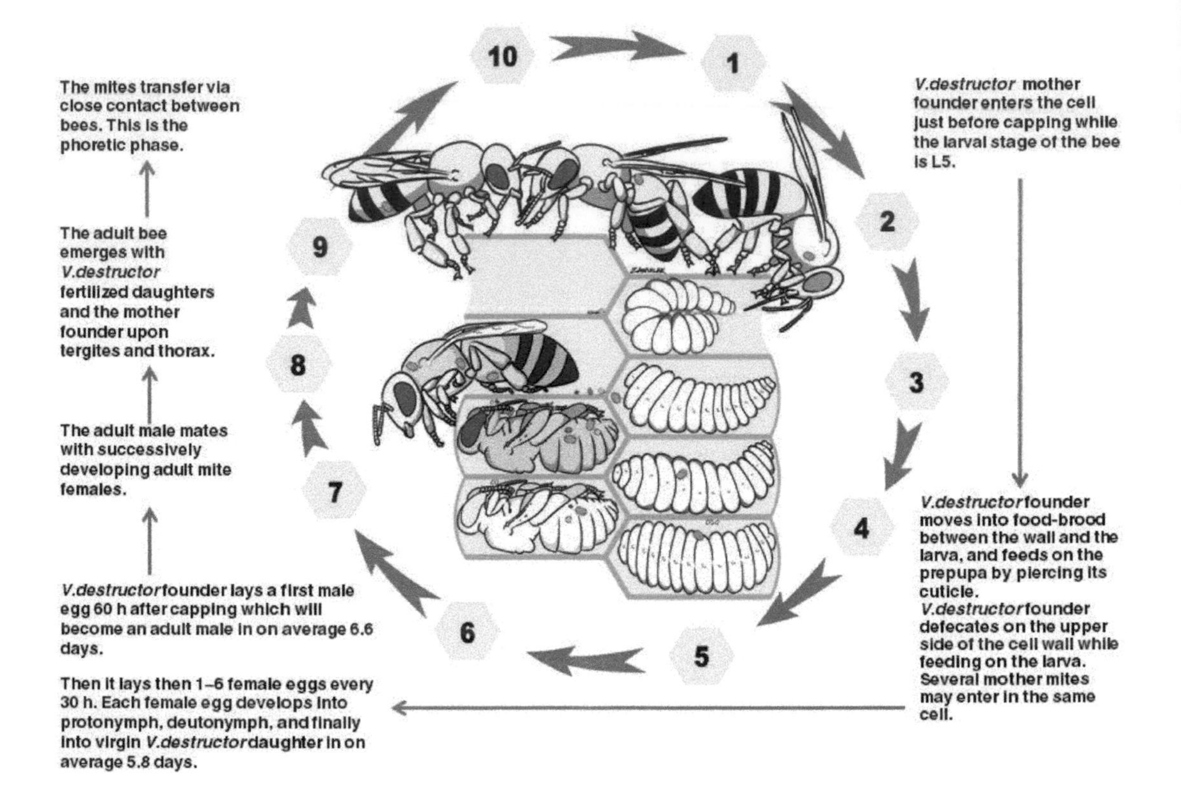

Figure 5.6 The life cycle of *Varroa destructor*. This cycle takes place in the brood cell. (Drawing © Jon Zawislak, University of Arkansas; text Nicolas Vidal-Naquet.)

are laid approximately every 30 hours and will develop into diploid females. In the worker brood, the mite may theoretically lay up to five eggs and in the drone brood up to six eggs, due to the longer capped brood period in drone cells than in worker cells (Rosenkranz *et al.*, 2010).

The development of the mite larva begins within the mite egg wall soon after oviposition. After hatching out of the egg, the protonymph and deutonymph stages occur, followed by the imaginal moult. Both these stages are divided into a mobile and an immobile pharate phase (Donzé and Guerin, 1994; Rosenkranz *et al.*, 2010). Ontogenesis lasts on average 5.8 days for female mites and 6.6 days for male mites (Rosenkranz *et al.*, 2010).

The development of *Varroa* eggs depends on brood homeostasis. Thus, outside a temperature range 31–37°C in the honeybee brood, *Varroa* eggs cannot develop and development of the bee brood is also impaired (Wendling, 2012). Mobile *Varroa* immature forms feed on the honeybee pupa through a single hole pierced in the cuticle by the mother mite. This hole is usually located on the fifth segment of the bee pupa. This feeding site is situated close to the 'faecal accumulation site' where the mites return to after feeding (Donzé and Guerin, 1994; Kanbar and Engels, 2003).

Varroa mites are sexually mature after the imaginal moult. The male matures before the female and waits at the faecal accumulation site for the first mature female to appear approximately 20 hours later. Then, the male starts mating with the first mature mite female. Several matings occur as further mature females appear. The spermatozoa are stored in the spermatheca of the *Varroa* females. Volatile female pheromones initiate mating behaviour and ensure the youngest females are the most attractive (Ziegelmann *et al.*, 2008; Rosenkranz *et al.*, 2010).

After the imaginal moult of the honeybee, female adult mites stay on one of the tergites before the emergence. After the emergence of the adult honeybee, only the mated female adult *Varroa* will survive and spread (Wendling, 2012). Immature females and males are not able to survive when the cell opens for the emergence of the young bee (Donzé, 1995; Martin, 1994)

Under natural conditions:

- A female *Varroa* can perform on average two to three reproductive cycles (Martin and Kemp, 1997; Rosenkranz *et al.*, 2010).
- The reproduction rate (number of viable adult offspring/mother mite) has been calculated to be 1.3–1.45 in a single infested worker brood and 2.2–2.6 in a single infested drone brood (due to the longer capping brood period) (Martin, 1994, 1995).

The success of *Varroa* female reproduction (and of reproduction rate) depends on (Rosenkranz *et al.*, 2010; Wendling, 2012):

- The survival of the female mite during the phoretic phase.
- The brood and in particular the drone brood.
- The fertility of female mites. Some *Varroa* female are infertile for reasons currently unknown. However, host factors, sexual maturity, and other factors are suspected.
- The number of mother mites infesting a single brood cell. In the case of multiple infestation of one cell, the reproductive rate per mother mite seems to be reduced (Mondragon *et al.*, 2006, Rosenkrantz *et al.*, 2010).
- The production and the maturation of at least one male and one female egg in the brood cell.
- The temperature (optimally between 36 and 38°C) and the humidity (optimally 70%; reproduction is impossible when the humidity level is higher than 80%).

1.4.4 *Varroa* population dynamics in honeybee colonies

The mite population in a honeybee colony increases after the first infestation. This population growth depends on several factors, including the initial mite population, the presence of brood, and other features of mite reproductive biology. The mite population also depends on 'reinfestation' due to drifting and robbing behaviours of bees during the beekeeping season.

In Europe and North America, a maximum threshold of 1,000–4,000 mites in a colony is considered as critical to colony health (Rosenkrantz *et al.*, 2010; Wendling, 2012; FERA, 2013b). A threshold of 1,000 mites is commonly used in the United Kingdom. In other parts of Europe, the average threshold is 2,000 mites per colony. Beyond this threshold, colonies face a significant risk of collapsing in the following months (Noireterre, 2011). This infestation level is known as the economic injury level (FERA, 2013a). The main fact to consider is that the increase in the *Varroa* population in a colony is a consequence of both reproduction of the mite within the capped brood cells and of new mites being introduced by robbing or drifting bees.

An infested colony may be reinfested by mites transported by drifting and robbing bees. This mainly occurs in areas with a high density of colonies.

Although some population dynamics models have been proposed, the evolution of the mite population from spring to autumn is quite difficult to predict due to the wide variety of factors influencing mite and colony biology and the mite–colony relationship (and in particular reinfestation by drifting and robbing behaviours). However, some authors have provided explanations for the increases in *Varroa* population (Martin, 1998; Noireterre, 2011; FERA, 2013b).

Modelling is important to understand the relationships between the mite, the colony, and environmental factors, and thus to set up prophylactic and control strategies to deal with *Varroa* (Martin, 1998, Wendling, 2012). The

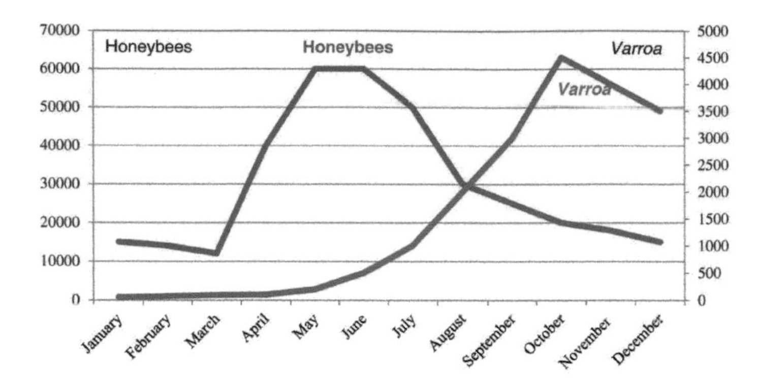

Figure 5.7 Annual population dynamics of *Varroa*. (Adapted from Noireterre, 2011; OIE, 2014b.)

mite population in a colony can double every 20 days in the spring and summer (Fries *et al.*, 1994).

Considering the entire beekeeping season in a temperate climate area, the number of *Varroa* increases slowly at the beginning, the maximum is reached late in the season (OIE, 2014a), and the mite population then decreases when wintering (when the brood rearing decreases and stops) (Figure 5.7).

However, the dynamics of the *Varroa* population in any given year depends on the number of mites present in a colony at the beginning of the season (Noireterre, 2011; FERA, 2013b).

At the beginning of a beekeeping season, before spring laying restarts following overwintering, it is usually considered that the infestation level in a colony should be less than a maximum threshold of 50 *Varroa* (Noireterre, 2011) (Figure 5.8). This threshold is also considered to be the maximum for a colony before wintering to limit the risk of winter colony mortality.

If the initial number of mites infesting a colony is higher, the risk threshold of 1,000–2,000 mites

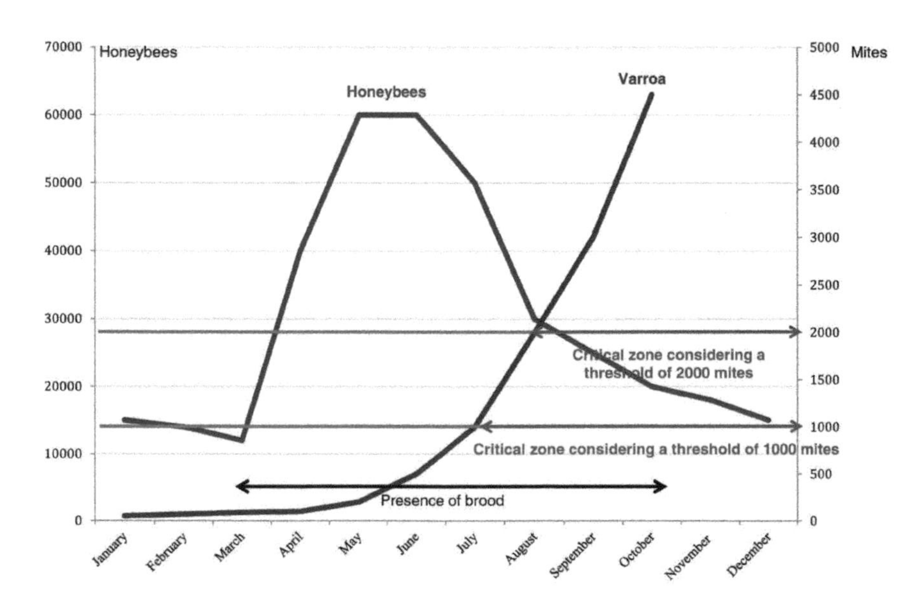

Figure 5.8 Population dynamics of *Varroa destructor* (from an initial 50 mites) within a colony of *Apis melliferra*. (Adapted from Noireterre, 2011.)

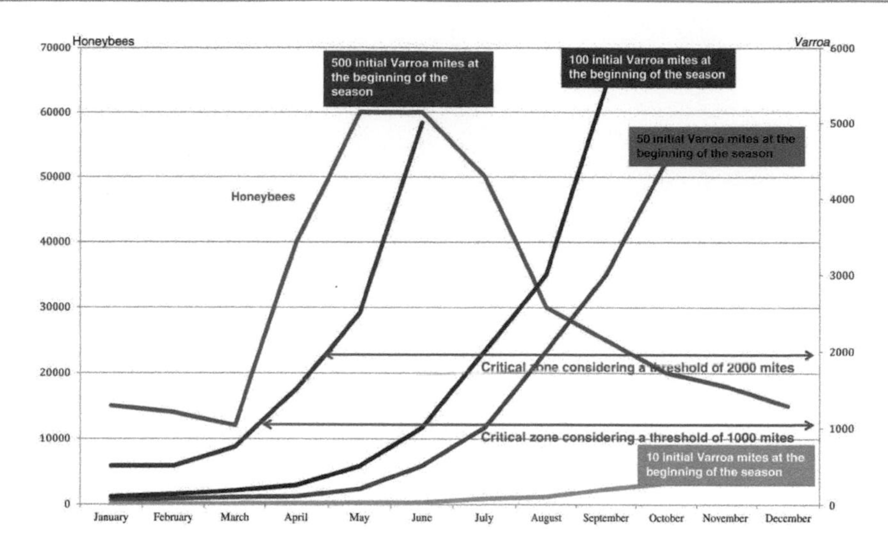

Figure 5.9 Consequences of different initial infestation levels of *Varroa* (10, 50, 100, and 500 mites) on the population dynamics and on the time to reach the critical threshold of 1,000 mites (UK) or 2,000 mites. (Adapted from Noireterre, 2011; FERA, 2013b.)

per colony (see above) will be reached sooner, posing a major risk to the colony's health and strength and therefore its productivity. The colony will also be at greater risk during the subsequent overwintering period (Figure 5.9).

In the event of 'reinfestation' during the season, the mite population may increase faster even if the initial infestation was below the 50 mites threshold (Figure 5.10) at the beginning of the season. Reinfestation may occur in areas

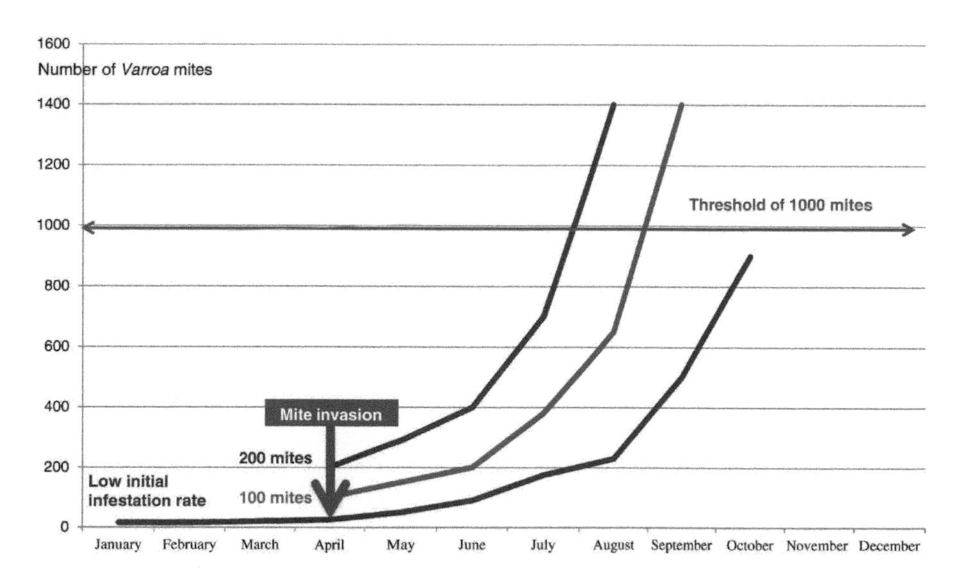

Figure 5.10 Effect of mite reinfestation during the season (from drifting and robbing bees) on subsequent mite population growth (adapted from FERA, 2013b). In the event of reinfestation, the risk threshold will be reached earlier within the season. This is a further important argument for monitoring *Varroa* infestation of colonies throughout the year.

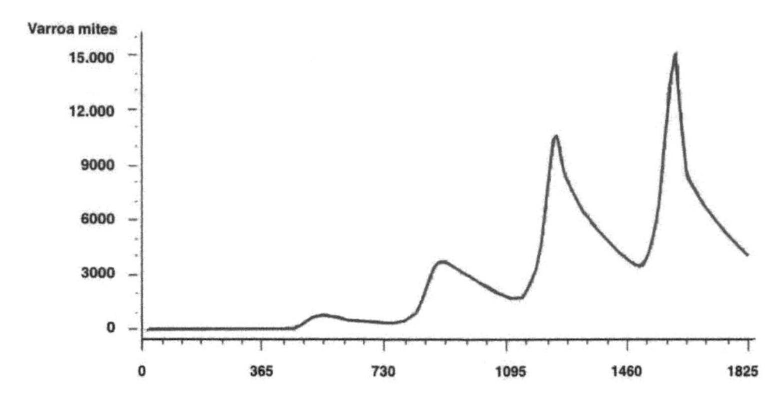

Figure 5.11 Mite population dynamics over 1,825 days (5 years). At D0, the population is 10 mites. (Fries *et al.*, 1994.)

with a high density of colonies by drifting or robbing behaviour. Reinfestation may also occur when control of *Varroa* infestation is inadequate or inefficient within an apiary or within neighbouring apiaries.

If several years elapse without any treatment and control measures, the dynamics of *Varroa* mite population will lead to an annually increasing harmful infestation of the colony far beyond the risk threshold (Figure 5.11).

In temperate climate regions, studies have shown that, due to the population dynamics of *Varroa*, colonies are at major risk of collapse from varroosis within 3–4 years after the initial infestation if nothing is done (Korpela *et al.*, 1993; Büchler, 1994, Rosenkranz *et al.*, 2010). However, in subtropical and tropical regions, *Varroa* infestation in *A. mellifera* colonies does not appear to impact colony size, health, and productivity (Muli *et al.*, 2014). Under tropical conditions, a low rate of *Varroa* growth in colonies has been reported (Rosenkranz *et al.*, 2010).

1.5 Varroosis

Varroosis is a disease of the honeybee *A. mellifera* due to the mite *V. destructor* affecting larvae, pupae, and adult bees (Grobov, 1976). Currently, varroosis must be considered as the consequence of *Varroa* infestation associated with the viruses this may transmit to the honeybees. The term 'bee parasitic mite syndrome' is probably more appropriate.

Infestation of honeybee colonies by *Varroa destructor* (and the resulting varroosis) is one of the OIE-listed diseases, infections, and infestations of honeybees (OIE, 2014a).

At the colony level, the clinical signs of varroosis are mainly weakening and collapse. Thus, pollination and honey production may be impaired.

1.5.1 Pathogenesis

The mite infestation is responsible for wide-ranging damage at both individual and colony levels, infesting and affecting both immature and adult forms.

Spoliage effect

Varroa is a haematophagous parasite of the honeybee. It has a spoliatory action on pupae and adult bees by damaging the cuticle to feed on haemolymph. Studies show lower protein concentrations in the haemolymph of infested bees (Bowen-Walker and Gun, 2001; Boecking and Genersch, 2008). In worker larvae, the reduction in the overall level of protein within the haemolymph is estimated at 27% and 50% in cases of single or double infestation (i.e. two mother founder mites infesting one cell), respectively. In drone larvae, the reduction in the overall quantity of protein within the haemolymph is reported to be lower, reaching approximately 12% irrespective of the infestation rate (Weinberg and Madel, 1985).

Effects on bee weight

Infestation by the mite induces a loss of weight of adult bees emerging from infested pupae. This weight loss depends on the number of mother mite founders and the level of mite reproduction (Rozenkranz *et al.*, 2010).

It has been reported that a single infestation within a brood cell induces a loss of body weight estimated to be 7–10% in adult honeybees emerging from such cells (De Jong *et al.*, 1982; Schatton-Gadelmayer and Engels, 1988; Kotwal and Abrol, 2009). When 3–5 mother mites infest a brood cell, the loss is estimated to be approximately 18% in newly emerging honeybees (Kotwal and Abrol, 2009). Infested bees are not able to attain their usual adult weight when infested during their development.

Reduction of lifespan

Varroa infestation is responsible for a reduction in the life expectancy of honeybees. It has been reported that adult workers from infested brood have shorter lifespans (Schneider and Drescher, 1987). In a colony, the lifespan of honeybees is reduced when the infestation increases (Kovac and Crailsheim, 1988; Ritter *et al.*, 1984). A study performed in Germany in 1984 reported that in colonies considered as weakly, averagely, or strongly infested, the life expectancy of workers was respectively estimated to be 15.6, 9.1, and 8.3 days between May and September (Ritter *et al.*, 1984). (The normal life span of workers in summer in temperate countries is considered to be up to 38 days (Winston, 1987).) Concerning drones, a study by Rinderer *et al.* (1999) has shown a reduction of their life expectancy too.

In summer, workers parasitized during their development have a significantly reduced lifespan and start their foraging activity earlier (Rozenkrantz *et al.*, 2010).

In the case of winter bees, infestation of the brood may prove a real problem for the strength of the colony for overwintering. Indeed, newly emerging bees from infested cells will not be able to ensure their role, in particular in the regulation of homeostasis during wintering. Thus, this will have negative consequences for the health and strength of the colony during overwintering and at the beginning of the next beekeeping season, and pose the risk of weakening and collapse (Amdam *et al.*, 2004; Wendling, 2012).

Morphological and anatomical deformities

Externally, the body of infested adult bees may appear shorter with a shortened abdomen and crippled wings (Figure 3.4). These deformities are considered to be the consequences of the transmission of DWV by *Varroa* at the larval or pupal stage (Rosenkrantz *et al.*, 2010).

Internally, the infestation of a pupa of a worker bee is responsible for a 15% reduction in the size of the hypopharyngeal glands (Schneider and Drescher, 1987), which can lead to problems with brood and queen nursing and can adversely affect the transformation of nectar into honey. It has been reported that the nursing stage is shortened (which may be linked to the earlier occurrence of the foraging task reported previously) (Janmaat and Winston, 2000).

Behavioural troubles

The learning and navigational abilities of parasitized foragers are impaired with consequences for orientation, flight, and successful return to the hive (Kralj *et al.*, 2007; Rosenkrantz *et al.*, 2010). These foragers may come back more slowly or not at all. In strongly infested colonies, there may be a major and rapid loss of foragers, soon leaving only the queen and a few hive workers (Wendling, 2012).

The infested foragers do not all die outside; some of them enter foreign hives, spreading the mite to other colonies (drifting behaviour). This behaviour is increased in strongly infested colonies (Sakofski *et al.*, 1990). Thus, the spread of the mite is potentiated by the impaired foraging behaviour.

Decrease in the reproductive potential of drones

Some authors report that the production and quality of spermatozoa are affected by *Varroa* infestation (Del Cacho *et al.*, 1996; Duay *et al.*, 2002). However, the main factor reducing reproductive ability is the loss of body weight of parasitized drones, leading to impairment of their flight performance, and rendering them unable to fertilize virgin queens (Duay *et al.*, 2002).

Immunosuppression effect on honeybees

Haemocyte concentration, which plays a role in immunity, is decreased in emerging workers parasitized during the pupal stage, but also in nurse bees in strongly infested colonies (Amdam *et al.*, 2004; Belaïd and Doumandji, 2010). Furthermore, *V. destructor* induces a reduction in the expression of the genes coding for antimicrobial peptides and enzymes linked to immunity, with consequences for the humoral and cellular immune response (Yang and Cox-Foster, 2005; Navajas *et al.*, 2008; Wendling, 2012). This mite-induced immunosuppression increases the sensitivity to pathogens and in particular viruses (Yang and Cox-Foster, 2005; Wendling, 2012).

Influence of mite infestation on gene expression

Varroa infestation is responsible for changes in the 'expression of genes related to embryonic development, cell metabolism and immunity' (Navajas *et al.*, 2008). Genes encoding antimicrobial peptides (abaecin, defensin, hymenoptaecin) and immunity-related enzymes (phenol oxidase, glucose dehydrogenase, glucose oxydase, lysozyme) are down-regulated (Yang and Cox-Foster, 2005). This immunosuppression probably favours the proliferation of pathogens and in particular DWV, causing cellular and molecular damage and consequently deformed abdomens, legs, and wings in bees. Furthermore, the expression of two genes (*slg* and *dlg1*) involved in development and metamorphosis is down-regulated by mite infestation (Navajas *et al.*, 2008). This down-regulation may be the consequence of the mite directly or via DWV.

The expression of the gene *pale* encoding tyramine hydroxylase and involved in dopamine synthesis is inhibited. This has consequences on neural development, in particular on behaviour, cognition, and learning (Navajas *et al.*, 2008). Searchers have also reported the down-regulation of genes involved in preventing progressive neural degeneration (*Dclic2* and *Atg18* gene enhancers of the blue cheese gene (*bchs*)) (Navajas *et al.*, 2008). Such inhibitions could explain, at least in part, the decrease in learning ability, the prolonged absences from the nest, and the lower rate of successful to return to the colony of foragers.

Vector of viruses (cf. Chapter 3)

Varroa destructor is a vector of viruses. The pathogenic effect of *Varroa* is considered as due to the combination of direct action by the mite and its role in transmitting viruses. Furthermore, the pathogenicity of some viruses in association or interaction with *Varroa* is increased (de Miranda *et al.* 2012).

The main viruses transmitted by *Varroa* are: ABPV (Figure 3.7), KBV, IAPV, DWV (Figure 3.4), and SBPV (Rosenkranz *et al.*, 2010). BQCV seems to be occasionally transmitted by *Varroa* (de Miranda *et al.*, 2012).

The clinical signs of varroosis affecting the brood and the morphological and behavioural symptoms leading to the weakening or collapse of a colony are the consequences of viral affects combined with the mite's pathogenic action. Currently, 'bee parasitic mite syndrome' is considered to be mainly the consequence of the combined pathogenic effects of *Varroa* and DWV.

Effects of varroosis at the colony level

Because the colony unit is a super-organism, all pathogenic effects on individuals may have major consequences for the strength and health of the colony.

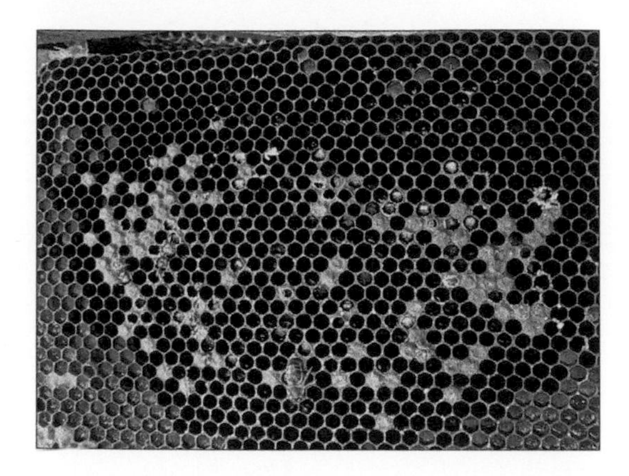

Figure 5.12 Appearance of a comb of a dead colony caused by varroosis. Note the reduced and scattered brood. (Photo courtesy © Lydia Vilagines, DVM.)

In a colony, *V. destructor*, via its damaging, mutilating, transmitting, and immunodeficiency-causing effects, increases mortality rate, reduces brood area, and adversely affects harvesting (Vidal-Naquet, 2011). The brood may appear mottled and scattered.

Infested honeybees are unable to maintain their social roles and labour activities. Thus, colonies may be weakened, allowing for an increased sensitivity to viral and bacterial diseases. A high mite infestation level leads to collapse of the colony. Thus, varroosis can have economic consequences, in particular by altering pollination activity and the production of honey.

1.5.2 Clinical signs of varroosis

The word varroosis is currently taken to cover both *Varroa* infestation and vectored virus infection ('bee parasitic mite syndrome'). The clinical signs of varrosis are as follows:

- When the mite infestation level is low, there are usually no clinical signs.
- In the case of moderate infestation level, the population of honeybees and the population dynamics are impaired. Honey production is also affected.
- When the *Varroa* infestation rate in a colony is high, the symptoms of varroosis usually observed are typical of 'bee parasitic mite syndrome' (Rosenkranz et al, 2010; Noireterre, 2011):
  - Adult honeybees with deformities, in particular wing deformities.
  - Crawling adult bees, crippled bees.
  - Scattered brood, due to the reproduction of *Varroa* within the cells.
  - Supersedure of queens.
  - Weakening of the colony and sometimes collapse and death of the colony as the final step of the disease. Dead colonies often contain a few living or dead bees, honey and pollen stocks, and some residual sealed brood.
  - The presence of mites on adult bees (phoretic *Varroa*) and in the uncapped brood cells.
  - A significant reduction in the bee population.

Therefore, given that *V. destructor* poses a major threat to colonies, fighting this mite is essential. To control infestation, treatments as well as beekeeping practices and selection are necessary.

1.5.3 Infestation threshold

The effect of infestation rate varies according to climate and season:

- Considering winter bees: under temperate conditions (e.g. Germany): a rate of 7% of winter bees infested by the mite may lead to colony collapse (Liebig, 2001). Before and during wintering, a threshold of 50 mites per colony is considered to be the highest infestation level acceptable in order to limit the risk of winter colony mortality and ensure as far as possible the expected development through the following beekeeping season.
- Considering summer bees: untreated colonies with approximately 30% of summer bees infested by *Varroa* will not survive to the following overwintering period (Fries *et al.*, 2003; Rosenkranz *et al.*, 2006, 2010).

- Control of *Varroa* infestation during the beekeeping season varies from region to region; the objective is to keep the *Varroa* population under 1,000 mites per colony in the UK, and from 2,000 to 4,000 in other parts of Europe and the US (Noireterre, 2011; FERA, 2013a). According to the Animal & Plant Health Agency, formerly FERA (FERA, 2013a), above 1,000 mites per colony there is a 'very significant' risk of 'bee mite parasitic syndrome' occurring. A threshold of between 1,000 and 2,000 mites per colony seems to be reasonable.

The following sections show that monitoring the infestation rate of the colonies throughout the year is crucial for optimal and adequate control of *Varroa*.

1.5.4 Diagnosis

Diagnosis of *Varroa* infestation is the consequence of the identification of the mite within the colony. *Varroa destructor* is quite easy to recognise. The female mite is dark reddish/brown with a flat, oval, crab-shaped body (1.1 mm × 1.5 mm) and can be seen with the nake eyes (Figure 5.1).

Differential diagnosis must consider:

- Other mites: *Tropilaelaps* spp. and *Melittiphis alvearius* (which is not a parasite of honeybee colonies, but a scavenger of pollen in beehives).
- The fly *Braula coeca*.

The methods of identification are:

- Debris examination.
- Examination of capped brood (mainly drone capped brood), by opening the capped brood with a honey uncapping fork.
- Examination of a sample of bees.

These methods are described in section 1.6.2 below.

However, qualitative diagnosis is not sufficient. Indeed, except for a few Varroa-free areas, all colonies in Europe and in many other regions are infested by *Varroa*. As previously described, it is crucial to evaluate and monitor the mite infestation level.

1.6 Control of *Varroa* infestation

Varroa is reported as a major cause in weakening and collapse of overwintering colonies in Europe and North America. Furthermore, according to Rosenkrantz *et al.* (2010), 'without any doubt, most of the colonies of *A. mellifera* in temperate climates will be damaged or even collapse within a few years if no control or inappropriate control methods are used'.

Controlling *Varroa* infestation means keeping the *Varroa* population under the threshold at which it becomes a threat to the colony (on average 1,000–2,000 mites in the beekeeping season). The fight against the mite involves the use of medicines (miticides) and biotechnical methods.

However, control of *Varroa* infestation needs to use scientifically proven methods performed with objectives as proposed, for example, by an integrated pest management (IPM) approach (FERA, 2013a). Management of *Varroa* infestation control involves knowledge of the *Varroa* life cycle and biology, and practical knowledge of the mite infestation rate obtained by monitoring colonies.

Finally, research on mite-tolerant bees suggests that using these for breeding might prove an effective method of control.

1.6.1 Good beekeeping practices

Proper control of *Varroa* infestation in an apiary requires in the first instance knowledge of and the respect for good sanitary beekeeping practices (cf. Chapter 8).

For a beekeeper, knowledge of *Varroa*'s biology and reproductive cycle, maintaining strong and vigorous colonies that exhibit good hygienic behaviour, and limiting robbing and drifting behaviours are essential practices (Spivak, 1996). Veterinarian practitioners in the field, for example while undertaking a sanitary audit of an apiary or when prescribing veterinary medicine products (VMPs), must advise that these good sanitary practices be followed.

1.6.2 Monitoring the colony parasite load (mite infestation)

Knowledge of the mite infestation rate in a colony, or a sample of colonies in a large apiary, is necessary for adequate and optimal control.

Several methods have been described. However, it must be taken into account that these are often time consuming. Thus, in the field, veterinarians and beekeeper must chose methods capable of implementation and best suited to the beekeeping management being practised.

Monitoring natural mite fall

The aim of this method is to estimate the natural mite fall (NMF). The NMF is defined as the number of mites per day falling naturally from the bees on to the floor of the hive. It is widely recognized that the NMF at a specific time is related to the *Varroa* infestation rate at that time (Fernández and Coineau, 2006; Coffey and Breen, 2013; FERA, 2013a).

In order to monitor NMF, a sticky floor (or fat-coated blanket) is unrolled under a wire-mesh floor in the hive. Then, the sticky floor or blanket is carefully examined and the mites counted each day (or every 5 days and converted to a daily NMF).

However, since the fall of mites depends on many factors (brood area, season, daily hive activity, etc.), this method sometimes gives results that are difficult to interpret (Martin, 1998; Vidal-Naquet, 2011).

According to the Animal & Plant Health Agency (FERA, 2013a), the level of infestation (low, medium, high) based on NMF can be interpreted as follows:

- From April to June:
  - Low infestation level: <2 NMF/day
  - Medium infestation level: 4–8 NMF/day
  - High infestation level: >8 NMF/day
- July:
  - Low infestation: 4–8 NMF/day
  - Medium infestation: 6–10 NMF/day
  - High infestation: >10 NMF/day
- August and September:
  - Low infestation: <4 NMF/day
  - Medium–high infestation: >4 NMF/day

Throughout the beekeeping season, from the early spring to autumn, it is considered that an NMF of >15 mites/day poses a serious threat to the colony and calls for urgent application of a miticide (FERA, 2013b). Some beekeeping stakeholders consider an NMF threshold of 10 mites/day to be more suitable.

After efficient treatment in the summer (or in winter, in brood-less colonies), an average of ≤1 NMF/day is considered to represent an infestation of 50 *Varroa* in the colony (Faucon, 2008; Noireterre, 2011; Vidal-Naquet, 2011), i.e. the threshold below which it is considered that the colony can overwinter with minimal risk in terms of *Varroa* infestation.

This method is considered to be sensitive, giving a quite precise indication of the *Varroa* infestation level of a colony. However, its implementation is time consuming, and may result in the accumulation of wax debris, attracting wax moths (FERA, 2013a).

Drone brood uncapping method

The aim of this method is to evaluate the percentage of drone pupae infested. This method is mainly performed in spring when the drone brood is present, and involves using a honey uncapping fork on an area of sealed drone brood at an advanced stage of development of the pupae (usually pink-eyed). If more than 5% of drone pupae are infested, the colony is considered endangered and at risk of collapse during the beekeeping season (FERA, 2013a). Unfortunately, this method is quite imprecise and only gives approximate results.

The drone brood uncapping method may be used to give useful snapshot of *Varroa* infestation level in a colony in spring. The precision of the results will depend on the number of cells uncapped. Determining the number of infested drone pupae found in a group of 50–100 uncapped cells provides a reliable estimate of the overall proportion of infested drone brood cells (FERA, 2013a).

The drone brood uncapping method may be used to decide immediate and appropriate measures in the field, for example during a spring inspection if some phoretic *Varroa* are observed during an examination of a colony, or if the colony is showing signs of weakening (Charrière *et al.*, 1998; FERA, 2013a).

This method is quick and easy to perform during routine colony inspections, and provides an approximate measure of the infestation level.

Evaluation of mite infestation by miticide application

The aim of this method is to estimate the total mite fall (TMF). It consists in the application of an authorized one-shot acaricide VMP (veterinary medicine product) into a hive and then counting the total mite drop (TMD) (Coffey and Breen, 2013). TMD refers to the total number of *Varroa* mites killed by a treatment (compared to the NMF, which refers to the daily natural fall of *Varroa* on to the floor of a hive). This method is mainly used for estimating the *Varroa* population in a brood-less colony (in particular because acaricides do not act on mites in capped cells).

Thus, this method provides an interesting way of evaluating the mite population before overwintering in brood-less colonies or/and before the beginning of the season.

In a temperate northern hemisphere climate, 50 *Varroa* in a colony is considered:

- Before overwintering as the maximal tolerance threshold, above which the colony will be in danger in winter.
- At the beginning of the beekeeping season as the maximal tolerance threshold, above which the colony will be in danger during the season (Faucon, 2008; Noireterre, 2011; Vidal-Naquet, 2011).

If there is no brood rearing in winter, the infestation level will not change (or may decrease by natural mite fall or if an acaricide is applied punctually).

Evaluation of mite infestation by sampling adult honeybees

The adult bee infestation rate provides an estimate of the parasitic pressure within a honeybee colony. This measurement can be performed in early spring to evaluate the parasitic pressure at the beginning of the season, during the season or in summer when the future winter bees are being reared, or in autumn to evaluate the mite infestation level in the brood-less colony before overwintering. Two methods that give reliable results are used to monitor mite infestation on adult honeybees: the flotation method and the powdered (iced) sugar method (Bak *et al.*, 2009).

First, 300 bees (100 ml = approximately 300 bees) are withdrawn from the hive into a small container (it is important to avoid withdrawing the queen). It is important to capture young adult bees living on a frame with open brood; indeed phoretic *Varroa* are much more prevalent on nurse bees than on bees in the supers (Lee *et al.*, 2010).

The flotation method consists in first freezing the bees, or killing them by submersion in alcohol (OIE, 2014a). The dead bees are then shaken in an alcohol or detergent solution which will dislodge the mites. The jars containing the samples are shaken by hand or with a shaking apparatus for 5 minutes. Centrifugation may also be used to dislodge *Varroa* mites from bees (Fakhimzadeh, 2000). The liquid is filtered through a sieve with 3 mm holes. Bees are also counted for a precise result. *Varroa* are collected in the solution and counted (De Jong *et al.*, 1982; Bak *et al.*, 2009; Vidal-Naquet, 2011; OIE, 2014a).

The powdered sugar shaking method preserves the bees alive and is performed in the field (Bak *et al.*, 2009). Dusting bees with icing sugar causes the mites to detach from the bees. It seems that the fine granules stick to the footpads of *Varroa* and render the mites unable to grip the surface to which they have been clinging. Approximately 300 bees are poured into a jar with a mesh cover (3–4 mm holes in the lid). Icing sugar is added. The jar is then gently shaken twice for 2 minutes with a 2 minute gap to cover the bees with the icing sugar. The jar is inverted and shaken over a bucket, into which the icing sugar and mites fall. Water is added: the sugar dissolves and the mites float to the surface and can be counted. (The bees can simply be released from the jar.)

The mite infestation rate on adult bees provides an estimate of the colony infestation rate (Fernández and Coineau, 2006).

The results of these methods can be interpreted as follows:

- If the mite infestation rate is <5%, the colony is considered to be weakly parasitized, and does not need immediate treatment.
- If the mite infestation rate is between 5–10%, treatment must be planned.
- If the mite infestation rate is >10%, the colony requires immediate treatment.

1.6.3 Control of *Varroa* infestation by application of veterinary medicines or officinal active substances

The aim of applying veterinary medicine to control *Varroa* infestation is to lower as far as possible the *Varroa* infestation level in a colony. Complete elimination and eradication of *Varroa* is impossible.

Currently, controlling *Varroa* infestation with chemicals, organic acids, or essential oils is necessary but not sufficient. Sanitary and biotechnological measures are major elements in managing the control of *Varroa*. Over the long term, it is hoped that medicine-less control of *Varroa* infestation will become possible, and this could come from bees tolerant of *V. destructor*. Many research teams are working on such honeybee strains.

Controlling *Varroa* infestation requires use of VMPs as well as sanitary and biotechnological measures.

Chemical control of *Varroa* infestation began in the 1980s with the use of acaricides efficient against *Varroa* and intended not to have strongly adverse effects on honeybee colonies (Weissenberger, 1988; Wendling, 2012).

Several points concerning VMPs are important for the veterinarian prescriber and the beekeeper user:

- VMPs must be prescribed by veterinarians according to local regulations.
- VMPs must not leave residues in the hive (or these must be lower than the residue maximal limit, RML) and must be applied out of honey-flow periods.
- VMPs must not be toxic to honeybees.
- VMPs must be used with care so as not to pose a risk to beekeepers and other operators. This is important for all VMPs and chemicals used for *Varroa* control. Suitable precautions must be taken when using organic acids, including the use of personal protective equipment (suit, gloves, glasses, etc.) against toxic chemicals.
- VMPs must be used according to the manufacturer's and veterinarian's instructions to achieve optimal efficacy.
- VMPs must be effective on phoretic *Varroa* (miticides, except formic acid, are not active on mites within cells)
- VMPs must result in a colony mite count of <50 *Varroa* before overwintering and at the beginning of the season. The infestation load must remain under the threshold of 1,000–2,000 *Varroa* mites during the season (Rosenkrantz *et al.*, 2010; Noireterre, 2011; Vidal-Naquet, 2011; FERA, 2013a).
- VMP use must be carefully assessed. A turnover of active substances employed in order to limit or avoid development of chemotherapeutic resistance is essential. Indeed, *Varroa* appears able to develop resistance to any chemical acaricide (FERA, 2013a).
- Chemicals used as miticides must be prescribed if permitted by legislation according to local regulation on veterinary medicines and the cascade principle (which allows veterinarians legally to prescribe medicines that are not authorized for the relevant clinical case or for the relevant species under treatment when there is no authorized VMP available: https://www.gov.uk/the-cascade-prescribe-a-veterinary-medicine-for-another-use).

Table 5.1 Main miticides and active substances used to control *Varroa* infestation

Active substance	Category	Regulation/ marketing authorization (MA)	Formulation	Mode of action
Amitraz (Apivar®)	Formamidine	MA in some European countries	Sustained-release formulation – strips hung between brood frames for 10 weeks. Strips should be repositioned at mid-treatment time	Octopaminergic agonist in arthropods
Flumethrin (Bayvarol®)	Synthetic pyrethroid	MA in some European countries	Sustained-release formulation – plastic strips hung between brood combs	Blocks the voltage-gated sodium and calcium channels
Tau-Fluvalinate (Apistan®)	Pyrethroid	MA in some European countries	Sustained-release formulation – strips hung between brood frames for 8 weeks	Blocks the voltage-gated sodium and calcium channels
Coumaphos (Asuntol®, Checkmite®, Perizin®)	Organophosphate	MA in some European countries	Strips (1.4 g coumaphos) hung between brood frames for 6 weeks	Inactivation of acetyl-cholinesterase
Oxalic acid (Bienenwohl®, Oxuvar®)	Organic acid	MA in some European countries	A single treatment: sugar syrup solution when brood is not present	Unknown
Formic acid (MAQS®)	Organic acid	MA in some European countries	Slow release pad: evaporation miticide. An empty super must be applied on the body of the hive during application.	Inhibits electron transport in the mitochondria/ neuroexcitatory effect
Thymol (ApiLifeVar®, Apiguard®, Thymovar®)	Monoterpenoid	MA in some European countries	Tablets or gel	Binds to octopamine or GABA receptors

A veterinary medicine may have MA in some countries and not in others. Prescribers and users
Sources: Quarles (1996), Rosenkranz (2010), Vidal-Naquet (2011), Gregorc (2012).

Period of treatment	Resistance/efficacy	Residues	Described toxicity of the active substance for bees
After the last honey harvest (summer to autumn according to region). Also in early spring before honey flow. Treatments are not to be applied during periods of honey flow. **Out of honey-flow period and supers removed**	Good efficiency. Resistance and lack of efficacy described	Residues detected in wax, pollen, and honey	Acute toxicity of amitraz solution has been shown experimentally
End of summer/autumn or early spring for 6 weeks. Treatments are not to be applied during periods of honey flow. **Out of honey-flow period and supers removed**	Pyrethroid-resistant mites reported. Mite cross-resistance to fluvalinate and flumethrin reported	Residues detected in wax, pollen, and honey	Increased mortality of aduts observed in the first days of application
Out of honey-flow period and supers removed	High resistance level and lack of efficacy described. Mite cross-resistance to fluvalinate and flumethrin reported	Residues detected in wax, pollen, and honey	Smaller queens when exposed to high doses of tau-fuvalinate
Out of honey-flow period and supers removed	Resistance and lack of efficacy described	Residues detected in wax, pollen, and honey	Bee mortality. Colony disorganization. Smaller queens, lower sperm viability in drones
At the beginning of winter as a complementary summer treatment, on brood-less colonies	High efficacy on brood-less colonies – no resistance described to date	Not described	Harmful effects on brood and bees following several applications at short intervals
Effective against phoretic and reproductive mites. Spring to autumn. Stop honey production if applied during honey flow and remove the honey supers. Temperature use: 10–29.5°C on day of application. Application should last 7 days	High efficacy reported. No resistance described to date	Hydrophilic – not described	Disorganization of the colony and induction of adult bee mortality and rejection of the queen. If temperatures exceed 29.5°C excessive brood and queen loss may occur.
Out of honey-flow period and supers removed. Temperature dependent, may cause disorders within the colony if temperature is too high	Efficacy reported to be between 66 and 90% on *Varroa*	Lipophilic – may affect the taste of the honey; generally recognised as safe for human consumption	Colony disorganization/ brood removal/queen mortality

must check regulations, dosages, and modes of usage before prescription and use.

- Chemicals (organic acids and thymol) must not be bought in hardware shops, etc., as is often done in beekeeping practice.

Miticides

Several miticides may be used to control *Varroa* infestation. The miticides presented here are the main ones prescribed and used in Europe (Table 5.1).

According to local regulation, miticides used in hives may have two different legal statuses: thus, they are considered as VMPs in the EU, or as biocides or pesticides in some other territories such as Canada and the US.

Amitraze (formamidine), tau-fluvalinate (pyrethroid), coumaphos (organophosphate) and flumethrin (pyrethroid) are synthetic acaricides used to control *Varroa* infestation. They are mainly used as sustained-release formulations because they do not have any efficacy on mites within capped brood cells. However, resistance and lack of efficacy have been described for these treatments (Rosenkranz *et al.*, 2010; Mallick, 2013).

Sustained-release amitraze has been reported to present a good efficacy (Faucon *et al.*, 2007). A field study performed in 2011 field by French beekeepers reported an efficacy of 95% or more in 77% of the colonies in which it was applied (Vandame, 2012). However, some cases of resistance to Amitraz from *Varroa destructor* have been reported in recent years (Maggi *et al.*, 2010).

Thymol and organic acids (formic acid, oxalic acid, and lactic acid) are miticides considered as natural compounds. VMPs containing formic acid, oxalic acid, and thymol exist. Unfortunately, not all EU countries (and worldwide) have marketing authorization for all these VMPs and, as a prescriber, a veterinarian has to follow local regulations and legislation on VMPs.

- Thymol is used as a sustained-release treatment but its use is temperature dependent.
- Formic acid exists as a sustained-release formulation and is interesting because it is effective against phoretic *and* reproductive mites in the capped brood (Imdorf *et al.*, 2003). It may cause disorder in the colony.
- Oxalic acid and lactic acid can be used in brood-less colonies as one-off treatments (i.e. for brood-less wintering colonies or for swarms). Oxalic acid must be applied only once: if it is applied several times at short intervals, it can harm adult bees, queen, and the brood. Organic acids must be used with great caution by veterinarians and beekeepers because of their high toxicity.

The use of thymol and organic acids is recommended for the following reasons:

- Their efficacy is reported as sufficient if they are correctly applied and managed with beekeeping and biotechnological practices.
- There is a low risk of problems with residues in products of the hive. Furthermore, oxalic and formic acids are natural ingredients of honey.
- There is a 'low probability of eliciting resistance after repeated treatments' (Rosenkranz *et al.*, 2010).

Treatment strategy

Because no miticides have 100% efficiency and eradication of *V. destructor* is impossible, and because managed colonies are food producers, treatment strategies must be set up and performed in association with biotechnological methods.

The treatment strategy depends on several factors: honey-flow period, meteorological conditions, geographic area, honeybee sub-species, production target, *Varroa* population growth, brood-less periods, beekeeping practices, and beekeepers (professional or non-professional). *The treatment strategy described here must be considered in combination with the sanitary and biotechnological measures described below.*

Basically, the treatment strategy aims to greatly reduce the mite population in the colony immediately after the final honey harvest in order to prevent, as far as possible, brood infestation (Wendling, 2012). The main objective is to ensure that the development of the future winter bees can occur in the best conditions with the lowest risk of bee parasitic mite syndrome. This strategy requires the application of sustained-release treatments (amitraze, tau-fluvalinate, thymol, or formic acid) within the colonies.

This strategy has a scientific basis:

- The mites endanger development of over-wintering bees, and viruses, and in particular DWV, transmitted by *Varroa* are a major threat for the colony.
- The mite reproductive cycle occurs within the capped brood.
- The dynamics of mite population favour this approach.

Recent work has shown that the lifespan of overwintering workers with high virus loads (DWV even if asymptomatic) seems to be shortened (Dainat *et al.*, 2012). Thus, a large reduction in mite population as soon as possible after the last honey harvest can potentially provide the greatest protection for the colony from *Varroa* and DWV. This will allow the colony to rear winter bees that are as strong as possible, which is essential if the colony is to overwinter in good condition.

The threshold of 50 *V. destructor* remaining within overwintering colonies is considered to be the objective. Monitoring may be performed by counting NMF or TMF.

If the treatment fails, another may be applied in the colony. A one-off treatment (e.g. oxalic acid) may be applied to a brood-less colony (just before the overwintering period and usually on a sunny, mild day in November) (Imdorf *et al.*, 2003).

Another method consists in applying a second treatment with another sustained-release treatment immediately before wintering or during the early spring period.

Thus, the treatment strategy involves the following steps:

- One sustained-release treatment immediately after removing the supers in summer.
- One second treatment (if necessary):
  - a one-off application of oxalic acid, e.g. in the brood-less colony after the summer treatment; or,
  - one sustained-release treatment before wintering or in early spring (withdrawing treatment before adding the supers to avoid residues in the hive products).

During the season, monitoring of the mite population (usually by measuring NMF or evaluation of mite infestation by sampling adult honeybees) is necessary (to detect significant increase, reinfestation, etc.) and another treatment may be required. This monitoring strategy is quite similar to the integrated pest management described in section 1.6.5 below.

One protocol may be followed based on assessing the NMF (Wendling, 2012; FERA, 2013a):

- May–July: NMF >3 mites/day – treatment with formic acid after honey spring harvesting (or sanitary measures such as withdrawing capped drone brood).
- End of July–August: NMF >10 mites/day – treatment with formic acid (after removing the honey supers).
- Throughout the season: NMF > 15 mites/day – the supers must be immediately removed and a treatment applied. The colony is endangered.

The treatment strategy requires a turnover of VMPs and chemicals to limit the risk of resistance. However, the chemical fight alone is not sufficient: no such treatment can completely and safely protect bees against *Varroa*.

Thus, the use of miticides is limited by various factors:

- No acaricide has a 100% efficacy.
- The use of miticides is potentially risky for the bees and for the consumers of hive products, due to residues in honey or wax. The year-on-year accumulation of residues within wax represents a major threat for honeybees and demands a regular renewal of the wax combs (usually every three years).

Hence such treatment must be considered in combination with beekeeping practices and biotechnogical control of *Varroa* infestation.

1.6.4 Biotechnological control methods

Biotechnological methods are an additional and necessary help for beekeepers attempting to control *Varroa* infestation. They are a part of good sanitary beekeeping practices (cf. Chapter 8).

These methods can be understood as additional to the use of VMPs in colonies. Eventually, these methods may temporarily replace the use of a VMP, e.g. during the active season to avoid contamination of the honey with residues.

Biotechnological methods can help beekeepers to reduce chemical use within hives as far as possible. They can also augment treatments with low or medium efficacy.

Both the reproductive cycle in the brood and the attractiveness of the drone brood for *Varroa* mites are the biological basis of these biotechnological measures.

Drone brood removal

Regular removal of capped drone brood may slow down mite population growth within the colony (Charrière *et al.*, 1998). This method can be performed in combination with routine colony health controls (FERA, 2013a). The efficacy of the drone brood removal method can be favoured by stimulating natural drone brood building with shallow comb (or a built comb from which the lower half has been removed). The frame must be placed inside the hive, in the brood chamber, when the queen begins to lay up drone brood. When the drone comb is full of capped cells, it must be removed from the hive before drone emergence and then destroyed. The *Varroa* mites within the cell will not be able to continue their life cycle and will be killed.

The frame can be replaced in the brood chamber immediately after brood removal. This technique may be repeated several times during the season. It is a useful, easy, quick but limited method. It is well tolerated by the colony.

The use of frames with sheets printed with drone foundations is an alternative to shallow combs. It will be necessary to remove and destroy all the frames when both surfaces of the comb are full of capped drone brood.

This method can be implemented in spring; however, spring is the reproductive season and removing drone brood can limit artificially drone rearing by the colonies. Thus, fertilization of virgin queens could potentially be affected. Hence, it is generally considered preferable to use this method in late spring/beginning of summer when the height of the reproductive season is over.

Queen trapping method: brood interruption

Caging the queen in a small trap on a brood comb at the centre of the hive body will halt ovipositioning (Lodesani *et al.*, 2014). This will lead to a complete interruption in brood production 24 days later (i.e. the time from egg laying to the emergence of drones).

By the end of this period of 24 days, all the new workers and drones have emerged and no more brood is then reared. The life cycle of *Varroa* is thus halted. The queen may then be freed. All the mites in the colony are at this point in time phoretic and a one-shot miticide (as oxalic acid) may be applied in the hive in order to kill most part of them. A colony can compensate for this loss of the brood within 8 weeks (Büchler, 2009).

This method is probably best implemented in July or August, according to the area and the climate. One drawback is that the loss of brood, though temporary, may weaken the colony.

Comb trapping method

The aim of this method is to trap the mites in capped combs of workers and then to remove these combs from the hive. The comb trapping method lasts at least 36 days and requires meticulous beekeeping skills (FERA, 2013a):

- At T0: in the brood chamber, the queen is confined to an empty worker comb (comb A) using a purpose-made comb-cage.

- At T0 + 9 days: the queen is confined to a second empty worker comb (B).
- At T0 + 18 days: the queen is confined to a third empty worker comb (C), and comb A, now capped, is removed from the hive.
- At T0 + 27 days, the queen is released into the brood chamber and comb B is removed from the hive.
- At T0 + 36 days, comb C is removed.

This is a very interesting and successful method; a 90% efficacy is reported (Wendling, 2012; FERA, 2013a). However, it is a time-consuming method that needs a series of manipulations that cannot easily be performed on a large-scale honeybee farm. This method must be implemented during the beekeeping season. Using the comb trapping method in late summer or autumn should be avoided as this endangers the production of winter bees.

Complete removal of the brood

The aim of the complete removal of the brood method is to separate the adult bees from the brood, giving the colony a 'brood-less' pause in the usual swarming period (Büchler, 2009). This method is similar to the queen trapping method as they are both based on brood interruption. Thus, the colony may be considered as a 'natural' swarm. While swarming, the colony is considered to leave behind in the hive some of its pathogenic agents and the brood. Furthermore, the reproduction cycle of *Varroa* is stopped.

This method is performed by a single and complete removal of the brood from the colony in June/July without summer-long sustained miticide application. The brood frames are replaced by frames with wax sheet foundations or by empty frames. However, a single application of formic acid or oxalic acid at the end of the process kills most of the phoretic *Varroa*. Colonies can compensate for this loss of brood within 8 weeks (Büchler, 2009). The new brood is reared in hygienic new combs with new wax. According to Büchler (2009), the complete removal of the brood does not provoke a decrease in the strength of the colony at the beginning of the overwintering or an impairment of honey production during the following year.

This method is similar in effect to the bee 'shock swarm method' (forming a naked swarm in a new hive) used in particular in the control of American and European foulbrood diseases.

Other techniques

Various other biotechnological methods have been described:

- Artificial swarm. This consists in setting up an artificial swarm from a parent colony during the swarming season (mainly before the end of May in temperate countries). The overall number of *Varroa* mites remains the same in the parent colony and the swarm but the *Varroa* infestation is reduced in each of them. It is reported that the parent colony will be strong enough to allow a honey gathering in July and the swarm to overwinter in good conditions (Wendling, 2012).
- The use of a wire-mesh floor can prevent fallen mites from returning to the bees within the hive. It improves hive ventilation and also helps in the fight against wax moth by preventing debris accumulating on the floor.

1.6.5 Integrated pest management (IPM) programme to control *Varroa* infestation

In agriculture, the aim of IPM is not to attempt to eradicate a pest but to keep infestation below the level where it is considered to cause significant harm (FERA, 2013a; Mallick, 2013). IPM combines monitoring, biotechnological control managements, and chemical controls throughout the year. Thus, treatments or pesticide inputs are reduced to the minimum level.

In the case of *Varroa*, because the aim of mite control is not eradication, which is impossible, but rather reducing the infestation as much as possible, IPM may be an interesting method in particular concerning the response to the issues raised by acaricide use (resistance, residues in the wax, toxicity for bees alone or in association with other residues, etc.).

Table 5.2 Example of integrated control methods: monitoring methods, biotechnological methods, and medicines used throughout the year (adapted from FERA, 2013b)

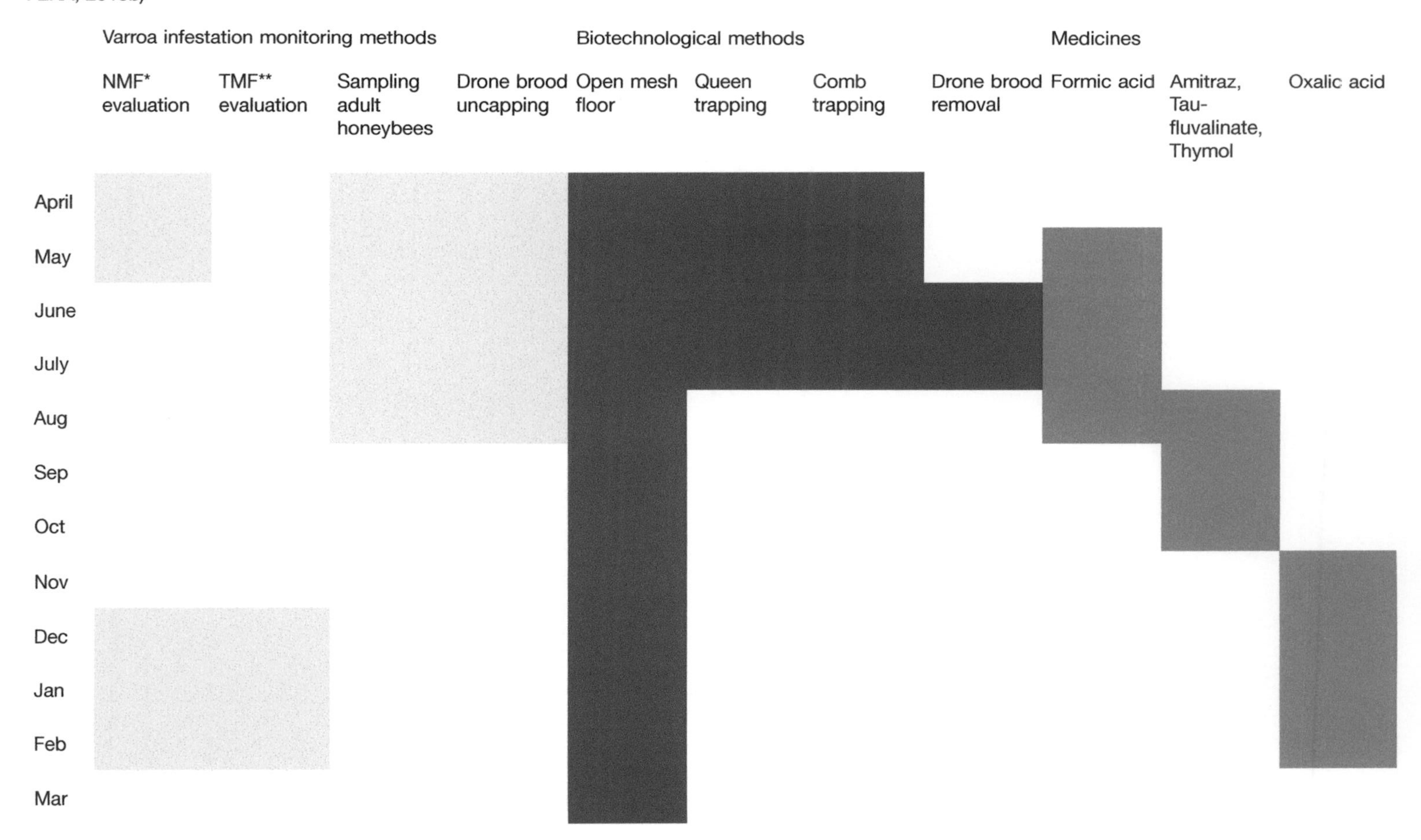

	Varroa infestation monitoring methods				Biotechnological methods				Medicines		
	NMF* evaluation	TMF** evaluation	Sampling adult honeybees	Drone brood uncapping	Open mesh floor	Queen trapping	Comb trapping	Drone brood removal	Formic acid	Amitraz, Tau-fluvalinate, Thymol	Oxalic acid
April											
May											
June											
July											
Aug											
Sep											
Oct											
Nov											
Dec											
Jan											
Feb											
Mar											

Example of integrated methods: Monitoring methods, Biotechnical methods, Medicines used throughout the year (adapted from FERA, 2013b).
*NMF, natural mite fall. **TMF, total mite fall.

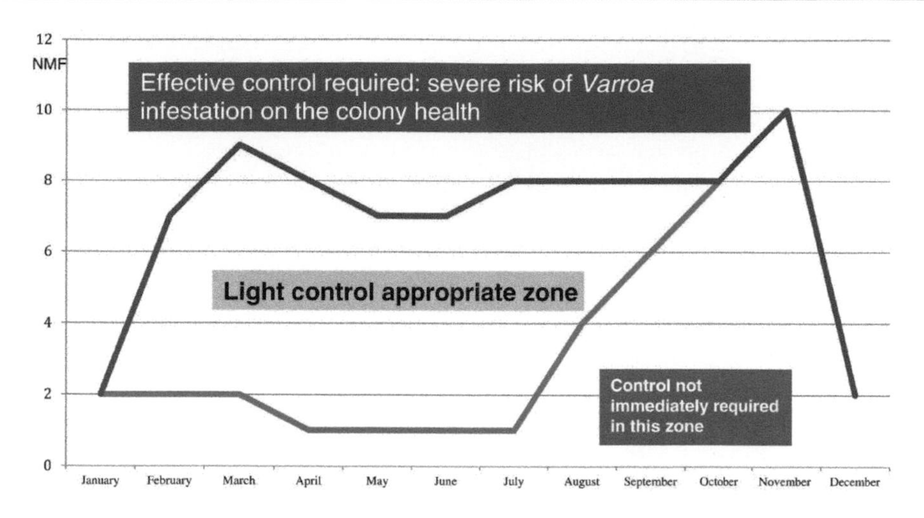

Figure 5.13 Using NMF to decide the level of controls to employ as proposed by the Food & Environment Research Agency (FERA, 2013a).

An IPM to maintain *Varroa* infestation under a defined harmful threshold within a honeybee colony involves the following elements:

- Application of good sanitary beekeeping practices.
- Application of monitoring and biotechnological methods that may help to reduce miticide use.
- Application of a sequence/rotation of miticides to limit occurrence of *Varroa* resistance.
- Choice of a miticide according to the level of infestation and the time of year.
- Application of a sustained-release miticide immediately after removing the supers in summer in order to give the colony the best conditions to rear strong and healthy winter workers.

Monitoring mite population is one pillar of the IPM program for *Varroa* infestation in colonies. Throughout the year, monitoring the level of mite infestation is necessary and enables decisions to be made as to what control method to apply. This will depend on the level of infestation in order to be under the thresholds usually recognized (50 *Varroa* during wintering in brood-less colonies; 1,000–2,000 *Varroa* during the beekeeping period).

Table 5.2 shows an 'example of IPM methods' adapted from the Food & Environment Research Agency (2013b) and provides information on some practical methods used by beekeepers to control *Varroa* infestation. This table lists appropriate methods of monitoring, appropriate biotechnological methods to control *Varroa* infestation, and appropriate medicines to use according to the time of the year (considering April as the beginning of the beekeeping season). It must be remembered that the beginning of the beekeeping season varies according to region (e.g. in southern territories, the beekeeping season may begin earlier and the table has to be adapted accordingly). It must also be taken into account that there is not one single IPM rule, but that the IPM must be the consequence of a well-considered plan, in particular according to the region, the environment, and the beekeeping farm.

Some IPM methods are proposed by the Animal & Plant Health Agency, formerly the Food & Environment Research Agency (FERA, 2013a). Using NMF to monitor the infestation level is time consuming. However, following NMF throughout the year is a way to decide the level of the control required (high, moderate, or light) (FERA, 2013a) (Figure 5.13).

Using only drone brood pupae infestation (DPI) may provide information to decide appropriate level of controls. According to the APHA (FERA, 2013a), the management of control according the infestation rate may be implemented as follows:

- April–June:
  - DPI < 2% (<1 mite/50 cells): it is not necessary to intervene.
  - 2% < DPI < 4% (1 mite/25 cells to 1 mite/50 cells): planning of a control management during the beekeeping season is necessary.
  - DPI > 4% (>1 mite/25 cells): it is necessary to consider a control management.
- June–July:
  - DPI < 3% (<1 mite/30 cells): it is not necessary to intervene.
  - 3% < DPI < 7% (1 mite/15 cells to 1 mite/30 cells): a light control is necessary
  - DPI > 7% (>1 mite/15 cells): the colony is endangered and application of a treatment is necessary.
- August:
  - DPI < 5% (<1 mite/20 cells): it is not necessary to intervene.
  - 5% < DPI < 10% (1 mite/10 cells to 1 mite/20 cells): a light control is necessary
  - DPI > 7% (>1 mite/15 cells): the colony is endangered and application of a treatment is necessary.

Any IPM involving *Varroa* monitoring, control methods and acaricide use must be adapted to each circumstance and may change during the year and from one year to the next for a colony or for an apiary. The IPM will depend on the beekeeping area, mite infestation level, mite reinfestation risk, honeybee sub-species and strains, climate and meteorological conditions, beekeeping practices, region, and country (Wendling, 2012; FERA, 2013a). The role of the veterinarian is to adapt the methods to each case according to the features of the apiary.

1.6.6 Other mite control management and perspectives for the future

The methods described in this section are currently areas of research and offer a possible future for the control of *Varroa* infestation. At present, the selection of honeybees that are tolerant of *Varroa* and biological control of *Varroa* infestation are not usable in beekeeping management.

Selection of honeybees tolerant of Varroa

The selection of *A. mellifera* that are tolerant of *V. destructor*, as observed in the relationship between *A. cerana* and *V. destructor*, is not yet a reality, though it offers promise as a method for control.

Research programmes have been undertaken to investigate the following factors in the quest to develop desirable inheritable features in honeybees (Rosenkranz *et al.*, 2010; Wendling, 2012):

- Population dynamics of *Varroa* in a colony.
- Control of mite reproduction.
- Hygienic behaviour (detection, uncapping, and removal of dead, diseased, or parasitized brood).
- Grooming behaviour (honeybee workers groom themselves (auto-grooming) and other nestmates (allo-grooming)). By grooming, honeybees remove mites from their body or from the bodies of other bees.

The most promising features seem to be hygienic behaviour and the population dynamics of *Varroa* in a colony (Wendling, 2012). Many research programmes are underway to create, for example, hygienic (HYG) bees and suppressed mite reproduction (SMR) bees (Rozenkrantz *et al.*, 2010). SMR bees are able to detect infested immature forms in the capped brood cell and remove them. A better proposed name is *Varroa* sensitive hygiene bees (VSH bees) (Harris, 2007). It seems that the removal of the infested pupae from the cells by VSH bees occurs mainly 1–5 days after capping. One hypothesis is that the detection and removal may be triggered by stimuli in cells containing 3- to 5-day-old pupae after capping (Harris, 2007).

However, if tolerant *Apis mellifera* is 'considered as the only long-term solution of the *Varroa* problem', there is currently no evidence of long-term inheritable features and tolerant honeybee *A. mellifera* lines (Rozenkrantz *et al.*, 2010).

Biological control

Biological control (bacteria and fungi) is considered by some authors as a promising approach to control *Varroa* infestation in colonies. However, biological control must be approached with care and caution.

Some bacteria (*Bacillaceae* and *Micrococcaceae*) are reported to have an in vitro pathogenic effect against *Varroa* (Tsagou *et al.*, 2004). However, at this time, there is no practical beekeeping application for these bacteria and further research is needed before a possible practical use can be realized.

Another field of research is entomo-pathogenic fungi. Some fungi (*Verticillium lecanii*, *Hirsutella* spp., *Paecilomyces* spp., *Beauveria bassiana*, *Metarhizium* spp., *Tolypocladium* spp.) have shown infectious and lethal effects on *Varroa* (Shaw *et al.*, 2002; Kanga *et al.*, 2003; Meikle *et al.*, 2008; Wendling, 2012). Practical use is not imminent and further study is needed.

In the conclusion of this chapter on *V. destructor*, the main point is to recall the damage caused by varroosis (bee mite parasitic syndrome) and the consequences for the colony. Moreover, controlling mite infestation is also essential for neighbouring colonies and apiaries.

2 Tracheal acariosis: infestation by the mite *Acarapis woodi*

Tracheal acariosis, also called acarine disease or acarapidosis, is a contagious parasitic disease of the adult honeybee (*A. mellifera* and other *Apis* species) (OIE, 2014a). It is caused by a mite living in the tracheae, *A. woodi* (Acari: Tarsonemidae). *Acarapis woodi* was first described on the Isle of Wight in 1919 after an epizooty responsible for dramatic colony losses. This discovery was the origin of the creation of the Buckfast honeybee strain by Brother Adam. (However, it was later reported that *A. woodi* was not responsible for 'Isle of Wight syndrome' (Bailey, 1964).) Tracheal acariosis has since then been described in many European countries.

Acariosis behaves as an enzootic. In the US, it spread as an epizootic in the 1980s (Bailey and Lee, 1959; Fernandez, 1999), causing devastating losses (Sammataro, 2012). It seems that honeybees in Europe present a better tolerance to *A. woodi* than those in the US (Fernandez, 1999). However, *A. woodi* infestation does not seem to be so harmful for honeybee colonies except in some cases of massive infestation (University of Florida, 2014). The productivity of managed colonies does not seem to be modified (Downey and Winston, 2001) or is reported to be affected only by higher levels of infestation (25–30%) within the colony (Fernandez, 1999).

According to Bailey and Perry (1982), the frequency of infestation of colonies has progressively decreased in England and in Wales from 1925 to 1980.

2.1 Regulatory status

Tracheal acariosis is a notifiable disease in some European countries (Appendix 2).

2.2 The pathogenic agent and its life cycle

This mite is an internal parasite of the respiratory system of the three castes of adult honeybees. Mated founder females that ensure spreading seem to have a certain attraction to drones in comparison to worker bees (Dawicke et al., 1992; Fernandez, 1999; OIE, 2014a).

The mites live in the tracheae, feeding on the haemolymph by puncturing the tracheal wall. The reproduction of these tracheal mites occurs in the tracheal system (OIE, 2014a).

The large prothoracic trachea is the main place where the mites live, feed, and reproduce. However, mites may sometimes be found in the

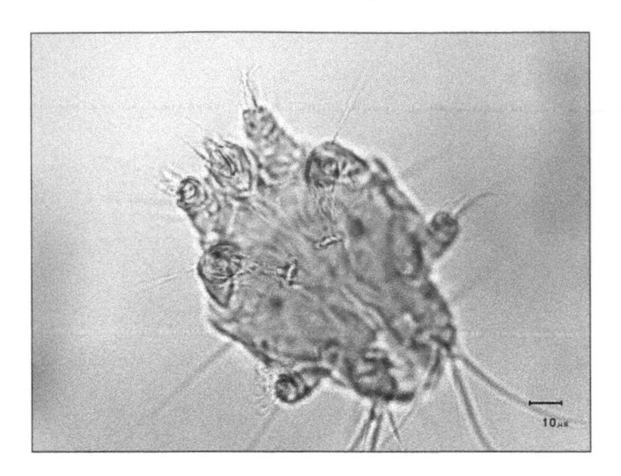

Figure 5.14 *Acaparis woodi* adult. (Photo courtesy © Monique L'Hostis, Oniris Veterinary School, Nantes.)

thoracic, abdominal, and head air sacs (Giordani, 1965, Wilson *et al.*, 1997).

The female is ovoid (140–175 µm × 75–84 µm) and the male is similar but smaller 125–136 µm × 60–77 µm (Figures 5.14 and 5.15) (Delfinado-Baker and Baker, 1984; University of Florida, 2014).

The reproductive phase occurs within the large thoracic trachea. Spreading occurs by migration of the female offspring from the parasitized honeybee to another bee. Young bees (1–3 days) are more attractive to *A. woodi* (after 9 days, spiracles are considered impassable) (Fernandez, 1999; OIE, 2014a). The mites enter through the spiracles within the bee trachea (through the prothoracic spiracle within the main thoracic tracheae).

Female mites lay 5–7 eggs in the trachea (other sources report 8–20 eggs) (OIE, 2014a). Development of male eggs takes 11–12 days while female eggs take 14–15 days. After mating, female offspring migrate to body hairs and then attach to other honeybees before entering the trachea within a spiracle (University of Florida, 2014).

The development cycle lasts at least 21 days (Fernandez, 1999). This fact may explain why, in the beekeeping season, *A. woodi* infestation is usually not severe: the summer honeybee's short lifespan and population renewal (25–35

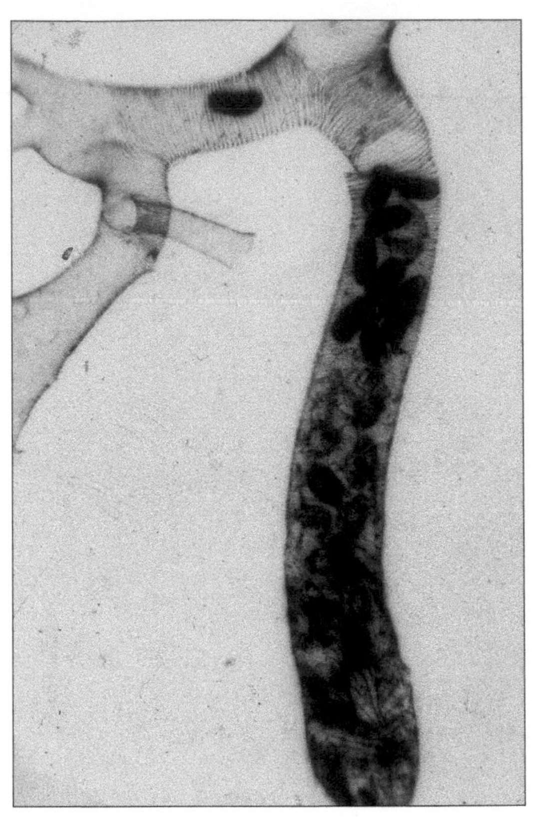

Figure 5.15 *Acarapis woodi* in tracheae (microscopic view). (Photo courtesy © Station de recherche, Agroscope Liebefeld-Posieux ALP, Switzerland.)

days) restricts the breeding possibilities of *A. woodi*. However, the longer lifespan of winter bees (which live through the overwintering period, sometimes 5–6 months) allows up to five or six generations of *A. woodi* to develop. Thus, the consequences of infestation of bees may be much more important and severe in winter.

2.3 Epidemiology

Only mated females leave the tracheae to contaminate other bees. Outside, *A. woodi* cannot survive for more than a few hours (Sammataro and Needham, 1996; Fernandez, 1999). Contamination occurs by contact between bees within the colony or between colonies by drifting and robbing within an apiary or between apiaries.

The mated female mites are more attracted to drones, which thus become the principal means of spreading *A. woodi* within the colony and also between colonies (Fernandez, 1999).

Commercial beekeeping, package bees, and/or queen trading and migration are the main causes of *A.woodi* infestation spreading.

Tracheal acariosis mainly spreads as an enzootic.

2.4 Pathogenesis

The consequences of *A. woodi* living, reproducing, and feeding in the tracheae (mainly prothoracic trachea) have both mechanical and physiological effects on the honeybee. Infestation may be unilateral or bilateral (Fernandez, 1999; OIE, 2014a).

Infestation leads to mechanical and physiological injuries:

- Partial or complete obstruction of the air ducts by filling the tracheae with coagulum, faeces, moulting debris, dead mites.
- Reduction of oxygenation of tissues linked to the prothoracic trachea, in particular flight muscles (on one or both sides) and brain.
- Loss of valuable haemolymph through the tracheal wall.
- Death of infested bees due to hunger, cold, and asphyxia.

Tracheal mites are also reported to act as a vector of some pathogens, in particular viruses, e.g. APV, CBPV, and KPV (Scott-Dupree *et al.*, 1995). Furthermore, parasitized bees seem to be more sensitive to pathogens, such as viruses (e.g. CBPV) (Bailey, 1965; Fernandez, 1999).

2.5 Clinical signs

The clinical signs of the disease are not really specific. They generally occur at the end of the overwintering period and in spring. Early signs of infection are frequently unnoticed, though it may be observed that some bees are unable to fly or are crawling; sometimes dead bees can be seen (Fernandez, 1999; OIE, 2014a).

When the infection is significant, the clinical signs become more apparent:

- At the individual level, dead bees, crawling bees, and paralyzed bees with dislocated wings (or K-wings) can be observed usually on the ground in the front of the hive (Sammataro, 2012). Bees are unable to fly and climb blades of grass. Overwintering capability can be altered by tracheal mite infestation. Indeed, parasitized winter bees are unable to produce heat (with their thoracic muscles) in order to maintain temperature within the cluster. Digestive signs, such as dysentery, may sometimes be observed.
- At the colony level, asymptomatic infestation is possible. However, in winter or early spring, depopulation, and even collapse, may be the consequences of acarine disease (Fernandez, 1999).

2.6 Diagnosis

The clinical signs cannot allow a diagnosis of acarapidosis because they are not really specific to the disease. However, a weakening colony with crawling bees climbing blades of grass, and paralysed bees displaying disjointed wings or K-wings on the ground in the front of the hive may be reasons to suspect acarapidosis.

However, these clinical signs are also observed in other diseases such as viral infections (CBPV, ABPV), nosemosis, and poisoning, which must be taken into account when making a differential diagnosis. The differential diagnosis list should also include other acarian diseases.

The diagnosis involves laboratory techniques and the identification of the mite.

Samples of the three castes can be used (the queen should be avoided); however, drones are more interesting because *A. woodi* are more attracted to them than to workers or queens (Fernandez, 1999; OIE, 2014a). A sample of 50 bees should be collected from a suspected colony (mainly crawling bees on the ground in front of the hive).

Direct microscopic examination of the prothoracic tracheae after dissection of the thorax is the best procedure. It can be done by the veterinarian practitioner or in a laboratory.

An ELISA test exists for diagnosis of tracheal mites; however, it is not a specific test and may give false-positive results (OIE, 2014a).

2.7 Prognosis

The prognosis may be severe in the case of high infestation level (>25%), in particular after the overwintering period and in spring (Fernandez, 1999). This is the consequence of the long lifespan of worker bees in winter allowing multiple development cycles in the respiratory system. However, such infestation loads are currently very rare and *A. woodi* is not considered to pose a real threat to colonies.

2.8 Control and management of *Acarapis woodi* infestation

No VMPs for tracheal acariosis are authorized for use in Europe (except for some rare exceptions). However, volatile acaricides used for *V. destructor* control are efficient against the tracheal mite. A VMP containing thymol, menthol, and camphor has shown 75% efficiency on *A. woodi* infestation in tropical conditions (Esquijarosa, 2003).

Thymol, menthol, formic acid, and amitraze are used in different countries and must be prescribed and applied according to local regulations in the frame of the cascade principle to prescribe a veterinary medicine for another use (Delaplane, 1992; Scott-Dupree and Otis, 1992; Vidal-Naquet, 2011). In 1984, menthol was used to control an epizootic outbreak of acariosis in the US (Delaplane, 1992).

The following are examples of the practical use of chemicals according to the FAO (2006) (these essential oils or organic acids must be officinal, coming from a veterinarian or a physician):

- Essential oils. Crystalline menthol (50 g) or thymol (15 g) is placed in a gauze bag on the top of the bars, and kept there for 1–2 months. External temperatures should be around 21°C; otherwise the menthol vapours will not reach the mites in the trachea.
- Formic acid (65%). Formic acid produces good results. A veterinary medicine with formic acid as the active ingredient exists on the market in some European countries.

Prophylaxis methods concern good beekeeping practices, in particular concerning the trade and exchange of honeybees. Selection of resistant strains is the best way to control tracheal acariosis and avoid the consequences of the disease. Resistant strains probably helped to manage the US epizootic in 1984 (Sammataro, 2012).

3 Tropilaelosis: infestation by the mites *Tropilaelaps clareae* and *Tropilaelaps mercedesae*

Tropilaelaps mites are parasites of immature stages of honeybees. Described initially in 1961, the mite *Tropilaelaps* is a haematophagous ectoparasitic mite (Delfinado and Baker, 1961; OIE, 2014a). Four species of this genus have been described: *Tropilaelaps clareae, T. koenigerum*, *T. mercedesae*, and *T. thaii* (Anderson and Morgan, 2007; Sammataro, 2012; OIE, 2014a). *Tropilaelaps clareae* was the first species discovered by an entomologist, G. Pangga, in 1961, and was first described by Delfinado and Baker (1961).

All these species are originally an ectoparasite of Asian honeybees (*Apis laboriosa* and *Apis dorsata*). *Tropilaelaps clareae* and *T. mercedesae* are damaging parasites of *A. mellifera*. *Tropilaelaps koenigerum* and *T. thaii* are not reported to be parasites of *A. mellifera* (Sammataro, 2012; OIE, 2014a).

Because apiculture has become a global 'industry', with international exchanges of bees and material, *Tropilaelaps* is a potential global threat, especially for non-infested regions (Pettis and Engelsdorp, 2010). For now (November 2014), *Tropilaelaps* remains in its original Asian and Indian subcontinental areas.

It is a worldwide regulated and reportable disease, requiring veterinary measures for safe trade in order to avoid spreading the mite (OIE, 2014a).

In uninfested regions, all stakeholders involved in apiculture (veterinarians, beekeepers, technicians) must be aware of this potential threat and be able to recognize or at least suspect *Tropilaelaps* spp. in colonies. Any suspect sample must be sent to the local reference laboratory for honeybee health (in the EU, the European Union Reference Laboratory for Honey Bee Health, Les templiers, 105 route des Chappes, BP 111, 06902 Sophia Antipolis Cedex, France).

3.1 *Tropilaelaps* infestation sanitary status

Tropilaelaps infestation is a notifiable disease in Europe and in many other countries worldwide and sanitary measures must be taken as soon as possible in the case of suspicion or/and positive diagnosis. It is a notifiable disease to the OIE (2014b) (Appendix 2)

3.2 *Tropilaelaps* species

The genus *Tropilaelaps* belongs to the class Arachnida, subclass Acari, order Mesostigmata, and to the family Laelapidae. Four species are currently known in this genus (Anderson and Morgan, 2007).

Tropilaelaps clareae's natural host is *Apis dorsata* (the large Asian honeybee) and its restricted home range is the Phillipines. It became a parasite of introduced *A. mellifera* in the Phillipines.

Tropilaelaps mercedesae is a parasite of the native *Apis dorsata* in mainland Asia and Indonesia (except Sulawesi Island) and *Apis laboriosa* in Himalayan countries (OIE, 2014b). *Tropilaelaps mercedesae* has become a parasite of introduced *A. mellifera* in those territories.

Tropilaelaps koenigerum is found on *A. dorsata* and *A. laboriosa*. The newly described species *Tropilaelaps thaii* has been found on *A. laboriosa* in mountainous Himalayan regions (Anderson and Morgan, 2007; OIE, 2014b).

The home ranges of these species are Asia and India, from western Iran to eastern Korea and from northern China to southern Indonesia and New Guinea.

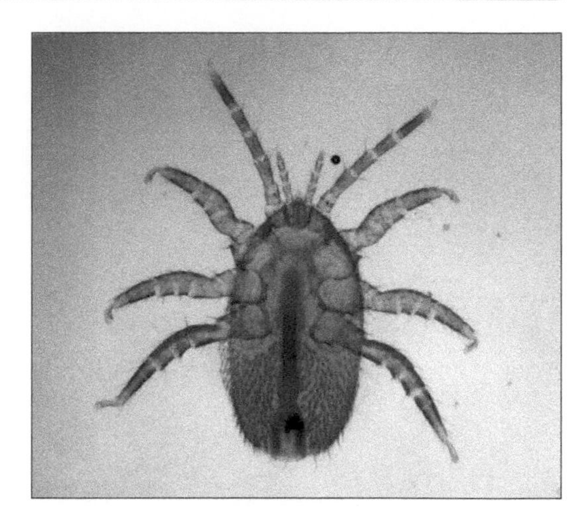

Figure 5.16 *Tropilaelaps* (×25). (Photo courtesy of © Anses Sophia-Antipolis.)

Currently, *T. clareae* and *T. mercedesae* are the two species reported to be able to infest *A. mellifera*.

3.3 Causative agents

Tropilaelaps is an oval-shaped Acari, with a light reddish-brown body. *Tropilaelaps clareae* size is about 1 mm × 0.5 mm. *Tropilaelaps mercedesae* is larger than *T. clareae* (Anses-FERA-FLI, 2013; FERA, 2013b) (Figure 5.16). Those two species are very similar and for long were considered a single species.

The mite is dorsoventrally flattened and is covered with bristles. Females are larger than males and their bodies are more sclerotized. They present a longitudinal ventral sclerotized furrow (Figure 5.16). Immature forms (eggs, larvae, protonymph, and deutonymph) develop within the brood cells.

In this chapter, the use of the word *Tropilaelaps* concerns only the two species infesting *A. mellifera*: *T. clareae* and *T. mercedesae*.

3.3.1 The adult female

The colonizing females (mother founders) reproduce in the sealed brood and feed on immature forms. They are not able to pierce the integument of adult honeybees and feed thereon. They have the ability to move quickly (on combs, adult bees, etc.). Their oval shape and rapid movement distinguish them from *Varroa*.

The idiosoma is composed of one dorsal scutum and several ventral scuta.

The dorsal scutum is entirely covered with fine and short bristles (also called setae). In the posterior region of the scutum, the setae are longer and thicker. The ventral part is composed of several scuta (sternal, genito-vental, anal, meta-sternal, and meta-podal), and two stigma extended by a perithreme (Delfinado and Baker, 1961).

There are four pairs of legs attached on the ventral shields. The first pair is drawn forward like antennae and is supposed to have a sensory role. The three pairs of hind legs are stocky and bent backwards; they participate in locomotion and attachment to bees. The legs are covered with bristles. On the extremity of the legs are tiny claws (Pierson, 2014).

The gnathosoma is almost entirely hidden by a dorsal extension of the body (bordered labrum). It carries the mouthparts: a pair of relatively short chelicerae with a not very powerful clip at their extremity, a pair of lateral pedipalps which have long bristles and simple claws, and an undeveloped hypostoma (Delfinado and Baker, 1961). The tritosternum, a Y-shaped sensory organ, is located on the ventral side, caudal to the gnathosoma (Pierson, 2014).

3.3.2 The adult male

The male *Tropilaelaps* is smaller and less sclerotized than the female. The dorsal scutum is covered with small bristles except for the posterior part where the bristles are longer and thicker (Delfinado and Baker, 1961; Baker et *al*., 2005). Compared to the female, the chelicerae are long and end in a thin and spiralled filament. The male uses the mobile parts of the chelicerae to introduce spermatozoa into the female genital tract (podospermy) (Rath *et al*., 1991). The male gonopore is situated in the rear of the gnathosoma.

3.3.3 The life cycle

The life cycle is quite similar to that of *Varroa*: a phoretic phase and a reproductive phase within the honeybee capped brood. The life cycle of Tropilaelaps is shorter than that of *Varroa* and its fertility is higher (FERA, 2013b).

The mother founder *Tropilaelaps* female enters the brood cell just before capping and lays 1–4 eggs (typically 3–4) within the cell. The reproductive phase occurs in both worker and drone brood, but drone brood is reported to have a higher attractiveness (though less marked than with *Varroa*) for mother founders (Burgett *et al*., 1983; OIE, 2014a).

The laid eggs will develop into one male and several females. After 12 hours, the eggs hatch into the larval stage that then develops into nymphs. Protonymph, deutonymph, and adults feed on the honeybee immature form. According to Kumar *et al*. (1993), the most parasitized stage of the host is the bright-red-eyed pupa stage, with larvae, protonymphs, deutonymps, and adults of *T. clareae* found in the cell.

The mating phase of the daughter mites occurs within the capped cell (Pierson, 2014). Mating has been observed in open cells after adult bee emergence or even outside brood cells (Wei, 1992; Woyke, 1994).

The reproductive cycle lasts about one week and is very short compared to that of *Varroa* (OIE, 2014a). Offspring (both female and male mites) and the original mother mite exit from the cell. This is different to the *Varroa* reproductive cycle in which only mated daughters and the founder emerge with the bee while the male dies (FERA, 2013b).

During the phoretic phase, *Tropilaelaps* mites attach to adult honeybees but are unable to feed on them. Thus, their lifespan outside the brood cell is very short. Because of their inability to feed on adult bees, after two days outside, mated females may die if they do not enter a new brood cell (Woyke, 1987). The phoretic phase is the means by which *Tropilaelaps* spread within the colony or between colonies (via the drifting, robbing, and swarming behaviour of adult honeybees).

The short life cycle with a very brief phoretic phase has two main consequences (FERA, 2013b; OIE, 2014b):

- The population of *Tropilaelaps* increases at a greater rate than that of *Varroa*.
- *Tropilaelaps* is not adapted to brood-less periods, e.g. overwintering periods. This feature may be used to control *Tropilaelaps* infestation.

3.4 Spreading and transmission

Natural spread occurs by drifting, robbing, and swarming (FERA, 2013b). In its phoretic phase, the mite can move quickly within the colony and honeybees spread the mites rapidly.

In terms of beekeeping activity, inappropriate management of combs and material, as well as migratory beekeeping, favour the spread of *Tropilaelaps* between colonies within an apiary and between apiaries. They also favour the spread of *Tropilaelaps* to non-infested areas.

Apiculture has become a global activity with trade and exchange of material, package bees, artificial swarms, nuclei, and queens. *Tropilaelaps* must be considered a major potential threat for non-infested regions.

3.5 Clinical signs of *Tropilaelaps* infestation: tropilaelosis

Tropilaelaps can cause the death up to 50% of honeybee larvae and consequently severe damage to heavily infested colonies. The clinical signs of tropilaelosis and varroosis are very similar.

The damage that occurs is mainly the consequence of features of the mite's life cycle:

- The life cycle occurs in the brood cell.
- It is very short, with adult *Tropilaelaps* unable to feed on adult bees and unable to survive more than two days.
- It leads to a large increase in *Tropilaelaps* population.

At the colony level, rapid weakening and collapse may occur. Some infested colonies swarm or abscond the hive as a natural means to control the infestation, favouring the spreading of the mite. At the entrance of the hive, some bees may be found crawling, unable to fly.

The brood appears irregular and poor, due to the death of the larvae. Some capped cells are punctured by cleaner workers trying to expel infested and dead larvae, pupae, and imagos. Cadavers of immature honeybees may be observed protruding from the cells (FERA, 2013b; OIE, 2014a).

Surviving adult bees emerging from infested larvae have a shorter lifespan.

The clinical signs on adult bees are:

- Lower body weight.
- Deformed abdomen.
- Deformed and shrunken legs and wings.

Like *Varroa*, *Tropilaelaps* is strongly suspected to be a vector of DWV. Indeed, DWV has been described associated with *T. mercedesae* infesting *A. mellifera* (Dainat *et al.*, 2009; Forsgren *et al.*, 2009; Sammataro, 2012).

3.6 *Varroa* and *Tropilaelaps* co-infestation

Co-infestation of both *Varroa* and *Tropilaelaps* is possible because they have the same host and the same ecological niche. In this situation, the mites fall into direct competition (Burgett *et al.*, 1983; Pierson, 2014).

During co-infestation of a brood cell by *V. destructor* and *T. clareae*, only female *T. clareae* seems to be able generate viable offspring (Burgett *et al.*, 1983). Another observation reports that when both mites are in the same cell, the reproduction of both mites declines (Ritter and Schneider-Ritter, 1988; OIE, 2014a). At the colony level, in the event of co-infestation, the increase in the population of *Tropilaelaps* is higher than that of *Varroa* (Burgett *et al.*, 1983).

3.7 Diagnosis

In infested countries, the detection and the monitoring of the *Tropilaelaps* are important to control the infestation, as must be done for *Varroa*.

In non-infested countries, importation of beekeeping material and bees must be highly regulated. In the case of introduction, detection of *Tropilaelaps* is crucial as soon as possible considering the risks for colonies: this will lead authorities to take sanitary measures to try to limit the spread of the mite and to try to eradicate it.

Diagnosis can be done by the same methods used for *Varroa* (OIE, 2014a):

- By collection of mites from honeybee samples.
- By examination of colony and brood: like *Varroa*, *Tropilaelaps* can be observed on adult bees. However, identification in the capped brood (in particular in drone capped brood) is the best and easiest means for diagnosis.
- By placing a mesh floor upon a sticky board in the hive.

Distinguishing between both mites is quite easy:

- *Varroa* mites are larger, oval- and crab-shaped, and move slowly.
- *Tropilaelaps* mites are smaller, elongated, and are fast running.

Differential diagnosis must also consider the fly *Braula coeca* (larger, rounder in shape with only three pairs of legs) and the mite *Melittiphis alvearius* (a scavenger of pollen in the hive) (Gibbins and van Toor, 1990; FERA, 2013b)

3.8 Control of *Tropilaelaps* infestation

Treatment with sustained-released acaricides (tau-fluvalinate, flumethrin, amitraze) or with carefully timed applications of formic acid, sulfur, and coumaphos is used in Asia to control *Tropilaelaps* infestation (Wilde *et al.*, 2000; OIE, 2014a).

Biotechnological methods are also used to control *Tropilaelaps* infestation. They are probably more efficient than for the control of *Varroa* infestation in particular because of the inability of *Tropilaelaps* to feed on adult bees and to live outside the cells longer than two days.

Biotechnological methods are based on biological features of the mite:

- The attraction of the mite to the brood.
- The inability to feed on adult bees.
- The short lifespan of mites outside the brood during the trophalactic stage (2 days).

Thus, husbandry methods leading to brood-less periods prevent *Tropilaelaps* from finding a host to support reproduction and survival (Woyke, 1984; Tangkanasing *et al.*, 1988; Wilde *et al.*, 2000). Such methods involve

- Removing all the brood combs from infested colonies.
- Removing the whole capped brood after caging the queen for 9 days (all the brood will be capped at this moment).
- Caging the queen for at least 21 days causes the brood surface to progressively decrease. The queen is released when all the brood-cells are empty and cleared (Woyke, 1984).

Because the mite is not able to survive a long brood-less period, *Tropilaelaps* infestation is probably 'relatively straightforward' to control using beekeeping methods (FERA, 2013b).

3.9 Preventing non-infested countries against *Tropilaelaps* mites

Global apiculture, with package bees, nuclei, artificial swarms on frames, and trade in queens and material (leading to exchange and movement of honeybees around the world) leads to a real and major risk of introducing *Tropilaelaps* in virgin territories. The mites have not yet been found the EU. '*Tropilaelaps* mites are statutory notifiable pests in the European Union. There is a legal requirement for any findings to be notified to regulatory bodies under EU legislation' (Anses–FERA–FLI, 2013).

The UK has developed a National Bee Unit to monitor apiaries for exotic threats, in particular concerning *Tropilaelaps* mites and the small hive beetle *Aethina tumida* (FERA, 2013b). This surveillance is performed by inspecting sentinel apiaries for exotic pests.

4 Infestation by the fly *Braula coeca*

Braula coeca is a flattened, blind, and wingless fly (Order: Diptera; Family: Braulidae). It is also (incorrectly) called 'bee louse' (Clément, 1905; Somerville, 2007), lice being a term given usually to Acarid parasites. It was first described by Réaumur (1734–42).

Adults live on the bodies of the three castes of honeybee. Larvae live in the honeycomb wax and tunnel through the wax capped honey cells. It is mainly considered as harmless to colonies. The bee louse is sometimes considered as a commensal insect of colonies (University of Florida, 2010). *Braula cœca* is described worldwide (Europe, Asia, Africa, South and North America and Tasmania). However, at least in Europe, the bee louse is now rarely observed in apiaries, probably because of the use of chemicals to control *Varroa* infestation. In some places where *Varroa* is not present, e.g. the island of Ushant off the coast of France, *Braula* is observed in many colonies.

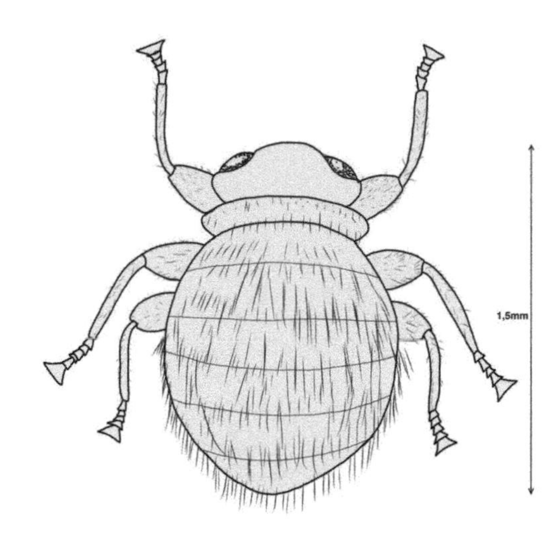

Figure 5.17 *Braula coeca* adult. (Drawing by Nicolas Vidal-Naquet, adapted from Paillot *et al.*, 1943.)

4.1 The fly *Braula coeca*

The *Braula coeca* adult is about 1.5 mm long, round-shaped, reddish-brown, and covered in spine-like hairs (Figure 5.17) (Clément, 1905; University of Florida, 2010). As an insect, it has three pairs of legs, and this may help to easily distinguish it from *V. destructor*. Tarsi, with a comb-shaped row of spines, allow it to hang upon the hairs of the adult honeybees (Dietz *et al.*, 1971). The adult bee louse moves around the bee with great agility (Dietz *et al.*, 1971).

Adults are found on the bodies of all three castes, with a preference for the queen (probably because of the frequency of feeding periods and because of the quality of the royal jelly). Up to 180 adult bee lice have been observed on a single queen (University of Florida, 2010). In order to feed, *Braula* moves near the mouth apparatus of the bee and steals the food provided by the nurse bees during trophallaxis (Clément, 1905; Somerville, 2007).

The female lays eggs in many places in the hive (empty cells, brood cappings, debris on the floor), but only the eggs oviposited on honey cappings will hatch.

The eggs are white and oval-shaped with two lateral flanges. The eggs measure on average 0.8 mm × 0.3 mm without the flanges and 0.84 mm × 0.42 mm with the flanges. The egg stage lasts 2–7 days (University of Florida, 2010). The larvae are maggot like. The larval development goes through three instars before pupation. The larval stage lasts 7–11 days. The pupae are creamy white in colour and measure 1.4–1.7 mm long × 0.5–0.75 mm wide (Sommerville, 2007).

The larva develops under the capping and burrows a 1 mm tunnel along the surface of the honeycombs, giving them a cracked appearance (Borchert, 1970; Somerville, 2007). The bee louse can live all winter long on the bees during the overwintering period. *Braula* spread via robbing and drifting honeybees.

4.2 Health impact of *Braula coeca*

Braula is mainly harmless and considered as innocuous for honeybee colonies.

It has been reported that in strongly infested colonies, the bee louse may disturb the egg-ovipositing of the queen (Ben Hamida, 1999).

The main economic impact of *Braula* fly infestation concerns the honeycombs (Somerville, 2007). The honeycombs appear cracked, burrowed, and are unstable. Their poor appearance renders them unsaleable (to honeycomb consumers). However, the honey within may still be extracted and sold.

4.3 Diagnosis

Diagnosis is made by identification of *B. coeca* on honeybees (workers, drones, and the queen). The flies are often found on the heads of the three castes of bees and particularly on the queen. A cracked appearance of the honeycombs is one of the clinical signs of infestation within the colony.

4.4 Control of *Braula* infestation

There is no treatment because the bee louse is not considered as a danger or a threat to colonies. However, medicines used against *Varroa* have a residual insecticidal property and thus are presumed to be efficient against *Braula*. Freezing the combs kills all stages of *B. coeca* (Somerville, 2007). Tobacco smoke is effective against *Braula* adults (Phillips, 1925; Ben Hamida, 1999). However, this treatment is not advisable because it is toxic to bees (and humans) and might contaminate the honey.

References

Alberti, G. and Hänel, H. (1986) Fine structure of the genital system in the bee parasite, *Varroa Jacobsoni* (Gamasida: Dermanyssina) with remarks on spermiogenesis, spermatozoa and capacitation. *Experimental and Applied Acarology*, 2: 63–104.

Alberti, G. and Zeck-Kapp, G. (1986) The nutrimentary egg development in the mite, *Varroa jacobsoni* (Acari, Arachnida), an ectoparasite of honey bee. *Acta Zoologica (Stockholm)*, 67: 11–25.

Amdam, G.V., Hartfelder, K., Norberg, K., Hagen, A., and Omholt, S.W. (2004) Altered physiology in worker honey bees (Hymenoptera: Apidae) infested with the mite *Varroa destructor* (Acari: Varroidae): a factor in colony loss during overwintering? *Journal of Economic Entomology*, 97: 741–747.

Anderson, D.L. and Trueman, J.W.H. (2000) *Varroa jacobsoni* (Acari: Varroidae) is more than one species. *Experimental and Applied Acarology*, 24: 165–189.

Anderson, D.L. and Morgan, M.J. (2007) Genetic and morphological variation of bee-parasitic *Tropilaelaps* mites (Acari: *Laelapidae*): new and re-defined species. *Experimental and Applied Acarology*, 43: 1–24.

Anses–FERA–FLI–European Union Reference Laboratory for Honey Bee Health (2013) *Tropilaelaps spp.* mites. Available at https://eurl-milk.anses.fr/en/minisite/abeilles/leaflet-tropilaelaps-beekeepers (accessed 31 July 2014).

Bailey L. (1964) The Isle of Wight Disease: the origin and significance of the myth. *Bee World*, 45: 32–37.

Bailey, L. (1965) Susceptibility of the honeybee, *Apis mellifera* Linnaeus, infested with *Acarapis woodi* (Rennie) to infection by airborn pathogens. *Journal of Invertebrate Pathology*, 7: 141–143.

Bailey, L. and Lee, D.C. (1959) The effect of infestation with *Acarapis woodi* (Rennie) on the mortality of honey bees. *Journal of Insect Pathology*, 1: 15–24.

Bailey, L. and Perry, J.N. (1982) The diminished incidence of *Acarapis woodi* (Rennie) Acari: Tarsonemidae) in honey bees, *Apis mellifera* L. (Hymenoptera Apidae), in Britain. *Bulletin of Entomological Research*, 72: 655–662.

Bak, B., Wilde, J., Siuda, M., and Kobylinska, M. (2009) Comparison of two methods of monitoring honeybee infestation with *Varroa destructor* mite. *Annals of Warsaw University of Life Sciences, Animal Science*, 46: 33–38.

Baker, R.A., Hick, A., and Chmielewski, W. (2005) Aspects of the history and biogeography of the bee mites *Tropilaelaps clareae* and *T. koenigerum*. *Journal of Apiculture Science*, 49: 13–19.

Belaïd, M. and Doumandji, S. (2010) Effet du *Varroa destructor* sur la morphométrie alaire et sur les composants du système immunitaire de l'abeille ouvrière *Apis mellifera intermissa*. *Lebanese Science Journal*, 11: 83–90.

Ben Hamida, T. (1999) Enemies of bees. In Colin, M.E., Ball, B.V., and Kilani, M. (eds), *Bee Disease Diagnosis, Options Méditerranéennes*, Series B: *Etudes et Recherches*. No. 25. CIHEAM Publication, Zaragoza, pp. 147–165.

Boecking, O. and Genersch, E. (2008) Varroosis – the ongoing crisis in bee keeping. *Journal of Consumer Protection and Food Safety*, 3: 221–228.

Borchert, A. (1970) *Les Maladies et Parasites des Abeilles*, trans. from German by J. Michelat. Vigot frères, Paris.

Bowen-Walker, P.L. and Gun, A. (2001) The effect of the ectoparasitic mite, *Varroa destructor* on adult worker honeybee (*Apis mellifera*) emergence weights, water, protein, carbohydrate, and lipid levels. *Entomologia experimentalis et applicate*, 101: 207–217.

Breguetova, N.G. (1953) The mite fauna of the Far East. *Parasitologuitcheskii Zbornik ZIN AN SSR*, 15: 302–338.

Büchler, R. (1994) Varroa tolerance in honey bees – occurrence, characters and breeding. *Bee World*, 49: 6–18.

Büchler, R. (2009) Des colonies saines grâce à un retrait complet du couvain. Available at: http://www.freethebees.ch/wp-content/uploads/2014/06/Brutentnahme-Francais-Print-13.6.2014.pdf (accessed 19 November 2014).

Burgett, M., Akratanakul, P., and Morse, R.A. (1983) *Tropilaelaps clareae*: a parasite of honeybees in south-east Asia. *Bee World*, 64: 25–28.

Charrière, J.D., Imdorf, A., and Fluri, P. (1998) Potentiel et limites de l'acaricide oxalique pour lutter contre *Varroa*. *Revue Suisse d'apiculture*, 95: 311–316.

Clément A.-L. (1905) Le *Braula cœca*. *La Nature*, 2e semester: 221–222.

Coffey, M.F. and Breen, J. (2013) Efficacy of Apilife Var® and Thymovar® against *Varroa destructor* as an autumn treatment in a cool climate. *Journal of Apicultural Research*, 52(5): 210–218.

Colin, M.E. (1982) La varroase. *Revue scientifique de l'Office International des Epizooties*, 1(4): 1177–1189.

Colin, M.E., Fernandez, P.G., and Ben Hamida, T. (1999) Varroosis. In Colin, M.E., Ball, B.V., and Kilani, M. (eds), *Bee Disease Diagnosis, Options Méditerranéennes*, Series B: *Etudes et Recherches*. No. 25. CIHEAM Publications, Zaragoza, pp. 121–142.

Dainat, B., Ken, T., Berthoud, H., and Neumann, P. (2009) The ectoparasitic mite *Tropilaelaps mercedesae* (Acari, Laelapidae) as a vector of honeybee viruses. *Insectes Sociaux*, 56: 40–43.

Dainat, B., Evans, J.D., Chen, Y.P., Gauthier, L., and Neumann, P. (2012) Dead or alive: deformed wing virus and *Varroa destructor* reduce the life span of winter honeybees. *Applied and Environmental Microbiology*, 78: 981–987.

Dawicke, B.L., Otis, G.W., Scott-Dupree, C., and Nasr, M. (1992) Host preference of the honey bee tracheal mite (*Acarapis woodi* Rennie). *Experimental and Applied Acarology*, 15: 83–98.

De Jong, D., De Jong, P.H., and Gonçalves, L.S. (1982) Weight loss and other damage to developing worker honeybees from infestation with *Varroa jacobsoni*. *Journal of Apicultural Research*, 21: 165–216.

Delaplane, K.S. (1992) Controlling tracheal mites (Acari: Tarsonemidae) in colonies of honeybees (Hymenotera: Apidae) with vegetable oil and menthol. *Journal of Economical Entomology*, 85: 2118–2124.

Del Cacho, E., Marti, J., Josa, A., Quilez, J., and Sanchez-Acedo, C. (1996) Effect of *Varroa jacobsoni* parasitization in the glycoprotein expression on *Apis mellifera* spermatozoa. *Apidologie*, 27: 87–92.

Delfinado, M.D. and Baker, E.W. (1961) *Tropilaelaps*, a new genus of mites from the Philippines (*Laelapidae* [s. lat.]: *Acarina*). *Fieldiana, Zoology*, 44: 53–56.

Definado-Baker, M. and Baker, E.W. (1984) Notes on honey bee mites of the genus *Acarapis* Hirst (Acari: Tarsonemidae). *International Journal of Acarology*, 8: 211–266.

Delfinado-Baker, M.D., Rath, W., and Boecking, O. (1992) Phoretic bee mites and honeybee grooming behavior. *International Journal of Acarology*, 18: 315–322.

de Miranda J., Gauthier L., Ribière M., and Chen Y.P. (2012). Honey bee viruses and their effect on bee and colony health. In Sanmarco, D. and Yoder J.A. (eds), *Honey Bee Colony Health Challenges and sustainable solutions*. CRC Press, Boca Raton, FL, pp. 71–102.

De Ruijter, A. and Kaas, J.P. (1983) The anatomy of the Varroa mite. In Cavalloro, R. (ed.), *Varroa jacobsoni Oud Affecting Honey Bees: Present Status and Needs*. A.A. Balkema, Rotterdam, pp. 45–47.

Dietz, A., Humphreys, W.J., and Lindner, J.W. (1971) Examination of the bee louse, *Braula cœca*, with the scanning electron microscope. *Apiacta*, 1.

Donzé, G. (1995) Adaptations comportementales de l'acarien ectoparasite *Varroa jacobsoni* durant sa phase de reproduction dans les alvéoles operculées de l'abeille mellifère *Apis mellifera*. Doctoral thesis, Université de Neuchâtel, Switzerland.

Donzé, G. and Guerin, P.M. (1994) Behavioral attributes and parental care of Varroa mites parasitizing honeybee brood. *Behavioral Ecology and Sociobiology*, 34: 305–319.

Downey, D.L. and Winston, M.L. (2001) Honey bee colony mortality and productivity with single and dual infestations of parasitic mite species. *Apidologie*, 32(6): 567–575.

Duay, P., De Jong D., and Engels, W. (2002) Decreased flight performance and sperm production in drones of the honey bee (*Apis mellifera*) slightly infested by *Varroa destructor* mites during pupal development. *Genetics and Molecular Research*, 3: 227–232.

Esquijarosa, E.M. (2003) Apilifevar and Apiguar: evaluation of two organic treatments against varroasis and acariosis of the Honeybee. In Apimondia. Standing Commission of Beekeeping Economy, XXXVIII Congress APIMONDIA, Ljubljana, Slovenia. Available at: http://www.apimondia.com/apiacta/slovenia/en/esquijarosa.pdf (accessed 29 July 2014)

Fakhimzadeh, K. (2000) A rapid field and laboratory method to detect *Varroa jacobsoni* in the honey bee (*Apis mellifera*). Available at: http://www.beekeeping.com/articles/us/detection_varroa.htm (accessed 2 October 2014).

FAO (2006) *Honey Bee Diseases and Pests: A Practical Guide*. Avalaible at: http://www.fao.org/3/a-a0849e.pdf (accessed 29 July 2014).

Faucon, J.P. (2008) Varroase et autres maladies des abeilles: causes majeures de mortalité des colonies en France. *Bulletin Académie Vétérinaire de France*, 161(3): 257–263.

Faucon, J.P., Drajnudel, P., Chauzat, M-P., and Aubert, M. (2007) Contrôle de l'efficacité du médicament APIVAR ND contre *Varroa destructor*, parasite de l'abeille domestique. [Control of the efficacy of APIVAR ND against *Varroa destructor*, a parasite of *Apis mellifera*.] *Revue de Médecine Vétérinaire*, 158(6): 283–290.

FERA: The Food & Environment Research Agency (2013a) Managing *Varroa*. The Food and Environment Research Agency, York.

FERA: The Food & Environment Research Agency (2013b) *Tropilaelaps* parasitic mites of the honey bees. The Food and Environment Research Agency, York.

Fernández, N. and Coineau, Y. (2006) *Varroa - The Serial Bee Killer Mite*. Atlantica, Biarritz.

Fernandez, P.G. (1999) Acarapidosis or tracheal acariosis. In Colin, M.E., Ball, B.V., and Kilani, M. (eds), *Bee Disease Diagnosis, Options Méditerranéennes*, Series B: *Etudes et Recherches*. No. 25. CIHEAM Publications, Zaragoza, pp. 107–115.

Forsgren, E., de Miranda, J.R., Isaksson, M., Wei S., and Fries, I. (2009) Deformed wing virus associated with *Tropilaelaps mercedesae* infesting European honey bees (*Apis mellifera*). *Experimental and Applied Acarology*, 47(2): 87–97.

Fries, I., Camazine, S., and Sneyd, J. (1994) Population dynamics of *Varroa jacobsoni*: a model and a review. *Bee World*, 75: 5–28.

Fries, I., Hansen, H., Imdorf, A., and Rosenkranz, P. (2003) Swarming in honey bees (*Apis mellifera*) and *Varroa destructor* population development in Sweden. *Apidologie*, 34: 389–398.

Garrido, C., Rosenkranz, P., Stürmer, M., Rübsam, R., and Büning, J. (2000) Toluidine blue staining as a rapid measure for initiation of oocyte growth and fertility in *Varroa jacobsoni* Oud. *Apidologie*, 31: 559–566.

Gibbins, B.L. and van Toor, R.F. (1990) Investigation of the parasitic status of *Melittiphis alvearius* (Berlese) on honeybees, *Apis mellifera* L., by immunoassay. *Journal of Apicultural Research*, 29: 46–52.

Giordani, G. (1965) Recherches au laboratoire sur *Acarapis woodi* (Rennie), agent de l'acariose des abeilles (*Apis mellifera* L.). Note 4. *Bulletin Apicole*, 8: 159–176.

Gregorc, A. (2012) A clinical case of honey bee intoxication after using coumaphos strips against *Varroa destructor*. *Journal of Apicultural Research*, 51(1): 142–143.

Grobov, O.F. (1976) La varroase de l'abeille mellifère. *Apiacta*, 11: 145–148.

Gunther, C.E.M. (1951) A mite from a beehive on Singapore Island (Acarina: Laelapidae). *Proceedings of the Linnean Society of New South Wales*, 76: 155.

Harris, J.W. (2007) Bees with Varroa Sensitive Hygiene preferentially remove mite infested pupae aged ≤ five days post capping. *Journal of Apicultural Research and Bee World*, 46: 134–139.

Imdorf, A., Charriere, J.D., Kilchenmann, V., Bogdanov, S., and Fluri, P. (2003) Alternative strategy in central Europe for the control of *Varroa destructor* in honey bee colonies. *Apiacta*, 38: 258–285.

Janmaat, A.F. and Winston, M.L. (2000) The influence of pollen storage area and *Varroa jacobsoni* Oud parasitism on temporal caste structure in honey bees (*Apis mellifera* L.). *Insectes Sociaux*, 47: 177–182.

Kanbar, G. and Engels, W. (2003) Ultrastructure and bacterial infection of wounds in honey bee (*Apis mellifera*) pupae punctured by Varroa mites. *Parasitology Research*, 90(5): 349–354.

Kanga, L.H.B., Jones, W.A., and James, R.R. (2003) Field trials using the fungal pathogen, *Metarhizium anis7opliae* (Deuteromycetes: Hyphomycetes) to control the ectoparasitic mite, *Varroa destructor* (Acari: Varroidae) in honey bee, *Apis mellifera* (Hymenoptera: Apidae) colonies. *Journal of Economic Entomology*, 96: 1091–1099.

Korpela, S., Aarhus, A., Fries, I., and Hansen, H. (1993) *Varroa jacobsoni* Oud. in cold climates: population growth, winter mortality and influence on survival of honey bee colonies. *Journal of Apicultural Research*, 31: 157–164.

Kotwal, S. and Abrol, D.P. (2009) Impact of *Varroa destructor* infestation on the body weight of developing honeybee brood and emerging adults. *Pakistan Journal of Entomology*, 31: 67–70.

Kovac, H. and Crailsheim, K. (1988) Lifespan of *Apis mellifera carnica* Pollm. infested by *Varroa jocobsoni* Oud. in relation to scason and extent of infestation. *Journal of Apicultural Research*, 27: 230–238.

Kralj, J., Brockmann, A., Fuchs, S., and Tautz, J. (2007) The parasitic mite *Varroa destructor* affects non-associative learning in honey bee foragers, *Apis mellifera* L. *Journal of Comparative Physiology A: Neuroethology, Sensory, Neural, and Behavioral Physiology*, 193: 363–370.

Kumar, R., Kumar, N.R., and Bhalla, O.P. (1993) Studies on the development biology of *Tropilaelaps clareae* Delfinado and Baker (Acarina: Laelapidae) vis a vis the threshold stage in the life cycle of *Apis mellifera* Linn. (Hymenoptera: Apidae). *Experimental and Applied Acarology*, 17(8): 621–625.

Langhé, A.B., Natzkii KV, and Tatzii, V.M. (1976) Klechtch *Varroa* (*Varroa jacobsoni*, Oudemans, 1904) i podkhody k razrabotke sredstv. *Ptchelovodstvo*, 13: 16–20.

Le Conte, Y., Arnold, G., Trouiller, J., Masson, C., Chappe, B., and Ourisson, G. (1989) Attraction of the parasitic mite *Varroa* to the drone larvae of honeybees by simple aliphatic esters. *Science*, 245: 638–639.

Lee, K.V., Moon, R.D., Burkness, E.C., Hutchison, W.D., and Spivak, M. (2010) Practical sampling plans for *Varroa destructor* (Acari: Varroidae) in *Apis mellifera* (Hymenoptera: Apidae) colonies and apiaries. *Journal of Economic Entomology*, 103(4): 1039–1050.

Liebig, G. (2001) How many Varroa mites can be tolerated by a honey bee colony? *Apidologie*, 32: 482–484.

Lodesani, M., Costa, C., Besana, A., Dall'Olio, R., Franceschetti, S., Tesoriero, D., and Vaccari, G. (2014) Impact of control strategies for *Varroa destructor* on colony survival and health in northern and central regions of Italy. *Journal of Apicultural Research*, 53(1): 155–164.

Lux, M. (1987) *Varroa jacobsoni* Oudemans ectoparasite de l'abeille *Apis mellifica* Linne. Etude physico-chimique et immuno-chimique de l'hémolymphe d'abeille saine ou parasitée. Thèse pour l'obtention du diplôme de l'École Pratique des Hautes Études. École Pratique des Hautes Études, Paris.

Maggi, M.D., Ruffinengo, S.R., Negri, P., and Eguaras, M.J. (2010) Resistance phenomena to amitraz from populations of the ectoparasitic mite *Varroa destructor* of Argentina. *Parasitology Research*, 107(5): 1189–1192.

Mallick, A. (2013) Action sanitaire en production apicole: gestion de la varroose face à l'apparition de resistance aux traitements chez *Varroa destructor*. Thèse pour obtenir le grade de Docteur Vétérinaire. Vetagro Sup, Lyon.

Martin, S.J., (1994). Ontogenesis of the mite *Varroa jacobsoni* Oud. in worker brood of the honeybee *Apis mellifera* L. under natural conditions. *Experimental and Applied Acarology*, 18: 87–100.

Martin, S.J. (1995). Reproduction of *Varroa jacobsoni* in cells of Apis mellifera containing one or more mother mites and the distribution of these cells. *Journal of Apicultural Research*, 34: 187–196.

Martin, S.J. (1998). A population model for the ectoparasitic mite *Varroa jacobsoni* in honey bee (*Apis mellifera*) colonies. *Ecological Modelling*, 109: 267–281.

Martin, S.J. and Kemp, D. (1997) Average number of reproductive cycles performed by *Varroa jacobsoni* in honey bee (*Apis mellifera*) colonies. *Journal of Apicultural Research*, 36: 113–123.

Meikle, W.G., Mercadier, G., Holst, N., Nansen, C., and Girod, V. (2008) Impact of a treatment of *Beauveria bassiana* (Deuteromycota: Hyphomycetes) on honeybee (*Apis mellifera*) colony health and on *Varroa destructor* mites (Acari: Varroidae). *Apidologie*, 39: 247–259.

Mondragón, L., Martin, S., Vandame, and R. (2006) Mortality of mite offspring: a major component of *Varroa destructor* resistance in a population of Africanized bees. *Apidologie*, 37: 67–74.

Moritz, R.F.A. and Jordan, M. (1992) Selection of resistance against *Varroa jacobsoni* across caste and sex in the honeybee (*Apis mellifera* L., Hymenoptera: Apidae). *Experimental and Applied Acarology*, 16: 345–353.

Muli, E., Patch, H., Frazier, M., Frazier, J., Torto, B., *et al.* (2014) Evaluation of the distribution and impacts of parasites, pathogens, and pesticides on honey bee (*Apis mellifera*) populations in East Africa. *PLoS ONE*. 9(4): e94459. doi:10.1371/journal.pone.0094459

Navajas, M., Migeon, A., Alaux, C., Martin-Magniette, M.L., Robinson, G.E., Evans, J.D., Cros-Arteil, S., Crauser, D., and Le Conte, Y. (2008) Differential gene expression of the honey bee *Apis mellifera* associated with *Varroa destructor* infection. *BMC Genomics*, 9: 301, doi:10.1186/1471-2164-9-301 (accessed 12 July 2014).

Noireterre, P. (2011) Biologie et pathogénie de *Varroa destructor. Bulletin des GTV*, 62: 101–106.

Official Journal of the European Union (2013) *Commission implementing decision of 11 October 2013 recognising parts of the Union as free from varroosis in bees and establishing additional guarantees required in intra-Union trade and imports for the protection of their varroosis-free status* (notified under document C(2013) 6599) L273/38–40.

OIE (2014a) Manual of Diagnostic Tests and Vaccines for Terrestrial Animals 2014. Apinae. Section 2.2. Available at: http://www.oie.int/en/international-standard-setting/terrestrial-manual/access-online/ (accessed 24 August 2014).

OIE (2014b) OIE Listed Diseases. Available at http://www.oie.int/en/animal-health-in-the-world/oie-listed-diseases-2014/ (accessed 29 April 2014).

Oldroyd B.P. (1999) Coevolution while you wait: *Varroa jacobsoni*, a new parasite of western honeybees. *Trends in Ecology and Evolution*, 14: 312–315.

Oudemans, A.C. (1904) On a new genus and species of parasitic Acari. *Notes from Leyden Museum*, 24: 216–222.

Paillot, A., Kirkor, S., and Granger, A.M. (1943) *L'abeille Anatomie, Maladies, Ennemis*. Imprimerie de Trévoux, Ain.

Pernal, S.F., Baird, D.S., Birmingham, A.L., Higo HA, Slessor, K.N., and Winston, M.L. (2005) Semiochemicals influencing the host-finding behaviour of *Varroa destructor*. *Experimental and Applied Acarology*, 37: 1–26.

Pettis, J. and Engelsdorp, D.V. (2010) Small hive beetles and *Tropilaelaps* mites, real problems for beekeepers. *Apimondia Proceedings*, p. 106.

Phillips, E.F. (1925) The bee louse *Braula cœca* in the United States. USDA Circular 334.

Pierson, L. (2014) *Tropilaelaps clareae* et *Aethina tumida:* deux arthropodes pathogènes pour l'abeille domestique (*Apis mellifera*), agents d'infestations inscrites sur la liste des maladies de première catégorie en France. Thèse pour le Doctorat Vétérinaire, Ecole Nationale Vétérinaire d'Alfort, Créteil.

Quarles, W. (1996) EPA exempts least-toxic pesticides. *IPM Practitioner*, 18: 16–17.

Rath, W., Delfinado-Baker, M., and Drescher, W. (1991) Observations on the mating behaviour, sex ratio, phoresy and dispersal of *Tropilaelaps clareae* (Acari: *Laelapidae*). *International Journal of Acarology*, 17: 201–208.

Réaumur, R.A. (1734–1742) *Mémoires pour servir à l'Histoire des Insectes*, Vol. 5. Imprimerie Royale, Paris.

Rinderer, T.E., De Guzman L.I., Lancaster V.A., Delatte G.T., and Stelzer, J.A. (1999) *Varroa* in the mating yard: I. The effects of *Varroa jacobsoni* and Apistan on drone honey bees. *American Bee Journal*, 139: 134–139.

Ritter, W., Leclercq, E., and Koch, W. (1984) Observations des populations d'abeilles et de Varroa dans les colonies à différents niveaux d'infestation. *Apidologie*, 15: 389–400.

Ritter, W. and Schneider-Ritter, U. (1988) Differences in biology and means of controlling *Varroa jacobsoni* and *Tropilaelaps clareae*, two novel parasitic mites of *Apis mellifera*. In Needham, G.R., Page, R.E., Jr, Delfinado-Baker, M., and Bowman, C.E. (ed.), *Africanized Honey Bees and Bee Mites*. Ellis Horwood, Chichester, UK

Rosenkranz, P., Kirsch, R., and Renz, R. (2006) Population dynamics of honey bee colonies and Varroa tolerance: a comparison between Uruguay and Germany. In Santana, W.C., Lobo, C.H., and Hartfelder, K.H. (eds), *Proceedings 7th Encontro Sobre Abelhas*. USP, Ribeirão Preto, Brazil.

Rosenkranz, P., Aumeier, P., and Ziegelmann, B. (2010) Biology and control of *Varroa destructor. Journal of Invertebrate Pathology*, 103: 96–119.

Sakofski, F., Koeniger, N., and Fuchs, S. (1990) Seasonality of honey bee colony invasion by *Varroa jacobsoni* Oud. *Apidologie*, 21: 547–550.

Sammataro, D. (2012) Global status of honey bee mites. In Sammatoro, D. and Yolder, J.A. (ed.), *Honey Bee Colony Health Challenges and Sustainable Solutions*. CRC Press, Boca Raton, FL, pp. 37–54.

Sammataro, D. and Needham, G.R. (1996) Host-seeking behaviour of tracheal mites (Acari: Tarsonemidae) on honey bees (Hymenoptera: Apidae). *Experimental and Applied Acarology*, 20: 121–136.

Schatton-Gadelmayer, K. and Engels, W. (1988) Blood proteins and body weight of newly-emerged worker honeybees with different levels of parasitization of brood mites. *Entomologia Generalis*, 14: 93–101.

Schneider, P. and Drescher, W. (1987) Einfluss der Parasitierung durch die Milbe *Varroa jacobsoni* aus das Schlupfgewicht, die Gewichtsentwicklung, die Entwicklung der Hypopharynxdrusen und die Lebensdauer von Apis mellifera. *Apidologie*, 18: 101–106.

Scott-Dupree, C. and Otis, G.W. (1992) The efficacy of four miticides for the control of *Acarapis woodi*

(Rennie) in a fall treatment program. *Apidologie*, 23(2): 97–106.

Scott-Dupree, C., Ball, B.V., Welsh, O., and Allen, M. (1995) An investigation into the potential transmission of viruses by the honeybee tracheal mite (*Acarapis woodi* R.) to honeybees. In *Canadian Honey Council Research Symposium Proceedings*, pp. 15–24.

Shaw, K.E., Davidson, G., Clark, S.J., Ball, B.V., Pell, J.K., Chandler, D., and Sunderland, K.D. (2002) Laboratory bioassays to assess the pathogenicity of mitosporic fungi to *Varroa destructor* (Acari: Mesostigmata), an ectoparasitic mite of the honeybee, *Apis mellifera*. *Biological Control*, 24: 266–276.

Somerville, D. (2007) *Braula* Fly. *Primefact* No. 649.

Spivak, M.S. (1996) Honeybee hygienic behavior and defense against *Varroa jacobsoni*. *Apidologie*, 7(4): 245–260.

Tangkanasing, P., Wongsiri, S., and Vongsamanode, S. (1988) Integrated control of *Varroa jacobsoni* and *Tropilaelaps clareae* in beehives in Thailand. In Needham, G.R., Page, R.E., Delfinado-Baker, M., and Bowman, C.E. (eds), *Africanized Honeybees and Bee Mites*. Ellis Horwood, Chichester, pp. 409–412.

Tofilski, A. (2012) Honey bee. Available from http://www.honeybee.drawwing.org. (accessed 10 July 2014).

Topolska, G. (2001) *Varroa destructor* (Anderson and Trueman, 2000); the change in classification within the genus *Varroa* (Oudemans, 1904). *Wiadomosci Parazytologiczne*, 47: 151–155.

Toumanoff, C. (1939) *Les ennemis des abeilles*. Editions IDEO, Hanoi.

Tsagou, V., Lianou, A., Lazarakis, D., Emmanouel, N., and Aggelis, G. (2004) Newly isolated bacterial strains belonging to Bacillaceae (*Bacillus* sp.) and Micrococcaceae accelerate death of the honey bee mite, *Varroa destructor* (*V. jacobsoni*) in laboratory assays. *Biotechnology Letters*, 26: 529–532.

University of Florida (2010) Bee louse. Available at: http://entnemdept.ufl.edu/creatures/misc/bees/bee_louse.htm (accessed 10 August 2014).

University of Florida (2014) Honey bee tracheal mite. Avalaible at: http://entnemdept.ufl.edu/creatures/misc/bees/tracheal_mite.htm#top (accessed 25 July 2014).

Vandame, J. (2012) Tests d'efficacité 2011 – Médicaments AMM de lutte contre Varroa. *La Santé de l'Abeille*, 249: 277–287.

Vidal-Naquet, N. (2011) Honeybees. In Lewbart, G.L. (ed.), *Invertebrate Medicine*, 2nd edn. Wiley-Blackwell, Chichester, pp. 285–321.

Wei, H.Z. (1992). Study on generative characteristics of *Tropilaelaps clareae* Delfinado et Baker (Acari: Laelapidae). *Proc. XIX International Congress of Entomology*. Abstracts XVIIP. Beijing, 9: 675.

Weinberg, K.P. and Madel, G. (1985) The influence of the mite *Varroa jacobsoni* Oud. on the protein concentration and the haemolymph volume of the brood of worker bees and drones of the honey bee *Apis mellifera* L. *Apidologie*, 16: 421–436.

Weissenberger, J. (1988). Contribution à l'étude de la lutte contre la varroase. Thèse de Doctorat Vétérinaire, École Nationale Vétérinaire d'Alfort, Maisons-Alfort.

Wendling, S. (2012) *Varroa destructor* (Anderson et Trueman, 2000), un acarien ectoparasite de l'abeille domestique *Apis mellifera* Linnaeus, 1758. Revue bibliographique et contribution à l'étude de sa reproduction. Thèse pour le Doctorat Vétérinaire, Ecole Nationale Vétérinaire d'Alfort, Créteil.

Wilde, J., Woyke, J., Neupane, K.R., and Wilde, M. (2000) Comparative evaluation tests of different methods to control *Tropilaelaps clareae*, a mite parasite in Nepal. In *Proceedings of the 7th International Conference on Tropical Bees and 5th AAA Conference*, Chaing Mai, pp. 249–251.

Wilson, W.T., Pettis, J.S, Henderson, C.E., Morse R.A. (1997) Tracheal mites. In *Honey Bee Pests, Predators and Diseases*, 3rd edn. AI Root Publishing, Medina, OH, pp 255–277.

Winston, M.L. (1987) *The Biology of the Honeybee*. Harvard University Press, Cambridge, MA.

World's Best Photos of *Varroa*, The (2014) Available at http://flickrhivemind.net/Tags/varroa/Interesting (accessed 15 October 2014).

Woyke, J. (1984) Survival and prophylactic control of *Tropilaelaps clareae* infesting *Apis mellifera* colonies in Afghanistan. *Apidologie*, 14(4): 421–434.

Woyke, J. (1987) Length of stay of the parasitic mite *Tropilaelaps clareae* outside sealed honeybee brood cells as a basis for its effective control. *Journal of Apicultural Research*, 26: 104–109.

Woyke, J. (1994). Mating behaviour of the parasitic honeybee mite *Tropilaelaps clareae*. *Experimental and Applied Acarology*, 18: 723–733.

Yang, X. and Cox-Foster, D.L. (2005) Impact of an ectoparasite on the immunity and pathology of an invertebrate: evidence for host immunosuppression and viral amplification. *Proceedings of the National Academy of Sciences USA*, 102: 7470–7475.

Ziegelmann, B., Steidle, H., Lindenmayer, A., and Rosenkranz, P. (2008) Sex pheromones trigger the mating behaviour of *Varroa destructor*. *Apidologie*, 39: 598.

6

Fungal and protozoan diseases

Several fungi generally regarded as beneficial, commensal, symbiotic, or opportunistic are found in bee colonies and their nests, in particular in the beebread (Foley *et al.*, 2012; Yoder *et al.*, 2013). However, some fungi are or may become pathogenic for *Apis mellifera* and hence able to damage colonies: these are fungi belonging to the division Ascomycota, namely *Ascosphaera apis* and *Aspergillus* spp. which are potentially pathogenic for the brood; and to the division Microsporidia, namely *Nosema apis* and *Nosema ceranae*, which are potentially pathogenic for adult bees.

This chapter describes the fungal and amoebal diseases affecting honeybee colonies:

- Fungal brood diseases (caused by *A. apis* and *Aspergillus* spp.).
- Microsporidial adult diseases (Microscoporidia belong to the kingdom Fungi). Microsporidial bee diseases caused by *N. apis* and *N. ceranae*.
- Amoebiasis caused by *Malpighamoeba mellificae.*

1 Chalkbrood disease: *Ascosphaera apis*

Chalkbrood disease, also called brood mycosis, is an invasive disease of the capped brood caused by the fungus *A. apis* (Spiltoir, 1955; Puerta *et al.*, 1997). The disease affects and is fatal to immature forms. Chalkbrood disease rarely causes collapse of the colony, but may weaken colonies by reducing the bee population and consequently may affect honey production (reductions of 5–37% have been reported) (Aronstein and Murray, 2010) and pollination activity.

Although chalkbrood disease is generally a minor problem for some beekeepers (e.g. hobby beekeepers), it is an economic issue for professional beekeepers.

The disease has been known since the beginning of the 1900s but was initially only distributed in Europe; however, in the mid-1960s it was also detected in the US (Aronstein and Murray, 2010). By the beginning of the 1970s, chalkbrood disease was reported to be having an economic impact in the US (Puerta *et al.*, 1997; Hitchcock and Christensen, 1972). *Ascosphaera apis* is now spread worldwide as a consequence of honeybee trade and global apiculture.

1.1 Regulatory status

Chalkbrood disease is not a notifiable disease to the OIE. However, it is a notifiable disease in Denmark, Norway, Portugal, and Romania (Appendix 2).

1.2 The fungus *Ascosphaera apis*

Ascosphaera apis is a fungus belonging to the phylum Ascomycota, the class Eurotiomycetidae, the order Onygenales, and the family Ascosphaeraceae (Skou, 1972, 1988; Lumbsch and Huhndorf, 2007; Aronstein and Murray, 2010).

This fungus was first described and named *Pericystis apis* by Maassen (1913). In 1955, its life cycle was described (Spiltoir, 1955) and the fungus was renamed *A. apis* (Spiltoir and Olive, 1955). The species of the genus *Ascosphaera* are insect pathogens (GBIF, 2014).

Ascosphaera apis is a heterothallic Ascomycota fungus with two morphologically identical and compatible haploid partners allowing for sexual reproduction. These partners can only be distinguished by their mating type (MAT) locus (Aronstein and Murray, 2010). On experimental culture, *A. apis* grows as a dense and white mycelium containing hyphae.

The reproductive process results in the formation of ascomata containing spherical-shaped asci in which ascospores are formed (Figure 6.1). The rupture of the ascoma allows the release of asci and ascospores, which are the transmissible form of the fungus.

The ascospores are on average 2.7–3.5 μm × 1.4–1.8 in size. The ascospores have a thick wall and a spore membrane providing protection against extreme environmental conditions (Aronstein and Cabanillas, 2010).

The germination of the ascospores depends on several specific factors found in the larval gut, in particular temperature, pH, and anaerobic conditions. The development and growth of *A. apis* depends on the larval food (Aronstein and Murray, 2010).

Ascospores are the resistant and transmissible form of the fungus. They may remain viable for 15 years in mummified bees, 4 years in the environment, and for extended periods in honey and wax.

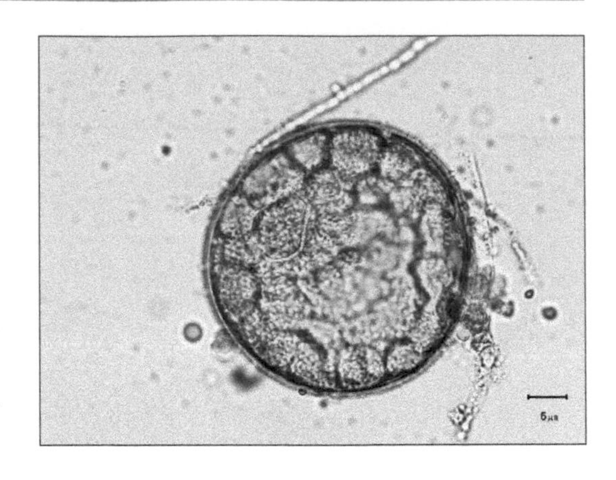

Figure 6.1 *Ascosphaera apis*: Ascoma containing asci in which spores are formed. (Photo courtesy © Monique L'Hostis, Oniris Veterinary School, Nantes.)

1.3 Spread, transmission, and contributing factors

The main routes of dissemination inside the colony are trophallaxis, food sharing, nursing tasks, and cleaning tasks. Between colonies and apiaries, drifting and robbing are responsible for the spread of the disease. Migratory beekeeping and trade as well as beekeeping practices (material exchange, etc.) are important means of dissemination between apiaries.

It is often considered that colonies are mainly asymptomatic in the presence of low levels of spores in the honey and pollen stored in the combs (Puerta *et al.*, 1999; Aronstein and Cabanillas, 2012).

The occurrence of contributing factors is necessary for the development of *A. apis* and the occurrence of chalkbrood disease.

The predisposing factors are various stressors of the colony (Puerta *et al.*, 1997; Flores *et al.*, 2005; Vidal-Naquet, 2011,12):

- Cold and dampness.
- Drop in brood temperature.
- Stress factors weakening colonies, e.g. viral diseases, *Varroa* infestation, foulbrood disease.
- Protein deficit.
- Beekeeping practices (e.g. using artificial swarms with a decreased worker/brood ratio, poor handling of materials).
- Honeybee strain susceptibility.
- Honeybees that exhibit poor hygienic behaviour.

1.4 Pathogenesis

Larvae are contaminated by ingestion of ascospores contained in the brood-food secreted by the food-producing glands of nurse workers. *A. apis* can infect the larvae of the three castes (workers, drones, queens). Larvae are more susceptible to being infected when they are young: 1–2 or 3–4 days old according to sources (Aronstein and Murray, 2010).

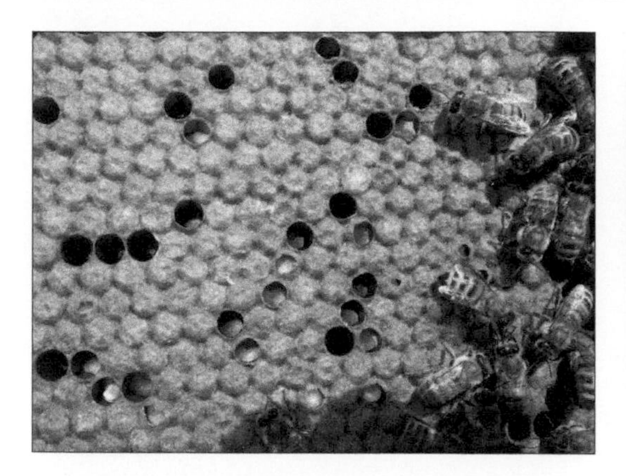

Figure 6.2 Brood affected by mycosis. The brood may appear mottled, with mummies present in the capped cells. Note the presence of white mummies in the uncapped cells here (the cappings have been removed by cleaner workers). (Photo courtesy of Lydia Vilagines, DVM.)

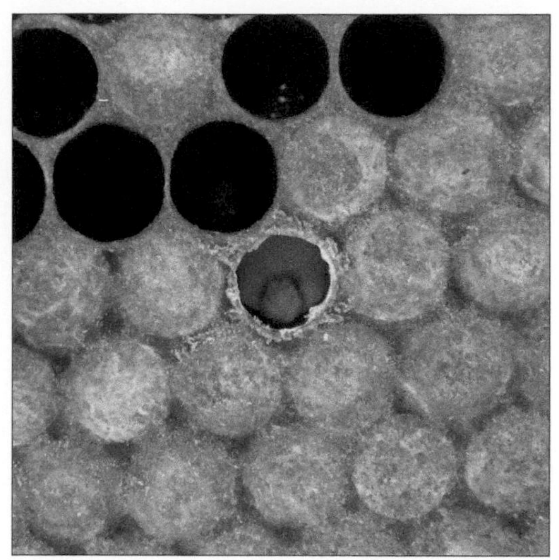

Figure 6.3 Mummy in an uncapped cell (the capping has been removed by cleaner workers). (Photo courtesy of Lydia Vilagines, DVM.)

Spores germinate in the gut lumen of the infected larva. After crossing through the peritrophic membrane and the digestive epithelium of the midgut, the mycelium grows and invades all larval tissues (Gochnauer and Margetts, 1979; Alonso *et al.*, 1993). Pupae are not affected.

The infested larvae die within the capped cells. They become pale yellow coloured, soft, and eventually covered with a fluffy white mycelium (Puerta, 1999).

Later, the dead larvae may dry and become white or black so-called chalkbrood mummies, depending of the presence or not of ascospores (Aronstein and Murray, 2010). Each black mummy contains 10^8–10^9 ascospores (Nelson and Gochnauer, 1982; Hornitzky, 2001). According to Aronstein and Murray (2010), white mummies do not contain ascomata and ascospores. It is mainly considered that young mummies are white, becoming black if the development of ascospores occurs (Puerta *et al.*, 1997).

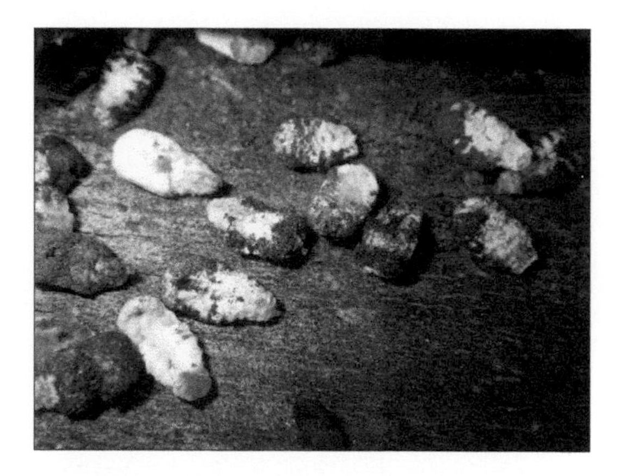

Figure 6.4 Black and white mummies. Black and white mummies on the front floor of a hive. The black mummies contain ascospores and the white mummies do not. (Photo courtesy of Lydia Vilagines, DVM.)

1.5 Clinical signs

Chalkbrood disease is exclusively a disease of the brood of honeybee colonies (Aronstein and Cabanillas, 2012). The clinical signs are the presence of mummies and, at the colony level, a 'progressive weakening of the colony' (Puerta *et al.*, 1997):

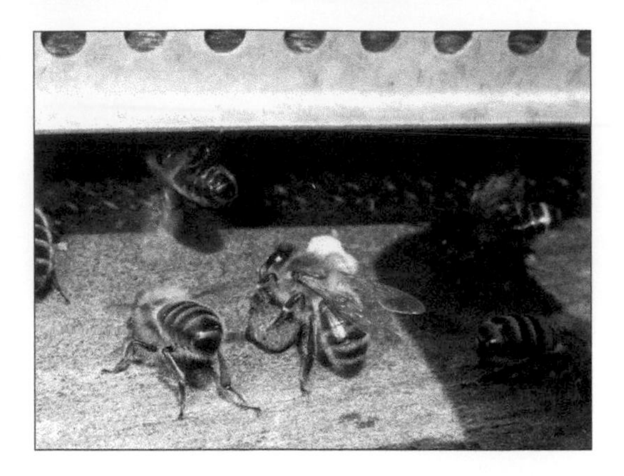

Figure 6.5 A cleaner bee removing a black mummy from the hive. (Photo courtesy of Lydia Vilagines, DVM.)

- The brood cells appear often punctured and mottled (a consequence of the labour of cleaner workers removing dead larvae) (Figure 6.2).
- In the cells, the presence of dead larvae covered by a fluffy white mould can be observed (hence the name of the disease). When the cadavers dry, they become white then black mummies (Figures 6.3 and 6.4).
- Mummies are observed inside brood cells or on the floor and in front of the hive after they have been removed from the cells by cleaner workers (Figure 6.5).

1.6 Diagnosis

The diagnosis of chalkbrood is mainly the consequence of a clinical examination and the observation of the following signs (Aronstein and Murray, 2010):

- Fluffy white mould in brood cells.
- White, grey, and/or black mummies at the entrance, on the floor of the hive, or in capped and uncapped brood cells.

Differential diagnosis is made in comparison with other brood diseases (sacbrood disease, European and American foulbrood diseases), in particular when there are no mummies in the hive.

Usually, the diagnosis is quite easy and does not necessarily require laboratory testing. However, the diagnosis must be associated with analysis of the predisposing factors of chalkbrood disease.

A positive diagnosis may be given by the microscopic observation of ascomata. Microscopic examination of ascomata requires 30–40× magnification, and visualization can be improved by staining with lactophenol cotton blue stain (LCBS) (Puerta *et al.*, 1997; Aronstein and Murray, 2010).

Direct microscopic examination of ascomata in black mummies confirms chalkbrood disease. If only white mummies are present, cultivation on agar medium is necessary to allow fungal growth, reproduction, and finally formation of ascomata.

In asymptomatic colonies, it may be valuable to detect covert infection.

Molecular identification of *A. apis* may be performed in this laboratory, though this is not a routine procedure.

1.7 Chalkbrood control and prevention

The management of chalkbrood disease in affected colonies mainly involves beekeeping practices and rearing honeybees that exhibit good hygienic behaviour, taking into account that spores may be found throughout the hive (beebread, honey, wax, wood, etc.) and can remain viable for many years.

If chalkbrood disease is detected, re-queening with queens that exhibit good hygienic behaviour potential and replacing combs may be sufficient, if prophylactic methods are established and predisposing factors corrected. It may be interesting to implement the shock swarm method to provide the colony with a pathogen-free hive. Strongly affected colonies should be eliminated and the material disinfected and sterilized.

There is no known treatment against brood mycosis. Some chemicals have been tested *in vitro* and *in vivo*, but none appear to control the disease sufficiently and safely (Aronstein and Murray, 2010). Antifungal drugs must not be used within colonies.

Certains natural compounds have been described as having some efficacy against chalkbrood. For example, the essential oil from *Satureja montana* has proven effective against chalkbrood at 0.01% in microcrystalline sugar candy (Colin *et al.*, 1989).

The management and prophylaxis of chalkbrood disease involves the following beekeeping practices:

- Hives must be well ventilated.
- Damp, cold, and shadowed apiary sites should be avoided. Particular attention must be given to the hive stand which must protect the hive against dampness from the soil.
- Hives must be kept as clean as possible and combs should be replaced annually in the case of overt disease (or at least every three years according to good sanitary beekeeping practice).
- Combs should not, as far as possible, be exchanged between hives, especially in cases of the disease.
- Avoid any pollen deficiency (Puerta *et al.*, 1997; Flores *et al.*, 2005). Supplementary feeding may be necessary, in particular in intensive apiculture.
- Honeybees must display good hygienic behaviour (Spivak and Reuter, 1998). Hygienic colonies seem be able to control chalkbrood disease sufficiently in most cases (Aronstein and Murray, 2010).

Sterilization of combs and beekeeping material with gamma-irradiation has been described but this method is not easily accessible in current apiculture.

2 Stonebrood disease: *Aspergillus* spp.

Stonebrood disease is a rare fungal infection of the brood caused by several fungi belonging to the genus *Aspergillus* (Shimanuki and Knox, 2000; Jensen *et al.*, 2013): *Aspergillus fumigatus*, *Aspergillus flavus*, and *Aspergillus niger*.

Stonebrood disease is a notifiable disease in Denmark, Norway, and Romania. It is not a notifiable disease to the OIE (Appendix 2).

Aspergillus is commonly found in the soil and in the environment (water, food, compost, mouldy hay, etc.). When *Aspergillus* spp. thrive principally as saprophyte fungi, they can become pathogenic for humans, mammals, birds, and insects, in particular in immune-deprived individuals, causing serious disease. In human and mammals, aspergillosis may affect the skin, eyes, and respiratory system from the nasal cavities to the lungs. The fungi can produce toxic and carcinogenic aflatoxins (Jensen *et al.*, 2013). Thus, beekeepers must be aware of this disease (despite its rarity) both for their own health and for the protection of consumers of hive products.

Stonebrood disease mainly occurs in weakened colonies, irrespective of the causes of this weakening.

Contamination is caused by ingestion of spores or by penetration through the cuticle of the larvae. Infected larvae become hardened and difficult to crush. They may turn yellow-green (*A. flavus*), grey-green (*A. fumigatus*), or black (*A. niger*) in colour. Adult bees may also be infected and die.

Diagnosis of stonebrood disease is not easy and requires laboratory identification.

Considering the risks to human health, precautions must be done to manage and control the disease. Strongly affected colonies should be eliminated and the material disinfected and sterilized. All the infected brood combs must be destroyed and good sanitary beekeeping measures implemented.

Prophylaxis against the disease requires strong colonies and good sanitary beekeeping practices.

3 Nosemosis: *Nosema apis* and *Nosema ceranae*

Nosemosis is a parasitical disease of *A. mellifera* adults affecting the three castes of honeybees (workers, drones, and queens) caused by two members of the phylum Microsporidia (kingdom Fungi):

- *Nosema apis* Zander (Zander, 1909; COLOSS Workshop, 2009; Higes *et al.*, 2010)
- *Nosema ceranae* (Fries *et al.*, 1996; Higes *et al.*, 2006; COLOSS Workshop, 2009).

Like all Microsporidiae, both *N. apis* and *N. ceranae* are obligate intracellular spore-forming parasites affecting exclusively the epithelial cells of the adult midgut (ventriculus). However, they cause two different diseases: Type-A nosemosis caused by *N. apis*, and Type-C nosemosis caused by *N. ceranae*, which each have their own and 'distinct epidemiological, clinical and pathological characteristics' (COLOSS Workshop, 2009; Higes *et al.*, 2010; Botias *et al.*, 2013).

Before 2005, *N. apis* was the only species of *Nosema* described in *A. mellifera* (Kilani, 1999b). In 2005, *N. ceranae* was described in colonies in Spain and then in other parts of Europe as well as in South and North America (Higes *et al.*, 2006; Klee *et al.*, 2007; Chen and Huang, 2010). Today, *N. ceranae* is found worldwide in *A. mellifera* colonies. *Nosema ceranae* was originally described as a parasite of the Asian honeybee, *Apis cerana* (Fries *et al.*, 1996). One hypothesis is that *N. ceranae* is currently replacing *N. apis* in certain populations of *A. mellifera* (Higes *et al.*, 2006; Chen and Huang, 2010; Fries, 2010).

In addition to *N. ceranae* shifting from *Apis cerana* to *A. mellifera*, studies have reported that a host shift has also occurred for *N. apis*, which has become a parasite of Asian honeybees. However, *N. ceranae* remains predominant in Asian honeybees (Chen and Huang, 2010). Global apiculture with trade and exchange, as well as migratory apiculture, may explain the worldwide spread of these Microsporidiae.

The pathogenicity of *N. apis* and *N. ceranae* infections is the subject of debate. Both *Nosema* species are often considered opportunistic pathogens, as are most Microsporidia (Weiss and Becnel, 2014). Although Type-A nosemosis is acknowledged to occur in certain conditions and with predisposing factors, Type-C nosemosis pathogenicity is a subject of discussion and debate among researchers (Colin *et al.*, 2008; Cox-Foster *et al.*, 2007). However, at this time, it seems that some evidence suggests that *N. ceranae* is harmful to the strength and health of honeybee colonies (with economic consequences on production) in the presence of predisposing factors such as temperature, climate, nutrition, parasite or host genetics, environmental contaminants, or other parasites (Higes *et al.*, 2008; Paxton *et al.*, 2007; Traver and Fell, 2011; Martín-Hernández *et al.*, 2012; Higes *et al.*, 2013; Botias *et al.*, 2013; Williams *et al.*, 2014).

This chapter attempts to present the current knowledge, based on research, of both types of nosemosis. The large body of published work dedicated to *N. ceranae* presents a range of sometimes diverse results; however, they tend to show a pathogenic effect of this agent when some of the above-mentioned predisposing factors are present (hence, this fungus can be defined as an opportunistic pathogenic agent).

3.1 Regulatory status

Type-A and Type-C nosemosis are notifiable diseases in many European countries. Type-A and Type-C nosemosis are not notifiable diseases to the OIE (2014b) (Appendix 2).

3.2 The microsporidians *Nosema apis* and *Nosema ceranae*

3.2.1 The spores

The spores, which are oval-shaped with a dark edge, are the infectious, resistant, and spreading form of *Nosema* spp. (OIE, 2014a; Chen and Huang, 2010) (Figure 6.6):

- The spores of *N. apis* are about 5–7 μm in length × 3–4 μm in width.
- The spores of *N. ceranae* are slightly smaller: 4–4.8 μm in length × 2.1–2.9 μm in width.

The internal structures of the spores of the two species are similar (Figure 6.7) (Chen and Huang, 2010; Dussaubat-Arriagada, 2012):

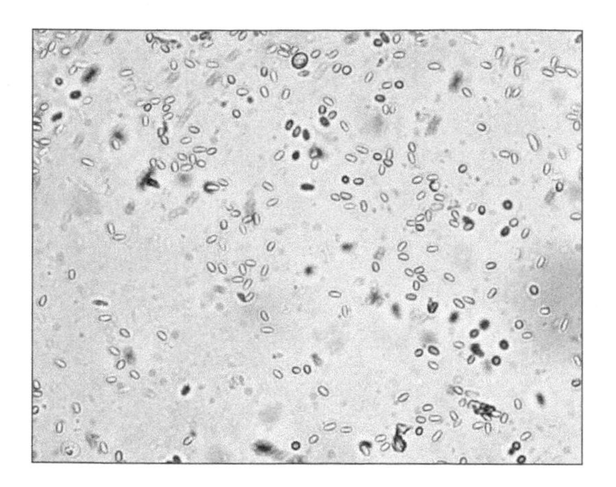

Figure 6.6 Spore of *Nosema* spp.: microscopy (×400). (Photo courtesy © Anses Sophia-Antipolis.)

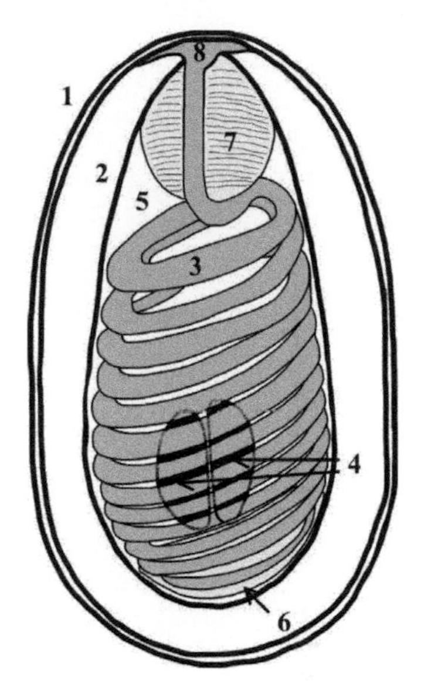

Figure 6.7 Spore of *Nosema*: (1) exospore; (2) endospore; (3) polar filament; (4) diplokaryotic nuclei; (5) cytoplasma; (6) posterior vacuole; (7) lamellar polaroplast; (8) anchoring disc. (Drawing: Nicolas Vidal-Naquet.)

- A thickened wall composed of an exospore layer and an endospore layer protecting the sporoplasm.
- Diplokaryotic nuclei.
- A long coiled polar filament around the diplokaryon. *Nosema apis* spores have more than 30 coils and *N. ceranae* between 18 and 21.
- Lamellar polaroplasts below an anchoring disc located in the anterior part of the spore.
- The posterior vacuole.

Differentiation between the spores of both species is difficult by microscopic identification and requires PCR analysis.

The spores of *N. apis* remain viable more than 1 year in faeces, 4 months in honey and wax, and up to 4.5 years in infected bee cadavers (OIE, 2014a). The spores of *N. ceranae* seem to be more resistant to desiccation and heat but very sensitive to freezing; however, the lifespan of the spores in the hive (honey, wax, bees, etc.) is unknown at this time (Fries, 2010). *Nosema ceranae* seems to be more prevalent in hot countries and territories.

3.2.2 The life cycle

After ingestion by adult bees, the spores of both species germinate in the midgut (ventriculus) of adult bees. The polar tube is everted and allows penetration through the cell membrane of the sporoplasm containing the genetic material into the bee epithelial cellular cytoplasm (Wittner and Weiss, 1999). There, the sporoplasm reproduces as numerous spores after the merogony and sporogony stages (see Figures 6.8 and 6.9). The cell dies and the spores are liberated in the lumen of the ventriculus (Figure 6.10a,b). It is reported that 30–50 million spores may fill the digestive tract. Those spores contaminate other cells, accumulate in the hindgut, and are evacuated in the faeces, allowing transmission to other bees.

After infection of an epithelial cell, the development of numerous mature spores takes 3 days in the case of *N. apis* and 4 days in the case of *N. ceranae* (Forsgren and Fries, 2010).

3.3 Type-A nosemosis

Type-A nosemosis is considered an opportunistic disease. It appears to be quite benign in the

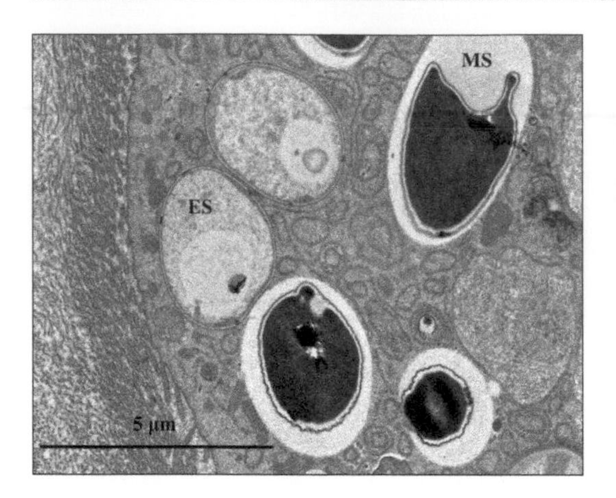

Figure 6.8 Electron microscope image of an infected ventricular cell filled with different parasitic stages: meronts, mature spores (MS), and empty spores (ES) (day 3 post-infection). (Photo courtesy © Mariano Higes, Centro Regional Apicola Marchamalo, Castilla-la-Mancha.)

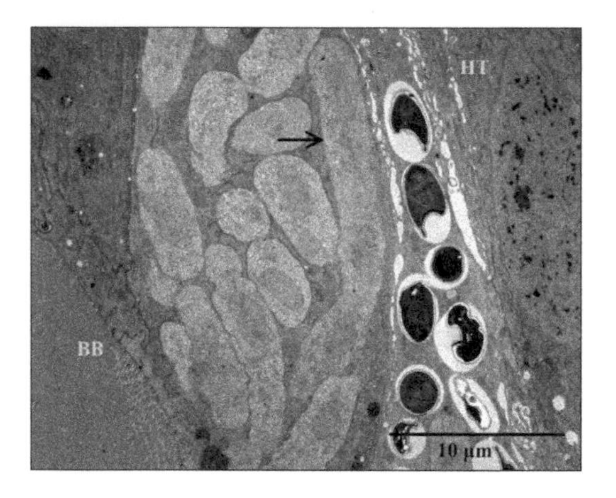

Figure 6.9 Electron microscope image of ventricular cells infected with *Nosema ceranae*. Merogonial plasmodia with four diplokarya (arrow). BB, brush border; HT, healthy tissue. (Photo courtesy © Mariano Higes, Centro Regional Apicola Marchamalo, Castilla-la-Mancha.)

absence of predisposing factors. However, if predisposing factors are present, Type-A nosemosis may lead to weakening and collapse of the infected colony (Fries, 2014).

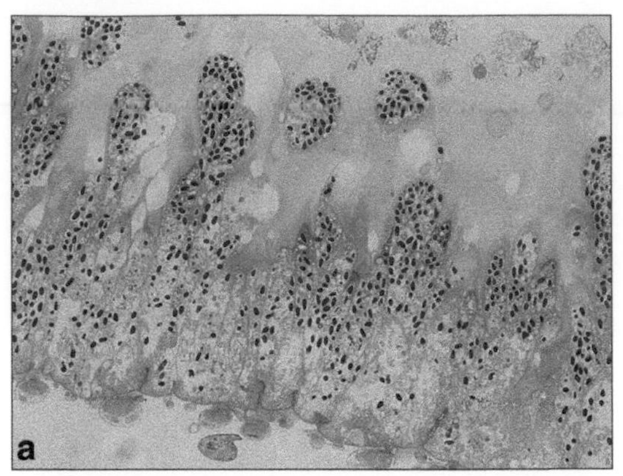

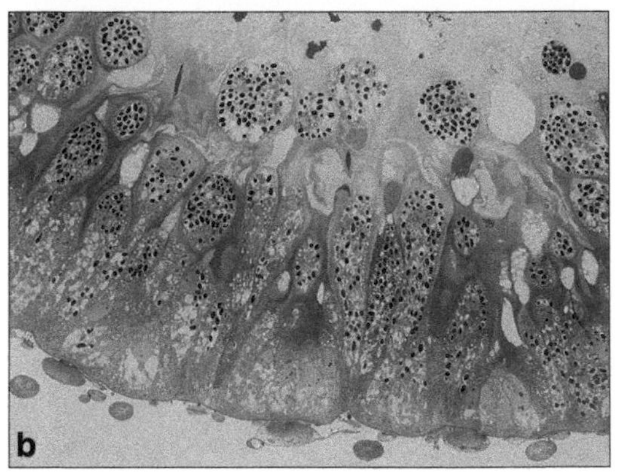

Figure 6.10 Epithelial cells infested by *Nosema* spp. (a) *Nosema apis*, day 15 after experimental infection (toluidine blue, 400×). (b) *Nosema ceranae*, day 15 after experimental infection (toluidine blue, 400×). (© Heike Aupperle.)

3.3.1 Epidemiology and transmission

Nosema apis is reported to be more prevalent in mild or temperate regions (Higes *et al.*, 2013). In temperate climates, there is a seasonal pattern of prevalence (Bailey, 1955; Fries, 2010; Higes *et al.*, 2013) characterized as follows:

- Low prevalence in summer (the disease is asymptomatic or hardly detectable).
- Small peak in autumn.
- Increasing slight prevalence in winter.
- Large peak in early spring and affecting winter bees.

Infection occurs after the ingestion of spores in the feed or water, via trophallaxis or perhaps after grooming of the body hairs (Webster, 1993). Combs contaminated with spores of *N. apis* (which remain viable for more than 1 year in faecal deposits) are reported to be the primary source of infection (Bailey, 1955, 1962). Thus, beekeeping practices and exchange of material may be responsible for *N. apis* spores spreading between colonies.

3.3.2 Pathogenesis

Contamination is the consequence of the ingestion of spores by adult bees. The infectious dose of *N. apis* is reported to be on average 100 spores per bee (Fries, 2010). The mean ID_{50} has been experimentally evaluated as 390 for *N. apis* (Forsgren and Fries, 2010).

Alteration of the digestive tract

The multiplication of *N. apis* occurs within the ventriculus epithelium cells (Fries; 1988). This leads to:

- An inflammation of the digestive tract with diarrhoea or constipation caused by obstruction by the numerous released spores (Kilani, 1999).
- The digestive function of infected bees becomes disorganized and nutrient uptake is impaired.
- The epithelial cells degenerate with large vacuoles and glycogen deposits, leading to lesions in the epithelioma. Ribosomes aggregate, leading to a reduction in RNA synthesis that alters the secretion of proteins and enzymes (Kilani, 1999).
- The consequence is a negative effect on fat bodies, protein metabolism, and protein levels in the haemolymph. The lesions in the digestive tract may be an entry point for other pathogens.

Alteration of the hypopharyngeal glands

Atrophy of hypopharyngeal glands in workers is observed in *N. apis* infection, affecting larval food production and brood rearing (Wang and Moeller, 1969). At the colony level, the consequence is a decrease in the honeybee population and in the production of honey (Fries, 2010).

Effects of Nosema apis on the immune response

The immune response of the honeybee is rapidly activated after *N. apis* infection.

The expression of antibacterial peptides (abaecin, defensin, and hymenoptaecin) and phenoloxidase (which favour nodulation, encapsulation, and phagocytosis) has been shown to increase respectively 4 days and 7 days after *N. apis* infection (Glinski and Jarosz, 2001; Antunez *et al.*, 2009).

Effects of Nosema apis on queen physiology

Type-A nosemosis alters the development of the queen's ovaries, leading to infertility and re-queening by supersedure (Fyg, 1964; Liu, 1992; Kilani, 1999).

Reduction of lifespan

Nosema apis-infected honeybees have been shown to have a reduced lifespan (Goblirsch *et al.*, 2013).

Colony organization changes

Nosema apis infection affects mainly winter bees, altering the nursing of brood at the end of the overwintering period. In normal conditions, this brood allows the emergence of a new generation of workers at the beginning of the season. If the egg laying and/or the brood rearing are impaired by a lack of worker bees, the new generation of bees at the beginning of the season will be affected, leading to weakening or collapse of the colony.

3.3.3 Contributing factors

Nosema apis is reported as commonly present in adult bees in apiaries as a covert infection without causing any damage (Kilani, 1999). However, at the present time, reports suggest that *N. apis* is being supplanted by *N. ceranae* and outbreaks of Type-A nosemosis seem less frequent. *Nosema apis* infection is favoured by some well-known predisposing factors. The factors known to affect outbreaks and severity of Type-A nosemosis are:

- Weather conditions: a long and rainy winter inducing hive confinement increases *N. apis* contamination of the colony (Kilani, 1999).
- A long rainy period and confinement favour Type-A nosemosis.
- Climate: *N. apis* infections are more prevalent in temperate regions.
- Age of the bees: overwintering bees are reported to be more susceptible to *N. apis*.
- Inherited features: Causasian and Italian bees are reported to be more susceptible to *N. apis* (Kilani, 1999).
- Beekeeping practices:
  - Wintering with forest honey (containing melezitose) as a food source. Melezitose can crystallize, causing midgut epithelial lesions potentially favouring development of *N. apis*.
  - Inadequate feeding with runny syrup may be the cause of diarrhoea and soiled combs when bees are confined.
  - Protein starvation, in particular before the overwintering period.
  - Inadequate preparation of the winter bees.
  - Inadequate management of beekeeping material (combs, supers, etc.).

3.3.4 Clinical signs of Type-A nosemosis

An outbreak of Type-A nosemosis exhibits the following colony-level symptoms:

- Weakening and mortality of colonies in winter or early spring.
- Reduced colony productivity.
- Occurrence of associated infections such as amoebiosis of the Malpighian tubules (Kilani, 1999) and viral infections. Thus, oral black queen cell virus (BQCV) infection is reported to depend strongly on co-infection with *N. apis*. Bee virus Y and filamentous virus are also considered to be dependent on *N. apis*.

At the individual level, the following clinical signs are observed (Kilani, 1999, Vidal-Naquet, 2011):

- Workers affected by dysentery: one of the main clinicals sign in the hive is the presence of pale to brown excreta covering the combs but also the front and the bottom of the hive.
- Workers may also be affected by constipation and present distended abdomens due to accumulation of spores within the rectum.
- Crawling bees unable to fly can be observed at the front of the hive.
- The queen may be infected in winter and her fertility can be altered, to the point of sterility. In this case, the colony may not be able to replace the queen and the colony can collapse.
- In spring, the infected queen is replaced by supersedure, if she is still capable of laying diploid eggs (Kilani, 1999).
- The first brood of the season may be affected by the decreased number of winter bees in charge of brood nursing at the end of overwintering period.

3.3.5 Clinical and differential diagnosis of Type-A nosemosis

The clinical pattern of overt Type-A nosemosis is not specific to the disease and only a presumptive diagnosis can be given.

In temperate regions, at the end of winter or in spring, the observation of colony collapse or the occurrence of colony weakening with diarrhoea and observation of crawling and/or dead bees in the front of the hives may be suggestive of Type-A nosemosis.

Furthermore, the suspected diagnosis must be associated with the evaluation of the predisposing factors, in particular taking into account meteorological and climatic factors, beekeeping practices, *Varroa destructor* control management, and nearby agricultural practices (in particular, pesticide use on crops).

Differential diagnosis must take into account acarapidosis (crawling bees with K-wings), amoebiosis (presence of sulphur-yellow diarrhoea), viral diseases but also poisoning and any cause of colony weakening (Kilani, 1999; OIE, 2014a).

In the field or at the veterinary clinic, a simple test may be performed on diseased bees: after sectioning the head, pulling on the rear end of the abdomen reveals the gut. In the case of Type-A nosemosis, the gut appears milky-white coloured and translucent. Bees non-infected with *N. apis* present a yellow to reddish coloured (pollen-coloured) gut.

Positive diagnosis will be confirmed by a laboratory test. Laboratory testing for both Type-A and Type-C nosemosis is described below in section 3.5.

3.4 Type-C nosemosis

Type-C nosemosis can be considered as an emerging disease. Much research has been, and continues to be, performed to understand the pathogenicity of this disease. The presence of *N. ceranae* may be asymptomatic in colonies and may not lead to adverse effects (Fernandez *et al.*, 2012; Traver *et al.*, 2012; Fries, 2014). Type-C nosemosis is mainly reported, in particular in Spain, to induce colony weakening and even collapse. Type-C nosemosis remains a widely debated disease and a subject of controversy between researchers in particular concerning the pathogenicity of *N. ceranae.*

3.4.1 Epidemiology and transmission

The seasonality pattern of *N. ceranae* infection is different from that of *N. apis.* In hot regions, there is no seasonal pattern for *N. ceranae* which can be detected throughout the year (Martin-Hernandez *et al.*, 2007, 2012; Traver and Fell, 2011; Higes *et al.*, 2013). In tropical and subtropical climates, the spore load of *N. ceranae* is negatively correlated with the average temperature (Dussaubat-Arriagada, 2012). In temperate climates, the peak of *N. ceranae* infection occurs between spring and early summer and sometimes in autumn (Oliver, 2011). In Germany, *N. ceranae* is reported to present two peaks of infection, in spring and autumn (Gisder *et al.*, 2010). The infection occurs after the ingestion of spores of *N. ceranae* with food or water (Chen and Huang, 2010).

The main spreading routes of *N. ceranae* seem to be different from those of *N. Apis.* Indeed, no dysentery is reported and consequently no soiled combs observed. Global apiculture, with its trade and exchange of package bees and queens, is supposed to be responsible of the worldwide spread of *N. ceranae.*

Mixed infection with both *Nosema* spp. is commonly observed (Paxton *et al.*, 2007; Chen *et al.*, 2009; Forsgren and Fries, 2010).

3.4.2 Pathogenesis: consequences of *Nosema ceranae* infection on the physiology of the honeybee

Contamination is the consequence of the ingestion of spores. The infectious dose is slightly lower for *N. ceranae* than for *N. apis* (Fries, 2010). The mean ID_{50} has been experimentally evaluated at 85 spores for *N. ceranae* (Forsgren and Fries, 2010).

At the physiological level, *N. ceranae* infection induces pheromonal, hormonal, metabolic, energetic, and immune effects in bees:

- *Pheromone.* Infected bees are reported to present higher levels of ethyl oleate (EO) than healthy ones. EO is the 'primer pheromone' found in foraging workers. EO regulates the behavioural maturation of bees, delaying their transition to foraging. In infected bees, the level of EO is close to that usually found in foragers (Dubaussat *et al.*, 2013). An increased level of EO is reported to be linked to the level of *N. ceranae* infection. Alteration of QMP levels in queens has been described in *N. ceranae* infection (Alaux *et al.*, 2011).
- *Vitellogenin.* Experimentally, infected bees present a modification of the normal evolution pattern of vitellogenin (Vg) transcript. Vg in uninfected bees usually presents a peak in 8-day-old workers (nurse bee age) and then decreases progressively up to the age of 16 days. In infected bees, Vg transcript has been shown experimentally to present an opposite pattern with a lower level in nurse-aged bees,

increasing after the 8th day of age (Goblirsch *et al.*, 2013).

- *Juvenile hormone.* In the haemolymph of 8-day-old infected bees (nurse age), a spike of juvenile hormone (JH) has been reported which is not observed in uninfected bees of the same age (Goblirsch *et al.*, 2013).
- *Energetic stress.* Infected bees are subjected to energetic stress, which induces unusual hunger and an increase of food consumption as well as a decrease in trophallactic exchanges (Mayack and Naug, 2009). The energy needs of infected bees are confirmed by studies showing a significant increase in enzymes involved in carbohydrate catabolism and energy transfer.
- *Oxidative stress.* Infected bees are subject to oxidative stress. This is highlighted by the abundant level of antioxidant proteins in the midgut of *N. ceranae*-infected bees. However, according to Vidau *et al.* (2014), the antioxidant system of bees is not able to protect the epithelial cells of the gut, leading to their degeneration and lysis as described in *N. ceranae*-infected bees (Higes *et al.*, 2007). Furthermore, vitellogenin is reported to protect bees from oxidative stress. The decreased level of vitellogenin probably has a negative effect on antioxidant protection (Goblirsch *et al.*, 2013).
- *Vitellogenin, oxidative stress, and QMP in queens.* Alterations in the levels of vitellogenin (which affects fertility and longevity), total antioxidant ability, and QMP have been described (Alaux *et al.*, 2011). This may explain the effect on queen health and re-queening by supersedure following changes in pheromonal production.
- *Immunity.* Unlike *N. apis* infection, *N. ceranae* infection is reported to impair and even suppress the immune response by reducing the expression of some genes involved in immunity. Experimentally, the expression of antibacterial peptides was not modified 4 days after *N. ceranae* infection and invasion in the ventricular epithelium (Higes *et al.*, 2007; Antunez *et al.*, 2009). Furthermore, 7 days after infection, the expression of the genes coding for abaecin, hymenoptaecin, and glucose dehydrogenase is decreased experimentally (Antunez *et al.*, 2009).
- *Hypopharyngeal secretion.* Infected bees present an atrophy of the hypopharyngeal glands. According to Vidau *et al.* (2014), the level of some proteins (major royal jelly protein (MRJP) 1, 2, and 3, and alpha-glucosidase III) involved in energy supply but also in the production of brood food by the hypopharyngeal glands is decreased in the midgut of infected bees. These four proteins play a major role, and their decrease is probably related to the negative effects of *N. ceranae* infection on the hypopharyngeal glands and trophallactic exchange (Vidau *et al.*, 2014).
- *Lifespan of worker bees.* The lifespan of infected worker bees is decreased. Experimental findings show that worker bees infected by *N. ceranae* live 9 days less than uninfected bees (Goblirsch *et al.*, 2013).

3.4.3 Pathogenesis: consequences of *Nosema ceranae* on the honeybee colony

At the colony level, considering the adult bee population, capped brood, and honey production as indicators of colony health (Meikle *et al.*, 2008), a recent study (Botias *et al.*, 2013) has shown that *N. ceranae* infection may impair:

- The size of the adult honeybee population in a colony.
- Brood production (evaluated by the uncapped and capped brood).
- Honey production.

Strongly infected colonies are characterized by a small population and a small brood area, together with significant impairment of brood rearing as well as forager death (Botias *et al.*, 2013). Severe infections are described as leading to colony collapse with no bees found in the hive (Botias *et al.*, 2013).

At the individual level, *N. ceranae* infection is more prevalent in forager bees than in nest bees (Higes *et al.*, 2008; Martín-Hernández *et al.*, 2012;

Botias *et al.*, 2013). One of the main individual features of Type-C nosemosis is the high level of forager death. Young bees are considered less likely to be infected by *N. ceranae*. Furthermore, the return-flight success after a foraging flight has been shown to be impaired and compromised in *N. ceranae*-infected foragers (Wolf *et al.*, 2014). One hypothetical explanation is that energetic stress due to *N. ceranae* infection is compromising the return-flight performance (Wolf *et al.*, 2014; Vidau *et al.*, 2014). Another unconfirmed hypothesis is that *N. ceranae* can cause disorientation (Kralj and Fuchs, 2010).

The lack of foragers induced by Type-C nosemosis is counterbalanced by the plasticity of the honeybee colony. In the colony, plasticity in the division of labour allows nest bees, and in particular nurse bees, to become foragers prematurely – however, this can lead to disorganization of the colony and consequently to a reduction in the average lifespan of workers (Huang and Robinson, 1992). Furthermore, *N. ceranae* infection has been shown to induce atrophy of hypopharyngeal glands as well as to reduce secretion from these glands (Alaux *et al.*, 2010; Vidau *et al.*, 2014).

It seems that the number of worker bees infected by *N. ceranae* may be considered as an important factor to understand Type-C nosemosis.

Considering the number of infected bees, it is possible to suggest that:

- If only a few workers are infected, the colony will be able to counterbalance the harmful effects of *N. ceranae* by the queen increasing her laying activity and by the plasticity of labour replacing lost bees to rear the brood (Goblirsch *et al.*, 2013).
- If the number of infected workers is high or severe, the colony will become disorganized and Type-C nosemosis will affect bee population, brood production, and honey production. The consequences will be weakening or even collapse of the colony. Because foragers are the main target of *N. ceranae*, if many of these are infected, the nest bee population will be adversely affected with an inbalance between brood and nurse bees. Hence, brood rearing will be impaired. The lack of food storage, impairment of brood-food production, and probable impairment of the homeostasis of the nest are reported to affect brood rearing and consequently may lead to the decline of the infected colony (Botias *et al.*, 2013).

3.4.4 Contributing factors

If environmental conditions, beekeeping practices, and food resources (flowering, honeydew, biodiversity) are favourable for honeybees, it is believed that colonies are able to defend themselves against *N. ceranae*.

However, *N. ceranae* infection (Type-C nosemosis) is at this time often described as pathogenic, potentially inducing colony weakening and collapse under certain conditions, especially when the temperature is high (Martin-Hernandez *et al.*, 2009; Botias *et al.*, 2013). At this time, the factors described to affect the occurrence and severity of Type-C nosemosis are:

- *Climate conditions. Nosema ceranae* is reported to be more prevalent in hot climates. The reproductive ability of *N. ceranae* increases with temperature (Martin-Hernandez *et al.*, 2009).
- *Age of the bees.* Forager bees are reported to be more susceptible to *N. ceranae*.
- *Genetics.* Genetic variants of *N. ceranae*, as well as genetic variants of honeybee strains, are suspected to play a role in the susceptibility of the bees to the parasite (Dussaubat *et al.*, 2013; Gomez-Moracho *et al.*, 2013; Williams *et al.*, 2014).
- *Food.* Lack of food, and in particular lack of pollen, may be a contributing factor for Type-C nosemosis (Eischen and Graham, 2008).
- *Pesticides.* Recent work has demonstrated interactions between imidacloprid and *Nosema*, causing an increased mortality (Alaux *et al.*, 2009). Another study has report that increasing prevalence of *N. ceranae* in

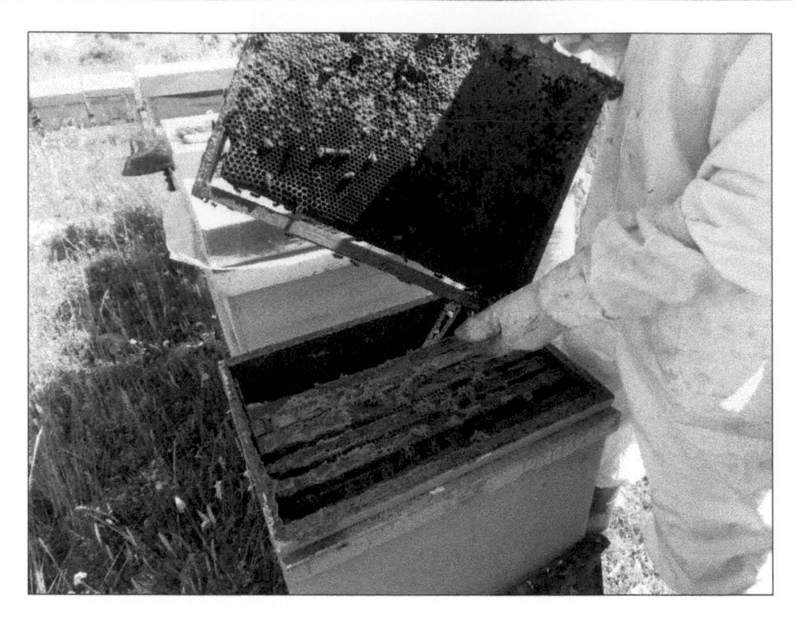

Figure 6.11 Colony severely affected by Type-C nosemosis. The colony collapses, leaving the hive without bees. (Photo courtesy © Mariano Higes, Centro Regional Apicola Marchamalo, Castilla-la-Mancha.)

apiaries associated with pesticide residues present in the hives (Fipronil and Thiacloprid) is able to cause colony depopulation (Vidau *et al.*, 2011).

- *Poor beekeeping practices* may greatly favour the development of *N. ceranae*:
  - Inadequate feeding: poorly nourished bees are more susceptible to *N. ceranae* than are well-nourished ones (Eischen and Graham, 2008).
  - Inadequate management of beekeeping material (combs, supers, etc.).

These contributing factors enable us to define *N. ceranae* as an opportunistic pathogenic agent.

3.4.5 Clinical signs of Type-C nosemosis

Type-C nosemosis features may be described by:

- At the individual level:
  - Homing failure and death of foragers.
  - Decrease in the nest bee population.
  - Premature aging of nest bees, and in particular nurse bees becoming foragers prematurely.
  - Decrease in the lifespan of adult honeybees.
  - Re-queening by *Nosema*-induced supersedure.
- At the colony level:
  - Decrease in the brood area (and impairment of brood rearing).
  - Decrease in the bee population.
  - Decrease of in storage and in particular honey production.

According to Botias *et al.* (2013), at the colony level, these three parameters should be considered as sub-clinical signs of Type-C nosemosis.

When the *N. ceranae* infection is severe or out of control, some colonies may collapse, leaving the hive without bees (Figure 6.11) (Higes *et al.*, 2008; Botias *et al.*, 2013).

Furthermore, *N. ceranae*, as a stressor that weakens colonies, may be a predisposing factor of diseases such as chalkbrood disease and foulbrood disease (Hedtke *et al.*, 2011; Botias *et al.*, 2013). Indeed, weakened colonies, imbalance between brood and nurse bees, and food deficiency potentially caused by *N. ceranae* are contributing factors of these fungal and bacterial diseases.

It must be remembered that *N. ceranae* may remain in colonies as a covert infection (Fernandez *et al.*, 2012), and if a few bees are infected, the colony will be able to compensate their loss and no clinical signs will be observed (Goblirsch *et al.*, 2013). Some studies performed in Spain, Uruguay, and Germany have shown that *N. ceranae* infection did not increase colony losses (Invernizzia *et al*, 2009; Fries, 2010).

3.4.6 Clinical and differential diagnosis of Type-C nosemosis

The clinical pattern of overt Type-C nosemosis is not specific to the disease; sub-clinical symptoms are considered to be a decrease in bee population, and a reduction in brood and honey production. Thus, considering the diseases or diverse causes that can result in these symptoms, differential diagnosis has to take into account all possible causes of colony weakening and collapse. Because foragers are the principal type of bee affected by Type-C nosemosis and die in the field due to their impaired homing ability, clinical examination of individuals for *N. ceranae* infection is generally impossible.

However, a clinical examination of the colony must be performed very carefully and accurately in order to highlight clinical signs to permit a diagnosis of any diseases that may be present.

In the case of Type-C nosemosis, the suspected diagnosis must involve the evaluation of all predisposing factors and in particular take into account geographic and climatic factors, beekeeping practices, *Varroa destructor* control management, food resources, feeding supplementation, and nearby agricultural practices (in particular pesticide use on crops).

A positive diagnosis of Type-C nosemosis requires laboratory testing, observation of clinical signs observed, and an health and environmental audit of the affected colony, in particular by studying the presence of predisposing factors.

3.5 Laboratory diagnosis of Type-A and Type-C nosemosis

3.5.1 Laboratory diagnosis and sampling choice

The standard laboratory method of diagnosis is to estimate the number of spores of *Nosema* spp. in a sample of 50–100 bees (Goblirsch *et al.*, 2013; OIE, 2014a).

The quality of the sampling is crucial. Samples must be representative and should be sent to the laboratory without delay in suitable packaging (Appendix 3). According to the OIE (2014a), 'for a reliable diagnosis, a number of bees in a sample should be examined. For example, 60 bees examined in a composite sample will detect a 5% infection level with 95% probability.'

Selection of the bees to be sampled is an important consideration. The OIE (2014a) standardization choice is a 'sample of older worker honeybees taken from the hive entrance or from peripheral frames if weather does not permit flight conditions'. However, when opening hives, all the worker bees, irrespective of their age group and task, tend to be found mixed together on the frames (Van der Steen *et al.*, 2012). Thus, selecting older bees for sampling is difficult. For a better result, sampling must be done immediately prior to the clinical examination. When opening the hives, older bees may be proportionally easier to find on the honeycomb storage (peripheral frames) or at the entrance of the hive (Van der Steen *et al.*, 2012).

Another approach to laboratory diagnosis involves estimating the proportion of infected bees in a colony. Indeed, in the pathogenesis of the disease, and in particular in Type-C nosemosis, the number of infected bees in a colony is thought to be linked to the symptoms observed at colony level (Goblirsch *et al.*, 2013). However, to date, no standard sampling or standard interpretation has been defined. In the same field, Mariano Higes proposes defining parameters such as the proportion of infected foragers to nurse bees to evaluate the prognosis of Type-C nosemosis (Higes *et al.*, 2010).

3.5.2 Laboratory methods

Microscopic identification

Microscopic examination allows identification of *Nosema* spp. spores. The spores of *N. apis* are slightly larger than those of *N. ceranae* and distinguishing the species by microscopy is not easy. The PCR method is the best way to distinguish the species.

Spore count

Laboratory estimates of infection level involve counting spores; the results are given as the number of spores/bees. Interpretation is difficult and the spore count has to be performed meticulously. Indeed, spore count results have been shown to be poorly correlated to qPCR results (Traver and Fell, 2011; Traver *et al.*, 2012): samples were found qPCR *N. ceranae* positive despite a lack of detectable spores. Spore count also depends on the samples and the bees sent.

PCR method

PCR is the most sensitive method for distinguishing *N. apis* and *N. ceranae.* Furthermore, qPCR is more sensitive than using spore counts and will detect infections 40% more frequently (Travers *et al.*, 2012).

Several PCR methods have been described in the scientific literature. OIE (2014) recommends multiplex PCR with *N. apis*, *N. ceranae*, and *Nosema bombi* (Martin-Hernandez *et al.*, 2007; Higes *et al.*, 2010; Fries *et al.*, 2013).

Interpretation of the results

PCR is the best method to identify the parasite and to quantitate levels of both *N. ceranae* and *N. apis* (Traver *et al.*, 2012). However, interpretation of the PCR results is not easy.

The interpretation of the results must take into account the following elements:

- The standard analytical scale supplied by the laboratory.
- The quality of the samples sent to the laboratory.
- The anamnesis (clinical history).
- The clinical data given by the clinical examination in the field and the evaluation of the predisposing factors (geographical area, climate, meteorology, beekeeping practices, nearby agricultural practices, etc.).
- The fact that the honeybee is a social insect and that the colony is considered as a super-organism and the bees are individual organisms (thus, a negative result, i.e. no spores found, does not necessarily indicate an infection-free colony, and a positive result does not necessarily mean a positive diagnosis).
- A positive detection of *N.apis* and *N. ceranae* is not necessarily a positive diagnosis of Type-A or Type-C nosemosis.

Complementary analysis

Given the fact that endocrine and chemical markers are modified in nosemosis, the evaluation of the health status of a colony as well as the ability of a colony to respond to an infection such as nosemosis can be evaluated by testing vitellogenin expression and JH level (Dainat *et al.*, 2012a; Goblirsch *et al.*, 2013). These factors should prove interesting for an evaluation of the prognosis for the affected colony, though it is unfortunately not feasible to measure these routinely.

Analysis of the chemical residues found in the hive may also prove interesting.

3.6 Prognosis

The prognosis of covert Type-A and Type-C nosemosis (asymptomatic colonies) can be considered as not serious if environmental, food resources, climate features, and beekeeping practices are favourable. However, colonies that are asymptomatic and healthy carriers of *Nosema* spp. can suffer from outbreaks of nosemosis, which cause severe damage and offer a poor prognosis.

The prognosis of overt Type-A and Type-C nosemosis tends to be severe, with weakening and even collapse of infected colonies likely. Both types of nosemosis may be responsible for a drop in honey production and economic losses. It is necessary to remember that covert infection may turn into overt infection mainly if predisposing and contributing factors are present. Thus, controlling both types of nosemosis by good beekeeping practices is a necessity.

3.7 Control of Type-A and Type-C nosemosis

3.7.1 Veterinary medicines

The antibiotic fumagillin is a veterinary medicine active against Microsporidia. It is recognized to be efficient against *N. apis* and *N. ceranae* (Williams *et al.*, 2008; Fries, 2010; Higes *et al.*, 2010), even though a recent study reported that *N. ceranae* may evade fumagillin control in honeybees in certain circumstances (Huang *et al.*, 2013).

The use of fumagillin is not authorized in the EU, mainly because no maximum residue limit (MRL) has been defined by European health authorities. In some other countries, e.g. the US and Canada, fumagillin is authorized to prevent and control *N. apis* infection. Treatment in autumn and in spring is officially advised. This may be related to a study performed in Spain showing that the control of *Nosema* infection in autumn and in spring can effectively ameliorate the negative effects of Type-C nosemosis on the strength, health, and productivity of colonies.

However, the use of fumagillin in the countries where it is authorized must be measured and associated with sanitary beekeeping practices. Indeed, this antibiotic is only efficient on the vegetative form of *Nosema* spp. and not on the spores. Consequently, a treatment will only whiten a colony while the spores remain in the wax, the honey, the pollen, or on the wood for a long time.

Alternative treatments are described as having an effect on *Nosema* infection, including plant extracts, algae extracts, thymol (a phenol found in thyme oil), and resveratrol (a polyphenol found in grapefruit and some other fruits) (Higes *et al.*, 2010).

Because of the lack of treatments available in Europe and because of the efficacy of fumagillin only on vegetative forms, good sanitary beekeeping practices and prophylaxis are the best means to control as far as possible both types of nosemosis.

3.7.2 Beekeeping practices and prophylaxis

Strongly affected colonies should be eliminated and the material disinfected and sterilized. If an affected colony is strong enough to survive, implementation of the shock swarm method (shaking bee method) is recommended.

In Europe, control of nosemosis currently involves good sanitary beekeeping practices and prophylactic methods based on the predisposing factors of the disease:

- Honeybees: local black honeybees adapted to their local environment should be reared by beekeepers.
- Healthy queens: the replacement of the queen yearly or every two years has become a necessity, especially in cases of nosemosis.
- Beekeepers must act to prevent nutritional deficiency. In the event of blossoming failure, protein deficiency due to pollen starvation, lack of biodiversity, or uncontrolled *Varroa* infestation, pollen or protein supplementation is urgently required.
- Precautions must be taken while feeding, in particular in winter and spring: feeding bees must not pose any risks to the digestive tract. For example, runny syrup may cause diarrhoea and should be used with caution.
- Apiary management must follow good sanitary beekeeping practices and suitable actions must be taken urgently if nosemosis is diagnosed in an apiary:
  - Replacement of combs as frequently as necessary.
  - Disinfection of the material to eliminate spores:
    - ► With a blowlamp for supers and hive bodies.
    - ► With acetic acid vapour for supers. The supers are stacked up to form a chimney

and a cup of 80% acetic acid (1 ml per litre of volume to disinfect) is placed at the base for 48 hours. The supers should then be aired well for 8 days before use (Kilani, 1999). Appropriate precautions must be taken by the users.
- In the case of *N. ceranae* infection, freezing the material may be used to kill the spores. The effect of freezing greatly reduces *N. ceranae* spore viability (Fries, 2010).
- Honey may be heated to 60°C and wax to 100°C for 30 minutes to eliminate *N. apis* spores (Kilani, 1999).

Nosemosis is not an easy disease to diagnose and Type-C nosemosis is quite difficult to assess. Interpretation and analysis of the laboratory tests can be difficult. The biology of the honeybee, environmental factors, food resources, *Varroa* control management, beekeeping practices, and crop management in the surrounding area must be taken into account for a positive diagnosis.

4 Amoebiasis of the Malpighian tubules: *Malpighamoeba mellificae*

Amoebiasis is a parasitic disease of adult honeybees caused by *M. mellificae* (Kingdom: Protozoa; Phylum: Amoebozoa), which develops in the Malpighian tubules. It is a disease described as often being found with Type-A nosemosis and perhaps with bee virus X (Bailey, 1968; Tanada and Kaya, 1993; Olivier and Ribière, 2006; AFSSA, 2008). This disease is more prevalent in Central Europe (AFSSA, 2008).

4.1 Regulatory status

Amoebiosis is not a notifiable disease to the OIE.

4.2 Pathogenic agent and life cycle

Malpighamoeba mellificae is an obligate parasite of adult honeybees. Infection occurs after the ingestion of cysts in soiled feed or water. *Malpighamoeba mellificae* cysts are spherical with an average size of 6–7 µm.

The first stage is the development of primary trophozoites in the midgut epithelial cells (Liu, 1985). These then reach the Malpighian tubes and develop into secondary trophozoites after multiplication by scissiparity (asexual reproduction) (Tanada and Kaya, 1993; AFSSA, 2008). Finally, mature cysts are produced and ejected with the faeces.

Malpighamoeba mellificae destroys Malpighian epithelia, inducing malfunction of the excretory system (Tanada and Kaya, 1993). Amoebiasis seems to be more severe when associated with other pathogenic agents in particular *Nosema* spp. (AFSSA, 2008).

4.3 Clinical signs

Amoebiasis is generally detected in the early spring when bees begin to venture outside the hive (Tanada and Kaya, 1993). Adult bees may be observed with a distended abdomen, unable to fly, at the front of the hives (Fluri *et al.*, 1998). The signs include also pale to sulphur-yellow diarrhoea and frequent defecation. The oldest bees are affected most by amoebosis.

In most cases *M. mellificae* does not cause obvious disease (Bailey, 1968). However, according to Fluri *et al.* (1998), depopulation and weakening of affected colonies may be observed. Co-infection with *N. apis* is often described.

Amoebiasis–nosemosis co-infection occurs in February and March. Affected bees present diarrhoea and the colony may weaken or even collapse within 10–20 days. Within the affected colonies brood, pollen, and honey remain. One of the major features of the co-infection is a wide imbalance between brood and adult population (Paillot *et al.*, 1943).

The diagnosis requires laboratory analysis with microscopic examination of the Malpighian tubules for cysts of *M. mellificae* (OIE, 2014a).

The dissemination and transmission of *M. mellificae* is the consequence of robbing, drifting, and inadequate sanitary management of colonies.

4.4 Control

There is no treatment known to date. Sanitary measures and good beekeeping practices constitute proper prophylactic management (Tanada and Kaya, 1993). Strongly infected and weakened colonies should be eliminated, and the hives and supers disinfected (Paillot *et al.*, 1943). The frames should be destroyed and burned. If an affected colony is strong enough to survive, implementation of the shock swarm method (shaking bee method) is recommended.

References

AFSSA Report (2008) Mortalités, effondrements et affaiblissements des colonies d'abeilles. [Mortality collapse and weakening of bee colonies.] AFSSA (Agence Française de Sécurité Sanitaire des Aliments).

Alaux, C., Brunet, J.L., Dussaubat, C., Mondet, F., Tchemitchen, S., Coucin, M., Brilard, J., Baldy, A., Belzunces, L., and Le Conte, Y. (2009) Interactions between *Nosema* microspores and a neonicotinoid weaken honey-bees (*Apis mellifera*). *Environmental Microbiology*, 3(3): 774–782.

Alaux, C., Folschweiller, M., McDonnell, C., Beslay, D., Cousin, M., Dussaubat, C., Brunet, J.L., and Le Conte, Y. (2011) Pathological effects of the microsporidium *Nosema ceranae* on honey bee queen physiology (Apis mellifera). *Journal of Invertebrate Pathology*, 106(3): 380–385.

Alonso, J.M., Rey, J., Puerta, F., Hermoso, M., Hermoso, J., and Flores, J.M. (1993) Enzymatic equipment of *Ascosphaera apis* and the development of infection by this fungus in *Apis mellifera*. *Apidologie*, 24: 383–390.

Antúnez, K., Martín-Hernández, R., Prieto, L., Meana, A., Zunino, P., and Higes, M. (2009) Immune suppression in the honey bee (*Apis mellifera*) following infection by *Nosema ceranae* (*Microsporidia*). *Environmental Microbiology*, doi:10.1111/j.1462-2920.2009.01953.x

Aronstein, K.A. and Murray, K.D. (2010) Chalkbrood disease in honey bees. *Journal of Invertebrate Pathology*, 103: S20-S29.

Aronstein, K.A. and Cabanillas, H.E. (2012) Chalbrood re-examined. In Sammatoro, D. and Yolder, J.A. (ed.), *Honey Bee Colony Health Challenges and Sustainable Solutions*. CRC Press, Boca Raton, FL, pp. 121–130.

Bailey, L. (1955) The epidemiology and control of Nosema disease of the honey bee. *Annals of Applied Biology*, 43: 379–389.

Bailey, L. (1962) Bee diseases. In *Report of the Rothamsted Experimental Station for 1961*. Harpenden, pp. 160–161.

Bailey, L. (1968) The measurement and interrelationships of infections with *Nosema apis* and *Malpighamoeba mellificae* of honeybee populations. *Journal of Invertebrate Pathology*, 12: 175–179.

Botias, C., Martin-Hernandez, R., Barrios, L., Meana, A., and Higes, M. (2013) *Nosema* spp. infection and its negative effects on honey bees (*Apis mellifera iberiensis*) at the colony level. *Veterinary Research*, 44: 25, doi:10.1186/1297-9716-44-25.

Chen, Y., Evans, J.D., Zhou, L., Boncristiani, H., Kimura, K., Xiao, T., Litkowski, A.M., and Pettis, J.S. (2009) Asymmetrical coexistence of *Nosema ceranae* and *Nosema apis* in honey bees. *Journal of Invertebrate Pathology*, 101: 204–209.

Chen, Y.P. and Huang, Z.Y. (2010) *Nosema ceranae*, a newly identified pathogen of *Apis mellifera* in the USA and Asia. *Apidologie*, 41: 364–374.

Colin, M.E., Duclos, J., Larribau, E., and Boué, T. (1989) Activité des huiles essentielles de Labiés sur *Ascosphaera apis* et traitement d'un rucher. *Apidologie*, 20: 221–228.

Colin, M.E., Gauthier, L., and Tournaire, M. (2008) L'opportunisme chez *Nosema ceranae*. *Abeilles & fleurs*, 690: 30–33.

COLOSS Workshop (2009) *Nosema Disease: Lack of Knowledge and Standardization* Proceedings of the Workshop, Guadalajara. Available at http://www.coloss.org/publications/Nosema-Workshop-Proceedings.pdf (accessed 23 August 2014).

Cox-Foster, D.L., Conlan, S., Holmes, E.C., Palacios, G., Evans, J.D., Moran, N.A., Quan, P.L., Briese, T., Hornig, M., Geiser, D.M., Martinson, V., VanEngelsdorp, D., Kalkstein AL, Drysdale, A., Hui, J., Zhai, J., Cui, L., Hutchison, S.K., Simons, J.F., Egholm, M., Pettis, J.S., and Lipkin, W.I. (2007) A metagenomic survey of microbes in honeybee colony collapse disorder. *Science*, 318: 283–286.

Dainat, B., Evans, J.D., Chen, Y.P., Gauthier, L., and Neumann, P. (2012) Predictive markers of honey bee colony collapse. *PLoS ONE*, 7(2): e32151. doi:10.1371/journal.pone.0032151

Dussaubat, C., Maisonnasse, A., Alaux, C., Tchamitchan, S., Brunet, J.L., Plettener, E., *et al.* (2010) *Nosema* spp. infection alters pheromone production in honey bee (*Apis mellifera*). *Journal of Chemical Ecology*, 36: 522–525.

Dussaubat, C., Maisonnasse, A., Crauser, D., Beslay, D., Costagliola, G., Soubeyrand, S., Kretzchmar, A., and Le Conte, Y. (2013) Flight behavior and pheromone changes associated to *Nosema ceranae* infection of honey bee workers (*Apis mellifera*) in field conditions. *Journal of Invertebrate Pathology*, 113: 42–51.

Dussaubat-Arriagada, C. (2012) Effets de Nosema ceranae sur la santé de l'abeille domestique Apis mellifera L. Changements physiologiques et comportementaux. Thèse pour obtenir le grade de Docteur de l'Université d'Avignon, Avignon.

Eischen, F.A. and Graham, R.H. (2008) Feeding overwintering honeybee colonies infected with *Nosema ceranae*. In Proceedings of the American Bee Research Conference. *American Bee Journal*, 148: 555.

Fernández, J.M., Puerta, F., Cousinou, M., Dios-Palomares, R., Campano, F., and Redondo, L. (2012) Asymptomatic presence of *Nosema* spp. in Spanish comercial apiaries. *Journal of Invertebrate Pathology*, 111: 106–110.

Flores, J.M., Guttiérez, I., and Espejo, R. (2005) The role of pollen in chalkbrood disease in *Apis mellifera*: transmission and predisposing conditions. *Mycologia*, 97(6): 1171–1176.

Fluri, P., Herrmann, M., Imdorf, A., Bülmann, G. and Charrière, J.-D. (1998) Santé et maladies des abeilles. Connaissances de base. Communication no. 33, Centre Suisse de Recherches apicoles, Station de Recherches Laitières, Liebefeld, Berne.

Foley, K., Fazio, G., Jensen, A.B., and Hughes, W.O. (2012) Nutritional limitation and resistance to opportunistic *Aspergillus* parasites in honey bee larvae. *Journal of Invertebrate Pathology*, 111(1): 68–73.

Forsgren, E. and Fries, I. (2010) Comparative virulence of *Nosema ceranae* and *Nosema apis* in individual European honey bees. *Veterinary Parasitology*, 170: 212–217.

Forsgren E. and Fries, I., (2013) Temporal study of *Nosema* spp. in a cold climate. *Environmental Microbiology Reports*, 5(1): 78–82.

Fries, I. (1988). Infectivity and multiplication of *Nosema apis* Z. in the ventriculus of the honey bee. *Apidologie*, 19: 319–328.

Fries, I. (2010) *Nosema ceranae* in European honey bees (*Apis mellifera*). *Journal of Invertebrate Pathology*, 103: S73-S79.

Fries, I. (2014) Microsporidia. In Ritter, W. (ed.), *Bee Health and Veterinarians*. OIE, Paris, pp. 125–129.

Fries, I., Feng, F., Da Silva, A., Slemenda, S.B., and Pieniazek, N.J. (1996) *Nosema ceranae* n.sp. (Microspora, Nosematidae), morphological and molecular characterization of a Microsporidian parasite of the Asian honeybee *Apis cerana* (Hymenoptera, Apidae). *European Journal of Protistology*, 365(3): 356–365.

Fries, I., Chauzat, M.-P., Chen, Y.-P., Doublet, V., Genersch, E., Gisder, S., Higes, M., McMahon, D.P., Martín-Hernández, R., Natsopoulou, M., Paxton, R.J., Tanner, G., Webster, T.C., and Williams, G.R. (2013) Standard methods for *Nosema* research. In Dietemann V., Ellis J.D., and Neumann P. (eds), *The COLOSS Beebook*, Vol. II: *Standard Methods for Apis mellifera Pest and Pathogen Research. Journal of Apicultural Research*, 52(1): http://dx.doi.org/10.3896/IBRA.1.52.1.14.

Fyg, W. (1964) Anomalies and diseases of the queen honey bee. *Annual Review of Entomology*, 9: 207–224.

Gisder, S., Hedtke, K., Mockel, N., Frielitz, M.C., Linde, A., and Genersch, E. (2010) Five-year cohort study of *Nosema spp.* in Germany: does climate shape virulence and assertiveness of *Nosema ceranae*? *Applied and Environmental Microbiology*, 76: 3032–3038.

Glinski, Z. and Jarosz, J. (2001) Infection and immunity in the honey bee *Apis mellifera*. *Apiacta*, 36: 12–24.

Goblirsch, M., Huang, Z.Y., and Spivak, M. (2013) Physiological and behavioral changes in honey bees (*Apis mellifera*) Induced by *Nosema ceranae* infection. *PLoS ONE*, 8(3): e58165. doi:10.1371/journal.pone.0058165.

Gochnauer, T.A. and Margetts, V.J. (1979) Properties of honeybee larvae killed by chalkbrood disease. *Journal of Apicultural Research*, 18: 212–218.

Gomez-Moracho, T., Maside, X., Martin-Hernandez, R., Higes, M., and Bartolomé, C. (2014) High levels of genetic diversity in *Nosema ceranae* within *Apis mellifera* colonies. *Parasitology*, 141: 475–481.

GBIF (2014) Ascosphaera L.S. Olive & Spiltoir. Available at: http://www.gbif.org/species/2595772 (accessed 14 August 2014).

Hedtke, K., Jensen, P.M., Jensen, A.B., and Genersch, E. (2011) Evidence for emerging parasites and pathogens influencing outbreaks of stress-related diseases like chalkbrood. *Journal of Invertebrate Pathology*, 108: 167–173.

Higes, M., Martin, R., and Meana, A. (2006) *Nosema ceranae*, a new microsporidian parasite in honeybees in Europe. *Journal of Invertebrate Pathology*, 92: 93–95.

Higes, M., Martín-Hernández, R., Botías, C., Garrido-Bailón, E., González-Porto, A.V., Barrios, L., del Nozal, M.J., Bernal, J.L., Jiménez, J.J., García-Palencia, P., and Meana, A. (2008) How natural infection by *Nosema ceranae* causes honey bee colony collapse. *Environmental Microbiology*, 10: 2659–2669.

Higes, M., Martin, R., and Meana, A. (2010) *Nosema ceranae* in Europe: an emergent type C nosemosis. *Apidologie*, 41: 375–392.

Higes, M., Meana, A., Bartolomé, C., Botias, C., and Martin-Hernandez, R. (2013) *Nosema ceranae* (Microsporidia), a controversial 21st century honey bee pathogen. *Environmental Microbiology Reports*, 5(1): 17–29.

Hitchcock, J.D. and Christensen, M. (1972) Occurrence of chalk brood (*Ascosphaera apis*) in honey bees in the United States. *Mycologia*, 64: 1193–1198.

Hornitzky, M. (2001) *Literature Review of Chalkbrood*. Publication No. 01/150. RIRDC, Kingston, Australia.

Huang, W.F., Solter, L.F., Yau, P.M., and Imai, B.S. (2013) *Nosema ceranae* escapes fumagillin control in honey bees. *PLoS Pathogens*, 9(3): doi:10.1371/journal.ppat.1003185.

Huang, Z.Y. and Robinson, G.E. (1992) Honeybee colony integration: worker-worker interactions mediate hormonally regulated plasticity in division of labor. *Proceedings of the National Academy of Sciences USA*, 89: 11726–11729.

Invernizzia, C., Abuda, C., Tomascoa, I., Harriet, J., Ramalloc, G., Campáb, J., Katzb, H., Gardiolb, G., and Mendozac, Y. (2009) Presence of *Nosema ceranae* in honeybees (*Apis mellifera*) in Uruguay. *Journal of Invertebrate Pathology*, 101: 150–153.

Jensen, A.B., Aronstein, K., Flores, J.M., Vojvodic, S., Palacia, M.A., and Spivak, M. (2013) Standard methods for fungal brood disease research. *Journal of Apicultural Research*, 52(1): doi:10.3896/IBRA.1.52.1.13.

Kilani, M. (1999) Nosemosis. In Colin, M.E., Ball, B.V., and Kilani, M. (eds, *Bee Disease Diagnosis, Options Méditérranéennes*. No. 25. CIHEAM Publications, Zaragoza, pp. 9–24.

Klee, J., Besana, A.M., Genersch, E., Gisder, S., Nanetti, A., Tam, D.Q., Chinh, T.X.,

Puerta, F., Ruz, J.M., Kryger, P., Message, D., Hatjina, F., Korpela, S., Fries, I., and Paxton, R.J. (2007) Widespread dispersal of the microsporidian *Nosema ceranae*, an emergent pathogen of the western honey bee, *Apis mellifera*. *Journal of Invertebrate Pathology*, 96: 1–10.

Kralj, J. and Fuchs, S. (2010) *Nosema* sp. influences flight behaviour of infected honeybee (Apis mellifera) foragers. *Apidologie*, 41: 21–28.

Liu, T.P. (1985) Scanning electron microscopy of developmental stages of *Malpighamoeba mellificae* prell in the honeybee. *Journal of Eukaryotic Microbiology*, 31(1): 139–144.

Liu, T.P. (1992) Oocytes degeneration in the queen honey bee after infection by *Nosema apis*. *Tissue Cell*, 24: 131–138.

Lumbsch, H.T. and Huhndorf, S.M. (eds) (2007) *Outline of Ascomycota*. The Field Museum, Department of Botany, Chicago. *Myconet*, 13: 1–58. Avalaible at: http://www.fieldmuseum.org/sites/default/files/Myconet_13a.pdf (accessed 14 August 2014)

Maassen, A. (1913) Weitere Mitteilungen uber der seuchenhaften Brutkrankheiten der Bienen. [Further communication on the epidemic brood disease of bees.] *Mitteilungen aus der Kaiserlichen Biologischen Anstalt fur Land- und Forstwirtscshaft*, 14: 48–58.

Martín-Hernández, R., Meana, A., Prieto, L., Salvador, A.M., Garrido-Bailón, E., and Higes M. (2007) Outcome of colonization of *Apis mellifera* by *Nosema ceranae*. *Applied and Environmental Microbiology*, 73(20): 6331–6338.

Martín-Hernández, R., Botías, C., Bailón, E.G., Martínez- Salvador, A., Prieto, L., Meana, A., and Higes, M. (2012) Microsporidia infecting *Apis mellifera*: coexistence or competition. Is *Nosema ceranae* replacing *Nosema apis*? *Environmental Microbiology*, 14: 2127–2138.

Mayac, C. and Naug, D. (2009) Energetic stress in the honeybee *Apis mellifera* from *Nosema ceranae* infection. *Journal of Invertebrate Pathology*, 100(3): 185–188.

Nelson, D.L. and Gochnauer, T.A. (1982) Field and laboratory studies on chalkbrood disease of honeybees. *American Bee Journal*, 122: 29–32.

OIE (2014a) *Manual of Diagnostic Tests and Vaccines for Terrestrial Animals 2014. Apinae*, Section 2.2. Available at: http://www.oie.int/en/international-standard-setting/terrestrial-manual/access-online/ (accessed 24 August 2014).

OIE (2014b) *OIE Listed Diseases*. Available at http://www.oie.int/en/animal-health-in-the-world/oie-listed-diseases-2014/ (accessed 29 April 2014)

Oliver, R. (2011) An update on the 'Nosema cousins'. *American Bee Journal*, 151: 1153–1158.

Olivier, V. and Ribière, M. (2006) Les virus infectant l'abeille Apis *mellifera*: le point sur leur classification. *Virologie*, 10(4): 267–278.

Paillot, A., Kirkor, S., and Granger, A.M. (1943) *L'abeille Anatomie, Maladies, Ennemis*. Imprimerie de Trévoux, Ain.

Paxton, R.J., Klee, J., Korpela, S., and Fries, I. (2007) *Nosema ceranae* has infected *Apis mellifera* in

Europe since at least 1998 and may be more virulent than *Nosema apis*. *Apidologie*, 38: 558–565.

Puerta, F., Flores, J.M., Ruiz, J.A., Ruiz, J.M., and Campano, F. (1999) Fungal diseases of the honeybee (*Apis mellifera* L.). In Colin, M.E., Ball, B.V., and Kilani, M (eds), *Bee Disease Diagnosis, Options Méditerranéennes*, Series B: *Etudes et Recherches*. No. 25. CIHEAM Publications, Zaragoza, pp. 61–68.

Shimanuki, H. and Knox, D.A. (2000) *Diagnosis of Honeybee Diseases*. United States Department of Agriculture (USDA), Agriculture Handbook No. 690.

Skou, J.P. (1972) Ascosphaerales. *Friesia*, 10: 1–24.

Skou, J.P. (1988) More details in support of the class Ascosphaeromycetes. *Mycotaxson*, XXXI(1): 191–198.

Spiltoir, C.F. (1955) Life cycle of *Ascosphaera apis* (*Pericystis apis*). *American Journal of Botany*, 42: 501–508.

Spiltoir, C.F. and Olive, L.S. (1955) A reclassification of the genus *Pericystis Betts*. *Mycologia*, 47: 238–244.

Spivak, M.S. and Reuter, G.S., (1998) Performance of hygienic honey bee colonies in a commercial apiary. *Apidologie*, 29: 291–302.

Tanada, Y. and Kaya, H.K. (1993) *Insect Pathology*. Academic Press, San Diego.

Traver, B.E. and Fell, R.D. (2011) Prevalence and infection intensity of *Nosema* in honey bee (*Apis mellifera* L.) colonies in Virginia. *Journal of Invertebrate Pathology*, 107: 43–49.

Traver, B.E., Williams, M.R., and Fell, R.D. (2012) Comparison of within hive sampling and seasonal activity of *Nosema ceranae* in honey bee colonies. *Journal of Invertebrate Pathology*, 109: 187–193.

Van Der Steen, J.J.M, Cornelissen, B., Donders, J., Blacquière, T., and Van Dooremalen, C. (2012) How honey bees of successive age classes are distributed over a one storey, ten frame hive. *Journal of Apicultural Research*, 51(2): 174–178.

Vidal-Naquet, N. (2011) Honeybees. In Lewbart, G.L. (ed.) *Invertebrate Medicine*, 2nd edn. Wiley-Blackwell, Chichester, pp. 285–321.

Vidal-Naquet, N. (2012) Tout sur la mycose du couvain d'*Apis mellifera* due à *Ascosphaera apis*. *La Semaine Vétérinaire*, 1498: 50.

Vidau C., Diogon M., Aufauvre J., Fontbonne R., Viguès B., Brunet J.L., Texier C., Biron D.G., Blot N., El Alaoui H., Belzunces L.P., and Delbac F. (2011) Exposure to sublethal doses of fipronil and thiacloprid highly increases mortality of honeybees previously infected by *Nosema ceranae*. *PLoS ONE*, 6(6): e21550. doi:10.1371/journal.pone.0021550.

Vidau, C., Panek, J., Texier, C., Biro, D.G., Belzunces, L.P., Le Gall, M., Broussard, C., Delbac, F., and El Alaoui, H. (2014) Differential proteomic analysis of midguts from Nosema ceranae-infected honeybees reveals manipulation of key host functions. *Journal of Invertebrate Pathology*, in press.

Wang, D.I. and Moeller, F.E. (1969) Histological comparisons of the development of the hypopharyngeal glands in healthy and *Nosema*-infected worker honey bees. *Journal of Economical Entomology*, 14: 135–142.

Webster, T.C. (1993) *Nosema apis* spore transmission among honeybees. *American Bee Journal*, 133: 869–870.

Weiss, L.M. and Becnel, J.J. (2014) *Microsporidia: Pathogens of Opportunity*. Wiley Blackwell, Oxford.

Williams, G.R., Sampson, M.A., Shutler, D., and Rogers, R.E.L. (2008) Does fumagillin control the recently detected invasive parasite *Nosema ceranae* in western honey bees (*Apis mellifera*)? *Journal of Invertebrate Pathology*, 99 : 342–344.

Williams, G.R., Shutler, D., Burgher-MacLellan, K.L., and Rogers, R.E.L. (2014) Infra-population and -community dynamics of the parasites *Nosema apis* and *Nosema ceranae*, and consequences for honey bee (*Apis mellifera*) hosts. *PLoS ONE*, 9(7): e99465. doi:10.1371/journal.pone.0099465.

Wittner, M. and Weiss, L.M. (1999) *The Microsporidia and Microsporidiosis*. ASM Press, Washington DC.

Wolf, S., McMahon, D.P., Lim, K.S., Pull, C.D., Clark, S.J., *et al.* (2014) So near and yet so far: harmonic radar reveals reduced homing ability of *Nosema* infected honeybees. *PLoS ONE*, 9(8): e103989. doi:10.1371/journal.pone.0103989.

Yoder, J.A., Jajack, A.J., Rosselot, A.E., Smith, T.J., Yerke, M.C., and Sammataro, D. (2013) Fungicide contamination reduces beneficial fungi in bee bread based on an area-wide field study in honey bee, *Apis mellifera*, colonies. *Journal of Toxicology and Environmental Health A*, 76(10): 587–600.

Zander, E. (1909) Tierische Parasiten als Krankenheitserreger bei der Biene. *Münch. Bienenztg.*, 31: 196–204.

7

Pests and enemies of honeybee colonies

The honeybee has numerous enemies that target the brood and adults, the nest (wax combs, wood of the hives), and the fruits of the colony's labour (honey, pollen). These predators belong to diverse animal groups: insects and other invertebrates, birds, and assorted mammals.

This chapter is devoted to these threats. In Europe, some have long been known, e.g. the greater and lesser wax moths. Others are invasive species such as the Asian hornet *Vespa velutina*, which was introduced into France in 2004 and first described in 2006, and has increased its distribution area steadily since then, and the small hive beetle introduced into the US, Australia, Cuba, and most recently Italy. Global apiculture and international trade and exchange of material are responsible for the introduction of these new invasive pests and enemies.

1 *Galleria mellonella*, the greater wax moth

Galleria mellonella is an insect of the order Lepidoptera belonging to the family Pyralidae. The larvae of *G. mellonella* are pests that attack the wax foundations of the combs, causing serious damage (Ben Hamida, 1999). The greater wax moth is more common than the lesser wax moth. It is a worldwide pest. According to the FAO (2006), the greater wax moth also causes damage in tropical and sub-tropical Asia. *Galleria mellonella* is unable to survive at low temperatures, and it does not cause damage at high altitudes (>1200 m) (Paddock, 1926).

Galleria mellonella has long been known. Aristotle describes a likely pest in *The History of Animals* (IX, 40): 'The diseases that chiefly attack prosperous hives are first of all the clerus. This consists in a growth of little worms on the floor, from which, as they develop, a kind of cobweb grows over the entire hive, and the combs decay' (trans. D'Arcy Wentworth Thompson, 1862).

1.1 Regulatory status

Galeria mellonella is not a notifiable pest.

1.2 The moth and its life cycle

Adult *G. mellonella* is a grey moth with reddish-brown anterior wings bearing mottling spots and pale cream-whitish hind wings. *Galleria mellonella* is 15 mm long with an average wingspan of 31 mm (Ellis *et al.*, 2013). The damage they do is caused by the caterpillars, which live and develop in galleries they create in the wax combs (Figure 7.1).

The colour of the larvae changes from creamy-white to grey as they grow. The first instars are 1–3 mm long, and 12–20 mm long (and 5–7 mm in diameter) when completely grown (Ellis *et al.*, 2013) (Figure 7.2). The caterpillars possess two well-developed mandibles, allowing them to tunnel into the combs.

The chrysalises develop within an off-white, parchment-thick cocoon and are yellow/reddish-yellow coloured (Williams, 1997).

The life cycle lasts between 4 weeks and 6 months (Ben Hamida, 1999) and occurs as follows:

- Adults live from 3 days to 1 month (Nielsen, 1971). During the evening, the day after mating with males in trees, the fertilized females enter the hive and lay eggs on the

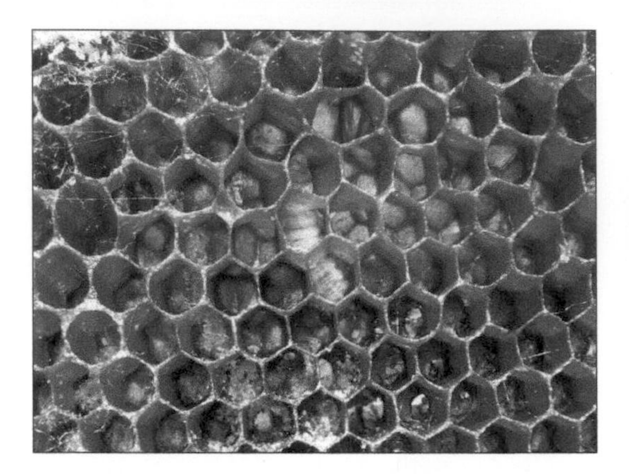

Figure 7.1 Caterpillar of *Galeria mellonella* burrowing a tunnel into the wax comb. (Photo courtesy of © Christophe Roy, DVM.)

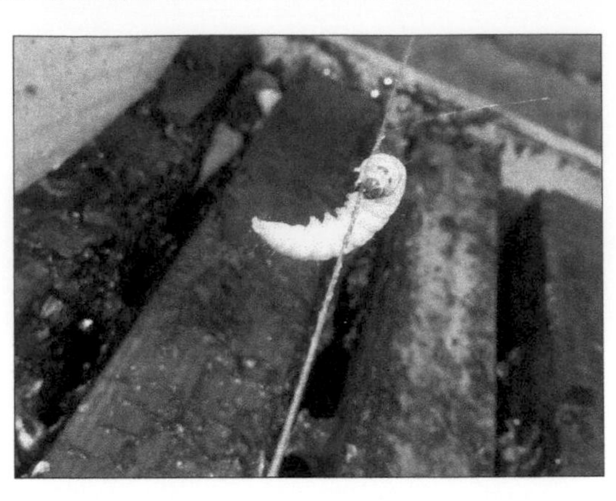

Figure 7.2 Caterpillar of *Galeria mellonella*. (Photo courtesy of © Christophe Roy, DVM.)

wax. In the morning, the females return to hide in the trees (Ben Hamida, 1999).

- The strongly adhered eggs are oviposited in clusters of 50–150 eggs in a location where bees cannot reach them (e.g. in dark cracks or crevices in combs, the edge of frames, or around the hives) (British Beekeepers Association, 2012; Ellis *et al.*, 2013). If moth females cannot enter the hive, they may lay eggs on the ground, and the larvae will reach the hives by gnawing their way through and into the hives (Toumanoff, 1939). Females can lay 300–600 eggs at a time and up to 1,800 during their lifetime (El Sawaf, 1950; Ben Hamida, 1999).
- Caterpillars grow and tunnel a gallery in the combs, consolidated this by spinning a silk thread (Figure 7.3). The webs thus created protect the caterpillars from worker bees. *Galleria mellonella* caterpillars feed on wax combs, larval skins, honey, pollen, residues, and impurities found in the cells (Ellis *et al.*, 2013). Their preference for wax means that they are most attracted by older dark combs. In those old combs, where the brood has been reared, are found moulting remains, pollen, and honey, and some other remnants (Shimanuki and Knox, 2000; Ellis *et al.*, 2013). The caterpillars can resist a food shortage, but in such cases the *G. mellonella* adults will be smaller (Marston *et al.*, 1975).
- Eighteen days after hatching, caterpillars begin to spin their cocoon, and the pupal phase begins.

1.3 Damage caused by the greater wax moth

The caterpillars of *G. mellonella* can affect live colonies and stored combs, often causing

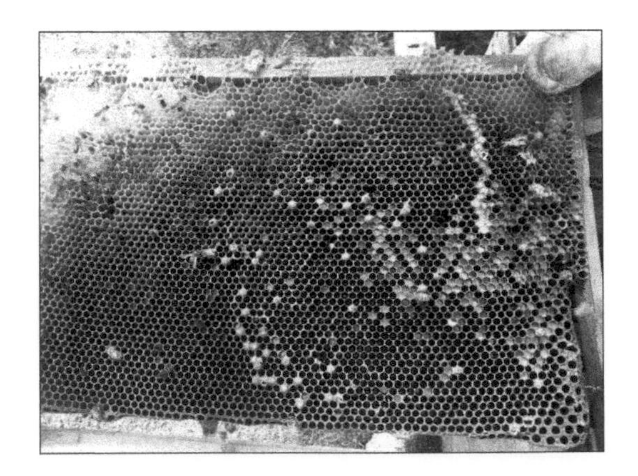

Figure 7.3 Silk-thread spun by a caterpillar of *Galeria mellonella* in a tunnel. (Photo courtesy of © Claire Beauvais, DVM.)

considerable damage (Vidal-Naquet, 2011). Combs stored in the honey house or elsewhere on the premises are at great risk of attack from these caterpillars.

In colonies, the greater wax moth causes gallieriosis (gallieriasis according to Ellis *et al.*, 2013). Strong colonies are able to manage the pest and even to eliminate it (Ben Hamida, 1999). The damage mainly affects weakened colonies.

The greater wax moth causes a range of damage:

- Caterpillars burrow tunnels into capped brood cells and feed on the midrib (the base of the comb on which the cells are constructed). The silk threads may trap the brood in the cells, altering its development (Figure 7.4). Immature forms may be trapped in the silk with the imago being unable to emerge, sometimes over a considerable surface of the brood comb (Williams, 1997, Ellis *et al.*, 2013). The wood of the frames, hive body, and supers may be damaged by the moth larvae. Indeed, the caterpillars chew the wood to make a cavity for cocoon attachment (Williams, 1997).
- The consequence of the development of the greater wax moth may be weakened colonies. In some cases infestation may lead colonies to abscond from the hive.
- The greater wax moth can also act as vector of brood disease, harbouring infectious pathogens, in particular *Paenibacillus larvae* spores (Toumanoff, 1939).

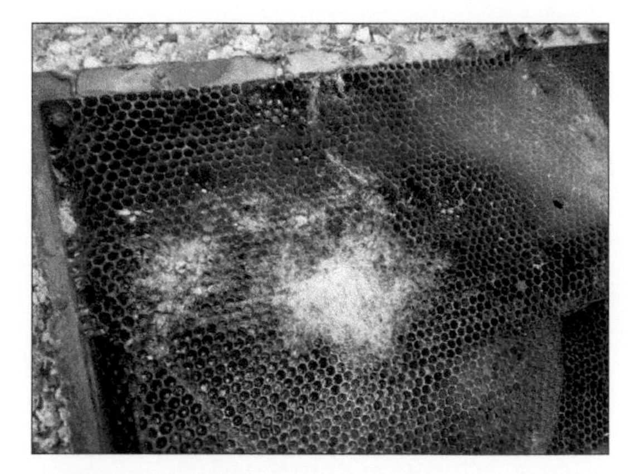

Figure 7.4 Extensive silk thread spun by caterpillars of *Galeria mellonella* on a comb. (Photo courtesy © Christophe Roy, DVM.)

Stored combs can be highly damaged, sometimes much more than live colonies, and become unusable for beekeeping. The wax foundations and comb may be severely damaged by the tunnels and extensive silky webbing left by the greater wax moth (Figure 7.4).

1.4 Control and management

The methods described here apply to both the lesser and greater wax moth.

1.4.1 Protecting colonies

Good sanitary beekeeping practices are the best way to control moth infestation. Strong and large colonies are able to manage the infestation.

During hive and apiary inspections, the removal of wax debris and scrapings from the floor and the vicinity of the hive is necessary.

1.4.2 Protecting stored material

Stored combs must be free of honey and pollen. Non-chemical methods offer the most effective protection when stored hive material is to be reused.

- *Air flow and light.* Stored combs are placed in supers. Supers are stacked in a criss-cross pattern to form a 2 m chimney open at the top and the bottom. This chimney should be well ventilated and able to be penetrated by light, minimizing wax moth infestation.
- *Low temperature.* Freezing combs and supers before placing them in plastic bags for storage provides a high level of protection against wax moths. Combs must be thawed and dried before storage. The freezing must last more than 24 hours at ≤0°C, 4.5 hours at −7°C, and 3 hours at −15°C (Cantwell and Smith, 1970; Charriere and Imdorf, 1999; Ellis *et al.*, 2013).

- *Use of strong colonies as comb protectors.* Strong colonies may be used to protect supers and combs (Ellis *et al.*, 2013). However, this method cannot be used when colonies are overwintering.
- *Chemicals.* Different active substances are or have been used to kill wax moths and protect the stored combs, including paradichlorobenzene (PDB), but this is a dangerous carcinogenic substance that can leave residues in wax and honey. Its use is completely unacceptable (Anses Agency, 2004).
  - The use of 'moth proofers' is dangerous for the bees and for consumers of hive products as residues of these insecticides persist in the wax.
  - The use of sulphur strips or acetic acid has been described to protect stored combs, super, and hives from the greater wax moth (British Beekeepers Association, 2012). It is essential to take stringent precautions when employing such products to protect both the bees and the users.
- *Biological methods.* Wax moths are sensitive to some viruses and bacteria, which can serve as a 'natural' epizootic (Metalnikoff, 1922). A serotype of *Bacillus thuringiensis* is able to infect and kill the greater wax moth (Barjac and Thomson, 1970). Using this bacterium as a biological agent can help to control the pest, but stringent precautions need to be taken with this insecticide-producing bacterium. It is administered as a concentration of bacterial spores. The correct dilution, as recommended by the supplying laboratory, is required to avoid bee toxicity. It can be a useful method for beekeepers with a small number of hives, such as hobby beekeepers. This method can be applied only if the product is suitably licensed.

2 *Achroia grisella*, the lesser wax moth

Achroia grisella is a Lepidopteran belonging to the family Pyralidae. The lesser wax moth is less widespread than *G. mellonella*.

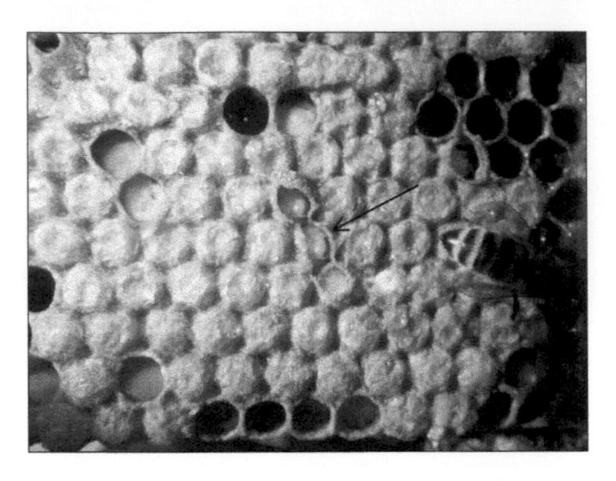

Figure 7.5 Bald brood. The *Achroia grisella* caterpillar burrows a straight gallery just below the surface of the capped brood cells, exposing adjacent pupae. (Photo courtesy © Lydia Vilagines, DVM.)

The adults have a silver body with a yellow head. The males are 10 mm long, while the females measure 12–14 mm with a wingspan of 16–24 mm. The female can lay between 250 and 300 eggs during her lifetime (Ben Hamida, 1999). The caterpillars are smaller than those of *G. mellonella*.

The damage to the hive inflicted by *A. grisella* is different to that caused by the greater wax moth. Caterpillars burrow straight galleries just below the surface of the capped brood cells. The cells are then uncapped and the pupae inside exposed. Clusters of adjacent cells are affected and the resulting brood defects are called 'bald brood' (Figure 7.5) (Borchert, 1974).

Control and management of the lesser wax moth is the same as for the greater wax moth.

3 *Aethina tumida*, the small hive beetle

The small hive beetle, *Aethina tumida* Murray, is a Coleopteran insect native to South Africa. It is an endemic pest and scavenger of Sub-Saharan colonies of African *Apis mellifera* species (Lundie, 1940; Neuman and Ellis, 2008; Vidal-Naquet, 2011). There, it does not cause severe damage to strong colonies because of the defence strategies developed by the native honeybees. This Coleopteran was first described in 1867 (Murray, 1867).

Global apiculture, with the trade and exchange of honeybees, is responsible for introducing this pest into a number of countries, where it has caused severe damage to infested European honeybee colonies and resulted in considerable economic loss.

In 1996, small hive beetles were found in European honeybee colonies in the US (Florida, South Carolina), and since then *A. tumida* has become an endemic species with an increasing distribution range.

In 2000, *A. tumida* was described in Egypt. In Australia, it was found in 2002 (Neumann and Elzen, 2004). In 2010, infestations were described in Canadian apiaries (Quebec and Ontario) near the border with the US (Ministry of Agriculture of British Columbia, 2012). In 2012, its presence was confirmed in Cuba.

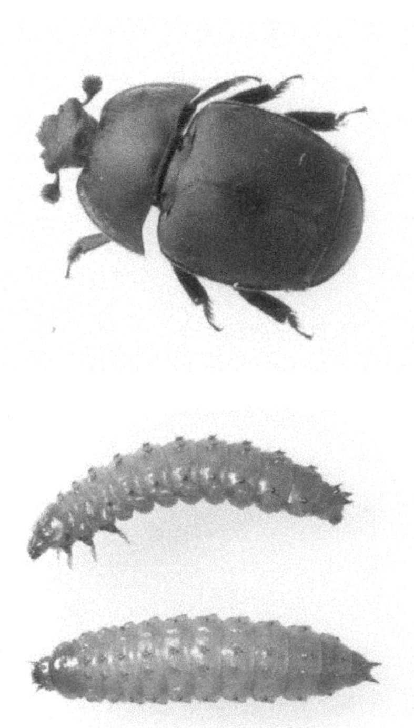

Figure 7.6 *Aethina tumida* adult and larva. (Courtesy © The Animal and Plant Health Agency (APHA), Crown Copyright.)

On 12 September 2014, *A. tumida* was discovered in an apiary in southern Italy in the province of Reggio di Calabria, near an important seaport. The Italian authorities took immediate measures, destroying the infested apiary and neighbouring apiaries, and using insecticides on the infested sites; a protection zone of 20 km and a surveillance zone of 100 km were established around the primary infested site. This was the first time that *A. tumida* had been described in Europe, except for an apparently brief introduction in Portugal where it was intercepted and eradicated in a consignment of queen bees from Texas (FERA, 2013). At the time of writing, 18 March 2015, despite the measures taken by the Italian authorities, *A. tumida* has been observed in 61 apiaries since 12 September, including apiaries in Sicily (Plateforme ESA, 2015).

In non-infested countries, beekeepers, as well as veterinarians and other professionals involved in apiculture, must be aware of the dangers posed by this pest. Thus, they must be able to recognize the species, and be ready to inform the authorities if an infestation is suspected. Sanitary measures must be taken immediately if an *A. tumida* infestation is suspected or diagnosed as described below for the present epizootic situation in southern Italy.

3.1 Regulatory status

Aethina tumida is a statutory notifiable pest to the OIE (OIE, 2014b). It is also notifiable to countries in the EU (Appendix 2).

3.2 Morphology and life cycle

3.2.1 Morphology

Aethina tumida is an insect belonging to the order Coleopteran and the family Nitidulidae. As a Coleoptera, it is characterized by thick elytra, the posterior membranous wings folded resting under the wing covers, and chewing mouthparts.

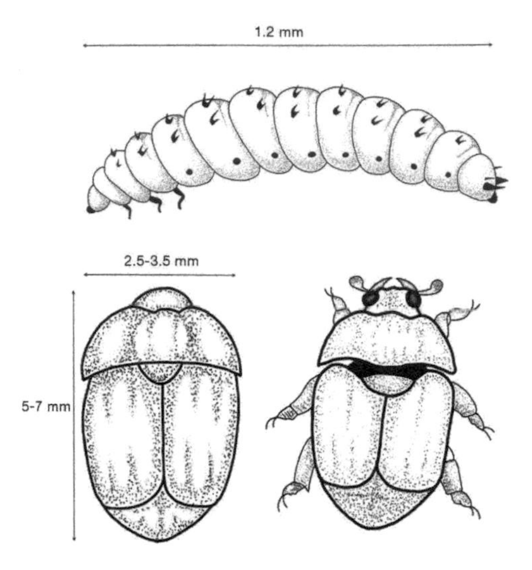

Figure 7.7 Drawing of *Aethina tumida* adult (showing on the left the head and antennae tucked down beneath the thorax as often observed in the hive) and larva. (Redrawn from Menier and Bertrand, 2014.)

The adult is a small, stocky beetle with a broad and dorsoventrally flattened body measuring approximately 5–7 mm long and 2.5–3.5 mm wide (Figures 7.6 and 7.7). Adult female small hive beetles (5.7 ± 0.02 mm × 3.2 mm) are slightly longer than males (5.5 ± 0.01 mm × 3.2 mm). One of the main morphological features of *A. tumida* is its club-shaped antennae that are common within the Nitulidae family (Figures 7.6 and 7.7). Under natural conditions the size of *A. tumida* may vary depending on environmental factors or diet (Ellis, 2004; University of Florida, 2013). The beetles are on average one-third the size of the bees.

The colour of *A. tumida* goes from light-brown to brown-black as the beetle matures and the exoskeleton sclerotises. The elytra do not cover the whole abdomen (the hind part of the abdomen is visible) and are covered with thin hairs.

The eggs are oviposited in the hives. They are pearly white and 1.4 mm long by 0.26 mm wide. They are usually laid in irregular clusters containing 10 to more than 30 eggs (Ellis, 2012; Cuthbertson *et al.*, 2013).

The larvae of *A. tumida* are creamy-white in colour (Figure 7.6). When they mature under favourable conditions, they may be up to 1.2 cm long, but tend to be smaller in the event of dietary deficiency. The larvae present three pairs of legs and two rows of spines, and have two large spines protruding from the rear (FERA, 2013).

The pupae live in the soil and are creamy-white coloured and darken as metamorphosis proceeds.

3.2.2 Life cycle (Figure 7.8)

Adults emerge from the soil where the pupal stage occurs. After emergence, adult *A. tumida* look for colonies to infest, attracted by colony odours and probably pheromones (Cuthbertson *et al.*, 2013). Field observations by US beekeepers show that the day after a colony has been inspected, cohorts of beetles are attracted there (FERA, 2013).

Aethina tumida depends on *A. mellifera* as a primary host. The beetle may also feed on fruits, such as certain Nutilidae (but reproduction on fruits has yet to be confirmed) (Ellis, 2012). The beetles seem to infest colonies at dusk (Neumann and Elzen, 2004).

When they find a colony, small hive beetles may face resistance from the colony guards (Ellis, 2012). Once inside the hive, the beetles tend to be confined by the bees to certain locations (cracks, crevices), limiting access to combs where they usually lay. However, if it is isolated from food resources, *A. tumida* may induce trophallactic behaviour in the bees, and feed directly from them.

According to Lundie (1940) and Ellis (2004), adults are sexually mature about 7 days after emergence from the soil. However, the mating behaviour of *A. tumida* is not well known (Ellis, 2012).

Several eggs are oviposited as typical irregular clutches in confined places. If *A. tumida* females escape confinement and are able to access the combs, oviposition occurs within pollen cells or brood cells. Each female is able to lay 1,000 eggs in her lifetime (Lundie, 1940).

After 3–6 days, the eggs hatch (Lundie, 1940; Cuthbertson *et al.*, 2013). Humidity seems to be a major factor for egg development and hatching as the eggs are very sensitive to desiccation if the humidity is <50% and draughts are present (Ellis, 2012). Temperature is also a factor influencing egg development and hatching.

Beetle larvae emerge from the eggs and immediately begin to feed on honey, pollen, and preferably brood (Neumann and Härtel, 2004; Ellis, 2012). Larval development depends on food and temperature, lasting on average 7–14 days though sometimes taking more than 30 days.

At the end of this feeding phase, the larvae leave the hive; this is the wandering phase defined by the end of feeding period and migration out of the hive to find a place in the soil to pupate (Ellis, 2012). The larvae seem to group together to move towards the soil, as an exodus from the colony. This wandering phase generally occurs at night (Cuthbertson *et al.*, 2013).

Thus, pupation occurs in suitable soil near the hive (on average within 90 cm, sometimes up to 20 m; in some rare cases, they can move up to 200 m to find a suitable soil to pupate). The

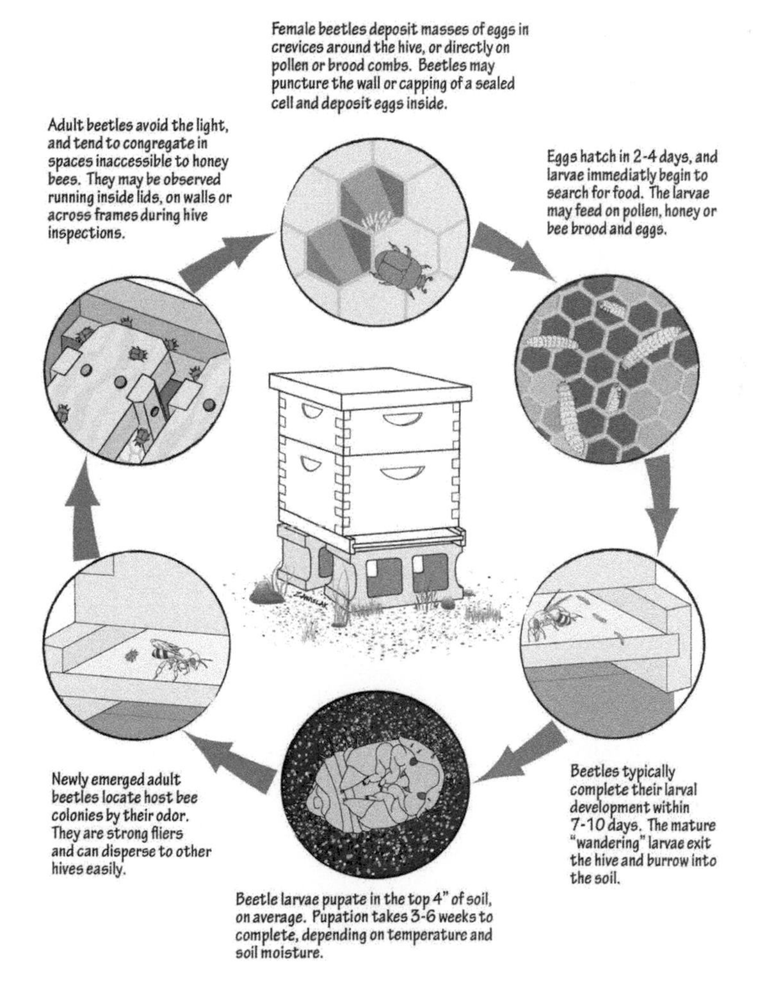

Figure 7.8 Life cycle of *Aethina tumida.* (Courtesy © Jon Zawislak, University of Arkansas.)

larvae burrow into the soil, usually to less than 10 cm (1–30 cm) from the surface, and build smooth-walled earthen cells in which to pupate (FERA, 2013). A moist soil favours the pupal stage while drier ones seem to lower pupation success (Cuthbertson *et al.*, 2013).

The pupal stage lasts between 2 and 12 weeks depending on temperature and humidity, but the majority of *A. tumida* adults emerge within 3–4 weeks (Ellis *et al.*, 2004; Ellis, 2012).

The period from the egg to the adult lasts approximately 4–6 weeks. Thus, in moderate climatic conditions, up to six generations of the beetle may occur in a year (Ellis, 2012).

The adult beetles leave the soil and are able to fly over long distances (5–10 km) to infest new colonies. High temperature and humidity are optimal for *A. tumida* (Ellis *et al.*, 2004). The adult beetle life span is 4–6 months (OIE, 2014a).

Aethina tumida may also infest and cause damages to bumblebee colonies and in particular commercial ones such as *Bombus impatiens*. Trade in bumblebees also poses a risk of introducing small hive beetle.

3.2.3 Damage caused by *Aethina tumida* infestation in colonies

Aethina tumida in Sub-Saharan countries

In Sub-Saharan countries, *A. tumida* is mainly a colony scavenger, feeding of pollen, honey, and brood. The beetle is a minor economic pest, affecting weak colonies and stored combs.

Strong colonies are able to fight and easily resist this insect (Neumann and Elzen, 2004):

- Guards fight by harassing beetles, preventing infestation.
- Bees fill cracks, crevices, and cavities with propolis.
- Bees remove larvae from the hive or build a structure from propolis to confine them.

In some circumstances (weak colonies), the small hive beetle may cause colony mortality or lead a colony to abscond (Ellis *et al.*, 2003; Ellis, 2012). When the colony absconds, honey, pollen, and brood remain behind. Before absconding, the queen usually continues to lay a few eggs and the workers consume pollen and honey (Winston, 1987). African bees have a tendency to abscond even in low-level cases of beetle infestation.

Aethina tumida in European honeybee colonies

Due to global apiculture, *A. tumida* has become an invasive species in Egypt, the US, Australia, Cuba, Canada, Mexico, Jamaica, and Europe (following its discovery in Italy in September 2014). It can cause severe damage to apiaries, and colony mortality is often observed following beetle infestation. The reasons for the extent of damage wrought by this beetle are not fully understood, as European honeybees present an aggressive behaviour against *A. tumida* invasion (biting and attacking beetles), and tend to confine the beetles as African honeybees do (Ellis, 2012). However, this defence behaviour of European honeybee colonies is not sufficient to control small hive beetle infestation.

Infestation by small hive beetle proceeds as follows (Ellis, 2012):

- Invasion of colonies by adult *A. tumida*.
- Accumulation of beetle population.
- Reproduction.
- Damage caused by larvae feeding on brood, pollen, and honey combs.
- Exodus of the larvae from the colony to nearby soil.
- Pupation in the soil and emergence of adults, which reinfest colonies.

The beetle larvae are mainly responsible for the damage that occurs in colonies as they burrow into combs, feeding on brood, honey, and pollen. A strong beetle infestation (>1,000 adult beetles per colony) can cause the colony to abscond.

All the colonies in an affected area are usually infested, but not all will die. According to Ellis (2012), some cases of colony collapse caused by *A. tumida* may originate due to other stressors such as parasites or pathogenic agents.

Faeces of *A. tumida* adults and larvae in honeycombs cause fermentation of the honey flowing out of the cells. The fermentation is due to SHB-infested yeasts and in particular to the yeast *Kodamaea ohmeri* (Schäfer *et al.*, 2009). This may occur in hives or in stored combs leading to economic losses as the honey becomes unfit for human and honeybee consumption and thus unsellable.

Ellis (2012) defines the small hive beetle as a 'secondary pest' of honeybee colonies in the US, as are the greater and lesser wax moths. *Aethina tumida* is reported to harbour and thus be a passive vector between bees and between colonies of pathogens such as the bacterium *Paenibacillus larvae* and the viruses DWV and SBV (see Chapter 3, sections 3 and 4) (Ellis, 2012).

3.2.4 Diagnosis

In uninfested countries, all the stakeholders involved in apiculture must be able to diagnose *A. tumida* or at least suspect it. This involves knowledge of the morphological features of eggs, larvae, and adults that may be found in hives.

Many non-dangerous Coleopteran species may be found in hives and a differential diagnosis needs to be done.

Sampling for laboratory examination is necessary, and is mandatory in countries where *A. tumida* is a notifiable pest. Notification to the relevant authorities is also mandatory, so that robust sanitary measures can be taken.

Laboratory examination can be done by binocular loupe identification of the species but also by the PCR method. Debris and other material in contact with bees may be analysed by this method, in particular in the case of package bees or when introducing queens from foreign countries (Ward, 2007; Vidal-Naquet, 2013).

3.2.5 Small hive beetle control

In non-infested countries

Aethina tumida is considered as a notifiable pest for the OIE and many countries. This requires sanitary measures when introducing bees (package bees, colonies, queens, etc.).

The following pathways present a risk of introducing *A. tumida*:

- Trade and movement of package bees, colonies, queens, alternative hosts such as bumblebees, and hive products. This also concerns movement of wax and materials, such as clothes used by apiarists.
- Importation of fruit (avocados, bananas, grapefruits, etc.) known to be an alternative host on which the beetles may feed and probably oviposit.

Importation of bees by beekeepers is regulated in the EU (Commission Decision 2003/881/EC; Commission Decision 206/2010). Importation of bees must be done through proper and legal channels and with a veterinary health certification. Current (May 2015) EU legislation prohibits imports of queens, package bees, and/or colonies from third world countries affected by *Aethina tumida* (small hive beetle) but also by American foulbrood and *Tropilaelaps* spp. (Tropilaelaps mite). Imports of package bees, colonies, and queens are only allowed from EU member states and New Zealand under a veterinary agreement between the EU and New Zealand. However, this legislation did not prevent the introduction of the small hive beetle into Italy in September 2014.

In the UK, a surveillance network has been developed to monitor exotic pests such as *A. tumida* and *Tropilaelaps* spp. According to the Animal and Plant Health Agency (FERA, 2013), 'the only chance for eradication will be early interception of exotic pests, so by targeting inspections to these areas we have a better chance of succeeding'.

Veterinarians (whether practitioners, officials, or researchers) play key roles in detecting these pests, and in defining and certifying sanitary measures to counter them.

Control measures in infested countries

In infested countries such as Australia and the US, chemical control measures were initially used. However, chemical control often proves inadequate, and poses risks of resistance, of toxicity for bees, and of residues occurring in hive products. It appears that the best way to fight the small hive beetle is to keep honeybee colonies strong and to employ mechanical traps to control the number of adult beetles infesting hives. If chemicals are used, they should be applied within an integrated pest management (IPM) framework:

- *Chemical measures* (Schäfer and Ritter, 2014). Permethrin is applied in the US to the soil around infested colonies. Within the hive, strips of coumaphos are used and placed on the underside of cardboard floor inserts. However, these two chemicals do not seem to be completely effective. Moreover, precautions must be taken to protect the bees and to avoid the risk of contaminating the honey and other hive products which may become unfit for consumption due to the presence of residues. Fipronil-treated cardboard placed in plastic boxes on the bottom boards of the hive and fipronil gels in traps are also sometimes used illegally by beekeepers in the US and Australia. This poses a major risk of poisoning the bees, as well as potentially compromising the safety of the hive products (honey, pollen, royal jelly, propolis, etc.) and hence consumer health.
- *Integrated pest management.* As in the *Varroa* IPM approach described in Chapter 5, *A. tumida* IPM combines chemical measures and beekeeping practices (Ellis, 2012; FERA, 2013). IPM will be more efficient if it involves all the stages of the small hive beetle's life cycle:
  - Standard good sanitary beekeeping practices to maintain strong colonies are necessary. This also involves the selection of colonies presenting good hygienic behaviour against the small hive beetle.
  - Moving colonies to new places periodically may help to limit any increase in the beetle population.
  - Some traps help to limit adult infestation.
  - Early honey extraction is necessary to limit the risk of contamination by small hive beetle faeces. In honey houses, humidity must be maintained at <50% to inhibit hatching of small hive beetle eggs (Ellis, 2012).
  - Biological control may be a (future) part of the IPM. Research is being done on bait containing the yeast *Kodamaea ohmeri* (mixed with pollen and honey) to attract the beetles into traps. In the soil, the action of certain nematodes seems to limit pupation of *A. tumida*.

In conclusion, small hive beetle can cause great damage to colonies and to production, leading to economic losses for honey farms. Although this beetle is now, like the moths, considered a secondary pest in the US, the appearance of *A. tumida* in 2014 in Italy represents a major threat to the whole of Europe.

Beekeepers and other apiculture stakeholders have a great responsibility to monitor their apiaries. Veterinarians, whatever their involvement, also have a major role to play, in particular in diagnosing *A. tumida* infestation, and in creating and implementing the sanitary measures which have to be taken when this pest, as any other, is introduced into new territories.

4 *Vespa velutina*, the Asian hornet

Twenty-two hornet species are listed worldwide (Rome *et al.* 2013; Natural History Museum, 2014; USAPHC, 2014). Two native species exist in Europe:

- *Vespa crabro*. Range area: northern and western Europe and northern Asia.
- *Vespa orientalis*. Range area: southern Europe, south-western Asia, north-eastern Africa and Madagascar.

Vespa crabro is not considered as a major predator in Europe. *Vespa orientalis* is a bee-hawking predator, and eastern *Apis mellifera* species have developed defence behaviours against this oriental hornet.

Hornets and wasps (*Vespa* spp., *Vespula* spp.) are known to be bee-hawking predators of *Apis* spp. worldwide. All Asian countries report damage to *Apis cerana* and *Apis mellifera* colonies attacked by hornets and wasps (FAO, 2006).

Vespa crabo was the only indigenous hornet living in France before 2004, when the Asian *Vespa velutina* Lepeletier was described in the Lot-et-Garonne *département* in south-west France (Haxaire *et al.*, 2006; Villemant *et al.*, 2006; Breton, 2012). *Vespa velutina nigrithorax*, a strictly Asian species, was the subspecies introduced. Overwintering queens have been accidently introduced into France, probably hidden within pieces of pottery from China. *Vespa velutina* has become acclimated in France, being able to nest and reproduce.

Since 2006, *V. velutina* has become an invasive species and has caused much damage to French apiaries, resulting in significant economic losses for the apiculture industry. Furthermore, *V. velutina* may potentially pose a danger to humans and may adversely affect the indigenous insect population on which it feeds (pollinators, scavangers, etc.).

4.1 Regulatory status

In France, *V. velutina* is a notifiable secondary pest.

4.2 Range distribution of *Vespa velutina nigrithorax*

Vespa velutina nigrithorax is adapted to areas with temperate to subtropical climates (Villemant *et al.*, 2011a). *Vespa velutina* is widespread in Asia (from north-eastern India to Indonesia, and in China, Nepal, Afghanistan, Bhutan, Laos, Malaysia, Taiwan, and Pakistan) (Archer, 1994). It was introduced into South Korea in 2002, where it has become an invasive species (MoonBo *et al.*, 2012).

To date, *V. velutina nigrithorax* is an invasive species found in France, Belgium, Italy, Spain, and Portugal. Since its introduction, the distribution range of *V. velutina* has increased each year. In 2014, it was detected in two-thirds of France, and in some parts of Belgium, Italy,

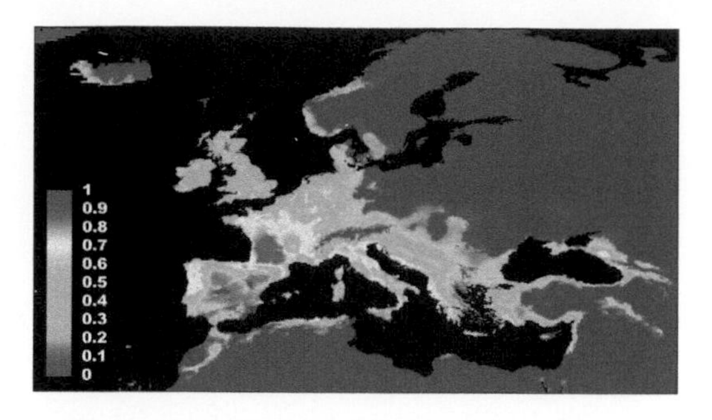

Figure 7.9 Predicting the risk of invasion by *Vespa velutina nigrithorax*; across Europe and the Middle East the invasion risk increases from blue to red. (Photo courtesy © Claire Villemant, MNHN; Villemant *et al.*, 2011a.)

Spain, and Portugal (Cabi, 2014). Its progress across Europe appears unstoppable.

Predictive studies suggest that countries susceptible to invasion by *Vespa velutina* are those situated along the Atlantic and northern Mediterranean coasts (Figure 7.9). The coastal areas of the Balkan peninsula, Turkey, and the Near East appear to be favourable for *V. velutina nigrithorax* (Villemant *et al.*, 2011a). Global trade poses the main risk of introducing the Asian hornet into countries currently free of this pest.

4.3 Morphology

The morphological features of female *V. velutina* are as follows (Haxaire *et al.*, 2006; Villemant *et al.*, 2006, 2011a,b):

- Workers and queens are morphologically uniform (Figure 7.10). Workers are up to 25 mm in length and the queens up to 30 mm.

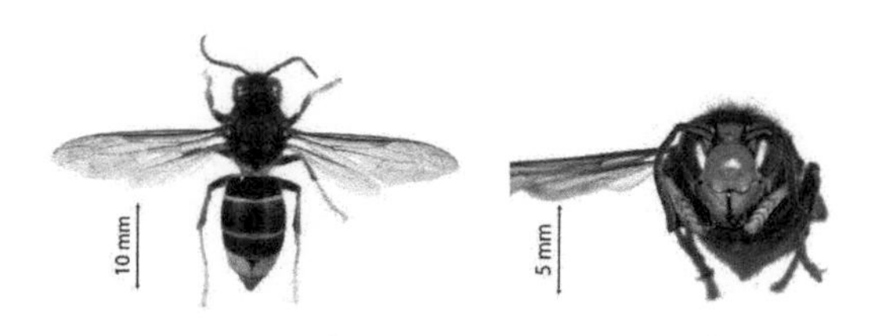

Figure 7.10 *Vespa velutina* female adult. (Photo courtesy © Claire Villemant, Museum National d'Histoire Naturelle, Paris.)

They are smaller than the European hornet *V. crabo*.

- The head is black with a yellow-orange face and mouthparts. The antennae are brown dorsally and yellow ventrally.
- The thorax is black with thin hairs; the wings are yellow.
- The legs are brown with a yellow end.
- The abdomen is brown with a thin yellow band on the hind part of the first segment, and a thin orange band on the second and third tergite. The fourth segment 'is almost entirely orange with a median basal triangular black marking'. The last segments (fifth and sixth) are more or less orange-brown. The ventral part of the abdomen is brown. Its stinger is not barbed and *V. velutina* does not die after stinging.

Male *V. velutina* are very similar to females only with longer antennae. The male hornets are stingless.

4.4 Structure of the nest

A primary nest is built up by a queen after overwintering. The primary nests are spherical and usually built low down. Little differentiable from other Vespidae (hornets, wasps) nests, they may be found everywhere – in eaves and fence posts, under sheds, and in empty hives, but very rarely in fresh soil or in holes in walls.

The secondary (mature) nests are hidden more than 10 m high in the foliage of leafy trees (Figures 7.11 and 7.12). They may also be found on the frames of sheds or in tree hedges. The secondary nests are on average 70 cm in diameter, oval-shaped, with a vertical axis. Some nests may reach 1 m in height and 80 cm in diameter. They have one lateral orifice through which the hornets enter or leave the nests (Villemant *et al.*, 2011b). The nests are made of paper (cellulose and water). Because of the need for water, these nests are often found near watercourses. The nests are often found empty after autumn. They are built for only one season.

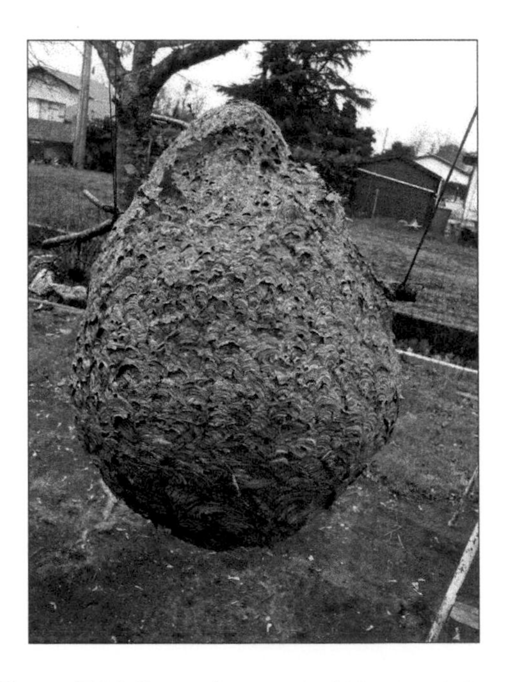

Figure 7.11 Secondary nest of *Vespa velutina*. (Photo courtesy © Raymond Saunier.)

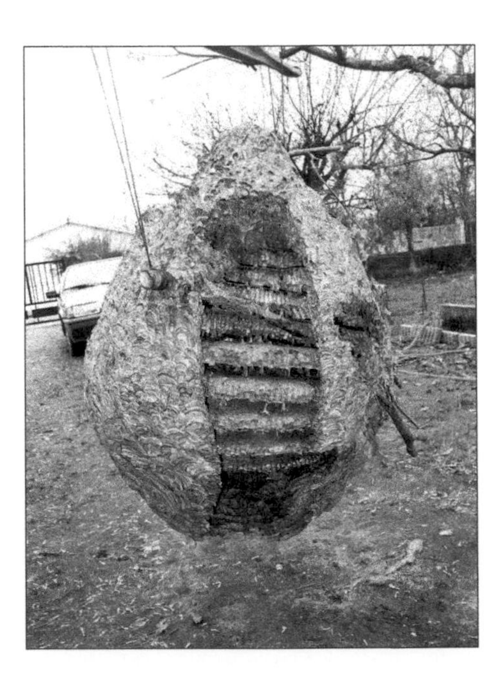

Figure 7.12 Secondary nest showing the internal structure. (Photo courtesy © Raymond Saunier.)

4.5 Life cycle

The cycle begins in spring after the overwintering period of a fertilized queen. Hibernation takes place in weather-protected shelters (under the bark of trees, under roof tiles, in plant pots, etc.).

When the temperature is favourable, the queen, called the 'founder' at this period of the cycle, builds a primary nest low down in order to rear the first workers.

In the middle of August, as the colony population increases, the queen may chose to relocate the colony with the first workers to a secondary nest at a higher location (e.g. a leafy tree) (Choi *et al.*, 2012; Rome et al., 2013). Up to 6,000 hornets are produced from a nest in a season. In a nest, there may be more than 2,000 individuals at any one time (Villemant *et al.* 2011b).

The more the colony increases, the longer the queen stays in the nest. Her only role will be laying eggs while the workers take charge of rearing the new larvae.

The colony population and its food needs increase, leading to more predation behaviour. Damage to honeybees then tends to become increasingly prevalent.

The sexual male and females emerge between mid-September and mid-October. The founder queen is usually dead when her sexual daughters (200–400) emerge (new future founders). Males and females mate usually in the tree canopy (Cabi, 2014). After mating, the males die and the fertilized females find a hibernation place to overwinter.

4.6 Nutrition

The adult diet is composed of sugar liquids, such as honey, honeydew, and nectar but also fruits and proteinaceous secretion delivered by the hornet larvae after stimulation.

The larvae are fed by workers. They have a 'carnivorous' diet: insects and in particular honeybees but also spiders, meat, and fish (this is why Asian hornets may be found flying around market stalls). Bees are butchered near the site of capture (hives). *Vespa velutina* removes the head, wings, legs, and abdomen and makes a meatball from the bee's thoracic muscles. The hornets bring these meatballs back to the nest to feed the larvae.

Hornet attacks on apiaries are numerous and frequent, particularly at the end of the honeybee season (September–December) when the production of new hornet queens increases food needs (Mollet and Torre 2006; CABI, 2014).

According to Villemant *et al.* (2011b), the diet of *V. velutina* varies according to the environment. In urban areas, *Apidae* represent 66% of the diet, while in agricultural and forest areas, *Apidae* represent only 35% of the diet. Thus, the high pressure is urban ranges may be because of the lack of insect–fauna diversity (Villemant *et al.*, 2011b).

4.7 Damage caused by *Vespa velutina* to honeybee colonies

Although in Asia *Apis cerana* has developed a behavioural defence strategy against the Asian hornet, this behaviour has not yet been observed in Europe with *Apis mellifera* (Figure 7.13). *Apis cerana* has developed a technique known as heat-balling to fight *V. velutina* (Papachristoforou *et al.*, 2007). During heat-balling, guard bees closely surround the attacking hornet and raise their thoracic temperatures. The core

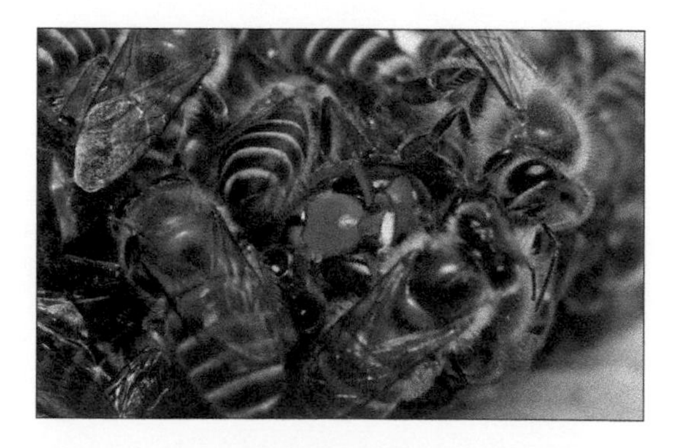

Figure 7.13 Heat-balling behaviour of *Apis cerana*. (Photo courtesy © Quentin Rome, Muséum National d'Histoire naturelle, Paris.)

temperature of the heat-balls reaches about 45°C, killing the hornet which cannot withstand such high temperatures (Tan *et al.*, 2012). However, in certain circumstances (e.g. when colonies are weakened), the Asian hornet may nevertheless be responsible for colony mortality.

Apis mellifera in Europe have not developed such an efficient defence behaviour, instead the guard bees group together to try to move the hornets away and attempt to sting the intruder. The predation behaviour of *V. velutina* may endanger honeybee colonies. Between July and December, the Asian hornet has high nutritional needs for brood rearing.

Hornets hover in flight around hives, waiting for returning foragers, which they catch and then carry off to a convenient location (Figure 7.14). Sometimes, before overwintering, hornets may enter the hive to feed on brood and honey.

In some places, up to 15 hornets can be found in front of each colony of an apiary (Breton, 2012; CABI, 2014). This level of predation of forager bees returning with nectar and pollen can seriously impair the food supply and weaken the colony, rendering it susceptible to infectious diseases.

Stress and defence behaviour increase energy consumption. Foraging may be reduced from July to October and preparation for the wintering period may be impaired. Thus, the bee-hawking Asian hornet may cause winter collapse of bee colonies that it attacks.

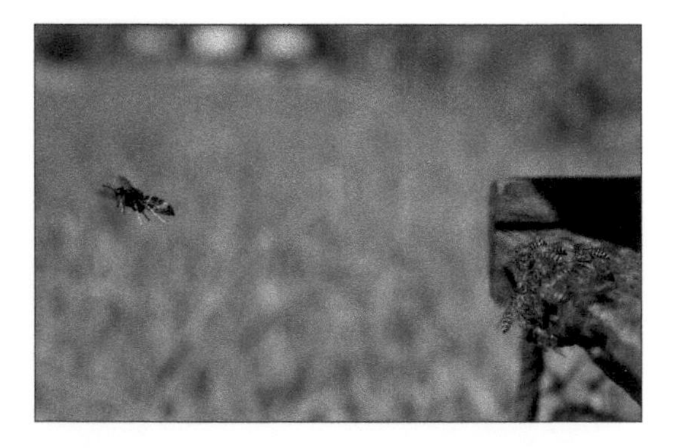

Figure 7.14 Hovering *Vespa velutina* waiting for foragers in front of a hive of *Apis cerana*. (Photo courtesy © Quentin Rome, Muséum national d'Histoire naturelle, Paris.)

In the south-west of France, it has been reported that 30% or more of annual colony mortality could be the consequence of Asian hornet predation (Breton, 2012).

Thus, *Vespa velutina* poses a major threat to honeybee colonies as is often the case with invasive species. In infested areas, it seems that *V. velutina* attacks mainly weakened colonies in an apiary; the largest and most populous colonies are less affected. In some places, colonies are suspected to develop fighting behaviour against *V. velutina* by propolizing the entrance of the hive and catching hornets there.

NB. Asian hornets are reported to be dangerous to humans if they approach nests (to <5 m), especially when the nest is well developed. The consequences of an Asian hornet attack are dangerous because of the number of hornets in a nest. Severe symptoms have been observed following several stings. De Haro states that 'a review of data from French Poison Control Centres showed only one envenomation clearly linked to *V. velutina*'. Since the arrival of the Asian hornet in France, there has been no increase in hymenoptera poisoning (de Haro et al., 2010).

4.8 Fighting *Vespa velutina*

Eradication of *V. velutina* from Europe is likely to be impossible. Beekeepers and authorities can only attempt to limit the damage caused by the Asian hornet. The fight against this hornet must be appropriate and as specific to the species as possible.

Counter-measures include:

- Protection of apiaries by bait trapping. Trapping must be performed *only* in the case of hornet attack and not as a preventive measure and the traps must be placed near the apiary to be efficient. The two types of bait are available:
  - Fermented old wax juice, which is used between July and November (Rome *et al.*,

2011). It is made from old brood comb + 1.5 l of water + 20 g of honey and left to stand for at least for 3 days to ferment.
  - Protein bait, usually made from fresh fish and used when hornets' food needs are increasing (between August and November when the future sexual adults are being reared).
- Protection of the hive:
  - By rearing strong and healthy colonies and implementing good beekeeping practices.
  - By reducing the size of the entrance to prevent Asian hornets from entering the hive (because of the size of the drones, this can only be done when there is no drone brood rearing).
  - By encouraging high blades of grass to grow in front of the hive.
  - By placing nets around the hives with a mesh size that allows the bees to pass through but stops the larger hornets.
- Setting up a surveillance network to monitor Asian hornet nests and oversee their destruction. This must be done according to local legislation. Based on the French experience, it is recommended that nest destruction is done before the emergence of sexual adults (October/November) and when workers are inside the nest (at daybreak or nightfall).
- By hive movement. It is considered necessary to change the location of a hive when more than five hornets are found attacking the colony. Indeed, beekeepers' experience has shown that finding five or more hornets in front of a hive can seriously endanger, or even kill, a colony.

Trapping founder queens is not a solution in the fight against *V. velutina*. Only 1% of the queens born in autumn will succeed the next year in founding a colony and producing a new sexual generation of Asian hornets (Edwards, 1980; Rome *et al.*, 2013): 95% of the founders die during the winter and 95% of the remainder die in spring during the competition for nesting sites. Thus, trapping founders will only decrease this usurping level and lead to a weakening of the young hornet colonies (Rome *et al.*, 2013). In France, it has been shown that spring trapping of founders is not an efficient means of controlling the Asian hornet population (Monceau *et al.*, 2012).

5 Other pests and enemies of the hives

Other insects, primarily those of the order Hymenoptera (ants, bees, hornets, and wasps among other winged insects), can be enemies of honeybee colonies and hives (Ben Hamida, 1999). According to the FAO (2006), ants are common predators of honeybees in tropical and subtropical Asia. There, they attack colonies en masse, removing everything they find within (bees, brood, and honey). In temperate countries, although certain species of ants are often found in hives, they do not cause major damage that endangers colonies. Coleopterans such as *Cetonia apaca*, *Cetonia morio*, and *Trichodes apiarius* may cause damage to hives, burrowing galleries into the combs (Toumanoff, 1939; Borchert, 1974). Some of these intruders lay eggs and reproduce in the hive.

Insectivorous birds (the European bee-eater is the major such predator in southern Europe, northern Africa, and western Asia; the green woodpecker and various tits also sometimes feed on bees) and mammals such as mice, hedgehogs, badgers, and of course bears are also enemies of bees and hives. Protecting apiaries with fences may be necessary – heavy-duty fences and electric fences are used in the US and Canada to keep bears out; plastic fences can prevent the green woodpecker gaining access to the hives.

In tropical and subtropical countries, amphibians (frogs and toads) and reptiles (geckos, skinks, lizards) may damage apiaries. Primates (monkeys) are also enemies of colonies, opening hives and feeding on honey and brood.

According to the FAO (2006), however, among the pests, including the primate pests, of honeybees, humans are 'probably the most destructive'.

References

Anses Agency (2004) Stratégie de réduction de risque consommateur pour le paradichlorobenzène. Available at: http://www.afssa.fr/ET/PPND0D9.htm?pageid=733&parentid=424 (accessed 20 November 2014).

Anses Agency (2014) Detection of *Aethina tumida* (small hive beetle) in southern Italy. Available at: https://sites.anses.fr/en/minisite/abeilles/detection-aethina-tumida-small-hive-beetle-southern-italy-0 (accessed 20 November 2014).

Archer, M.E. (1994) Taxonomy, distribution and nesting biology of the *Vespa* bicolor group (Hym., Vespinae). *Entomologist's Monthly Magazine*, 130: 149–158.

Barjac, H. and Thomson, J.V. (1970) A new serotype of *Bacillus thuringiensis*: *Bacillus thuringiensis* var. *thompsoni* (serotype 11). *Journal of lnvertebrate Pathology*, 15: 141–144.

Beebase. European Union (EU) Legislation http://www.nationalbeeunit.com/index.cfm?pageid=102 (accessed 18 March 2015).

Ben Hamida, T. (1999) Enemies of bees. In Colin, M.E., Ball, B.V., and Kilani, M. (eds), *Bee Disease Diagnosis, Options Méditerranéennes*, Series B: *Etudes et Recherches*. No. 25. CIHEAM Publication, Zaragoza, pp. 147–165.

Borchert, A. (1970) *Les Maladies et Parasites des Abeilles* (traduit de l'allemand par Michelat, J.). Vigot frères, Paris.

Breton, V. (2012) Le frelon asiatique, gestion au quotidien. In SNGTV (ed.), *Proceedings of the Journées nationales des GTV.* Nantes, pp. 841–846

British Beekeepers Association, The (2012) *Wax Moth in the Apiary*. Available at: http://www.bbka.org.uk/files/library/wax_moth_l020_(data)_r2_1342860174.pdf (accessed 26 August 2014).

Cabi (2014) Invasive Species Compendium. *Vespa velutina*. Available at: http://www.cabi.org/isc/datasheet/109164 (accessed 2 September 2014).

Cantwell, G.E. and Smith, L.J. (1970) Control of the greater wax moth, *Galleria mellonella* in honeycomb and comb honey. *American Bee Journal*, 110: 263.

Charrière, J.D. and Imdorf, A. (1999) Protection of honey combs from wax moth damage. *American Bee Journal*, 139(8): 627–630.

Choi, M.B., Martin, S.J., and Lee, J.W. (2012) Distribution, spread, and impact of the invasive hornet Vespa velutina in South Korea. *Journal of Asia-Pacific Entomology*, 15: 473–477.

Cuthbertson, A.G.S., Wakefield, M.E., Powell, M.E., Marris, G., Anderson, H., Budge, G.E., Mathers, J.J., Blackburn, L.F., and Brown, M.A. (2013) The small hive beetle *Aethina tumida*: a review of its biology and control measures. *Current Zoology*, 59(5): 644–653.

Edwards, R. (1980) *Social Wasps: Their Biology and Control.* Rentokil Limited, East Grinstead.

Ellis, J.D. (2004) The ecology and control of small hive beetle (*Aethina tumida* Murray). PhD thesis, Rhodes University, Grahamstown, South Africa.

Ellis, J.D. (2012) Small hive beetle (*Aethina tumida*) contributions to colony losses. In *Honey Bee Colony Health Challenges and Sustainable Solutions*. CRC Press, Boca Raton, FL, pp. 135–144.

Ellis, J.D., Hepburn, H.R., Delaplane, K.S., Neumann, P., and Elzen, P.J. (2003) The effects of adult small hive beetles *Aethina tumida* (Coleoptera: Nitidulidae), on nests and flight activity of Cape and European honey bees *Apis mellifera*. *Apidologie*, 34: 399–408.

Ellis, J.D., Hepburn, H.R., Luckmann, B., and Elzen, P.J. (2004) The effects of soil type, moisture, and density on pupation success of *Aethina tumida* (Coleoptera: Nitidulidae). *Environmental Entomology*, 33: 794–798.

Ellis, J.D., Graham, J.R., and Mortensen, A. (2013) Standard methods for wax moth research. COLOSS honey bee research association. *Journal of Apicultural Research* 52(1), available at: http://www.coloss.org/beebook/II/wax-moth (accessed 26 August 2014).

El Sawaf, S.K. (1950) The life-history of the greater wax moth (*Galleria mellonella* L.) in Egypt, with special reference to the morphology of the mature larva. *Bulletin la Société Fouad Premier d'Entomologie*, 34: 247–297.

FAO (2006) *Honey Bee Diseases and Pests: A Practical Guide*. Available at: http://www.fao.org/3/a-a0849e.pdf (accessed 29 July 2014).

FERA: The Food & Environment Research Agency (2013) *The Small Hive Beetle: A Serious Threat to European Apiculture*. The Food and Environment Research Agency, York.

Haxaire, J., Bouguet, J.P., and Tamisier, J.P. (2006) *Vespa velutina* Lepeletier, 1836, une redoutable nouveauté pour la faune de France (Hym., Vespidae) *Bulletin de la Société Entomologique de France*, 111(2): 194.

Lundie, A.E. (1940) The small hive beetle *Aethina tumida*. Union of South Africa Department of Agriculture and Forestry, Entomological Series 2. *Science Bulletin 220*. Government Printer, Pretoria, South Africa.

Marston, N., Campbell, B., and Boldt, P.E. (1975) Mass producing eggs of the greater waxmoth,

Galleria mellonella L. US Department of Agriculture Technical Bulletin 1510. Available at: http://naldc.nal.usda.gov/naldc/download.xhtml?id=CAT75662587&content=PDF (accessed 20 november 2014).

Menier, J. and Bertrand, C. (2014) *Aethina tumida*: Ne joue-t-on pas avec le feu? Available at http://www.beekeeping.com/sante-de-labeille/articles/aethina_tumida.htm (accessed 25 October 2014).

Metalnikoff, J. (1922) Une épizootie chez les chenilles de *Galleria mellonella. Académie des Sciences (France)*, 175: 68–70.

Mollet, T. and de la Torre, C. (2006) *Vespa velutina*. The Asian Hornet. *Bulletin technique Agricole*, 33(4): 203–208.

Monceau, K., Bonnard, O., and Thiéry, D. (2012) Chasing the queens of the alien predator of honeybees: a water drop in the invasiveness ocean. *Open Journal of Ecology*, 2: 183–191. doi: 10.4236/oje.2012.24022.

MoonBo, C., Martin S.J., and JongWook, L. (2012) Distribution, spread, and impact of the invasive hornet *Vespa velutina* in South Korea. *Journal of Asia-Pacific Entomology*, 15(3): 473–477.

Murray, A. (1867) List of Coleoptera received from Old Calabar. *Annals and Magazine of Natural History*, 19: 167–179.

Natural History Museum (2014) *Vespa crabo* (hornet). Available at: http://www.nhm.ac.uk/nature-online/species-of-the-day/collections/our-collections/vespa-crabro/ (accessed 2 September 2014).

Neumann, P., and Ellis, J.D. (2008) The small hive beetle (*Aethina tumida* Murray, Coleoptera: Nitidulidae): distribution, biology and control of invasive species. *Journal of Apicultural Research*, 47: 181–183.

Neumann, P. and Elzen, P.J. (2004) The biology of the small hive beetle (*Aethina tumida*, Coleoptera: Nitidulidae): gaps in our knowledge of an invasive species. *Apidologie*, 35(3): 229–247.

Neumann, P. and Härtel S. (2004) Removal of small hive beetle (*Aethina tumida*) eggs and larvae by African honeybee colonies (*Apis mellifera scutellata*). *Apidologie*, 35(1): 31–36.

Nielsen, R.A. (1971) Radiation biology of the greater wax moth, *Galleria mellonella* (L.): effects on developmental biology, bionomics, mating-competitiveness, and F1 sterility. PhD thesis, Utah State University, Logan, UT.

OIE (2014a) Manual of Diagnostic Tests and Vaccines for Terrestrial Animals 2014. Apinae. Section 2.2. Available at: http://www.oie.int/en/international-standard-setting/terrestrial-manual/access-online/ (accessed 24 August 2014).

OIE (2014b) OIE Listed Diseases. Available at http://www.oie.int/en/animal-health-in-the-world/oie-listed-diseases-2014/ (accessed 29 April 2014).

Paddock, F.B. (1926) The chronological distribution of the beemoth. *Journal of Economical Entomology*, 19, 136–141.

Papachristoforou, A., Rortais, A., Zafeiridou, G., Theophilidis, G., Garney, L., Thrasyvoulou, A., and Arnold, G. (2007) Smothered to death: hornets asphyxiated by honeybees. *Current Biology*, 17, R795–R796.

Plateforme ESA, http://www.plateforme-esa.fr/index.php?option=com_content&view=article&id=439:infestation-par-aethina-tumida-petit-coleoptere-de-la-ruche-au-sud-de-litalie&catid=159:actualites-internationales-aethina-tumida&Itemid=328 (accessed 18 March 2015).

Rome, Q., Muller, F., Théry, T., Andrivot, J., Haubois, S., Rosensthiel, E., and Villemant, C. (2011) Impact sur l'entomofaune des pièges à bière et à jus de cirier utilises dans la lute contre le frelon asiatique. In Barbançon, J.-M. and L'Hostis, M. (eds), *Journée Scientifique Apicole*, Arles, pp.18–20.

Rome, Q., Sourdeau, C., Muller, F., and Villemant, C. (2013) Le piégeage du frelon asiatique Vespa velutina nigrithorax. Intérêts et dangers. In *Proceedings Jornées Nationales GTV*. Nantes, pp. 783–788.

Schäfer, M.O. and Ritter, W. (2014) The small hive beetle (*Aethina tumida*). In Ritter, W. (ed.), *Bee Health and Veterinarians*. OIE, Paris, pp. 149–156.

Schäfer, M.O., Ritter, W., Pettis, J.S., Teal, P.E.A., and Neumann, P. (2009) Effects of organic acid treatments on small hive beetles, *Aethina tumida*, and the associated yeast *Kodamaea ohmeri. Journal of Pest Science*, 82(3): 283–287

Shaw, K.E., Davidson, G., Clark, S.J., Ball, B.V., Pell, J.K., Chandler, D., and Sunderland, K.D. (2002) Laboratory bioassays to assess the pathogenicity of mitosporic fungi to *Varroa destructor* (Acari: Mesostigmata), an ectoparasitic mite of the honeybee, *Apis mellifera. Biological Control*, 24: 266–276.

Shimanuki, H. and Knox, D.A. (2000) *Diagnosis of Honeybee Diseases*. United States Department of Agriculture (USDA), Agriculture Handbook No. 690.

Tan, K., Yang, M.X., Wang, Z.W., Li, H., Zhang, Z.Y., Radloff, S., and Hepburn, R. (2012) Cooperative wasp-killing by mixed-species colonies of honeybees, *Apis cerana* and *Apis mellifera. Apidologie*, 43: 195–200.

Toumanoff, C. (1939) *Les ennemis des abeilles*. Editions IDEO, Hanoi.

University of Florida (2013) Small hive beetle *Aethina tumida* Murray. Available at: http://entnemdept.ufl.edu/creatures/misc/bees/small_hive_beetle.htm (accessed 27 August 2014).

USAPHC (2014) Oriental Hornets. Available at: http://phc.amedd.army.mil/PHC%20Resource%20Library/Oriental%20Hornet%20FS%2018-074-0311.pdf (accessed 24 October 2014).

Vidal-Naquet, N. (2011) Honeybees. In Lewbart, G.L. (ed.), *Invertebrate Medicine*, 2nd edn. Wiley-Blackwell, Chichester, pp. 285–321.

Vidal-Naquet, N. (2013) *Aethina tumida* et *Tropilaelaps clareae*, parasites exotiques de l'abeille domestique *Apis mellifera* L. *Bulletin des GTV*, 70: 105–111.

Villemant, C., Haxaire, J., and Streito, J.C, (2006) Premier bilan de l'invasion de *Vespa velutina* Lepeletier en France (Hymenoptera, Vespidae). *Bulletin de la Société entomologique de France*, 111(4): 535–538.

Villemant, C., Barbet-Massin, M., Perrard, A., Muller, F., Gargominy, O., Jiguet, F., and Rome, Q. (2011a) Predicting the invasion risk by the alien bee-hawking yellow-legged hornet *Vespa velutina nigrithorax* across Europe and other continents with niche models. *Biological Conservation*, 144: 2142–2150.

Villemant, C., Muller, F., Haubois, S., Perrard, A., Darrouzet, E., and Rome, Q. (2011b) Bilan des travaux (MNHN et IRBI) sur l'invasion en France de *Vespa velutina*, le frelon asiatique prédateur d'abeilles. In Barbançon, J.-M. and L'Hostis, M. (eds), *Journée Scientifique Apicole*, Arles, pp. 3–12.

Ward, L., Brown, M., Neumann, P., Wilkins, P., Pettis, J., and Boonham, N. (2007) A DNA method for screening hive debris for the presence of small hive beetle (*Aethina tumida*). *Apidologie*, 38: 272–280.

Williams, J.L. (1997) Insects: Lepidoptera (moths). In Morse, R. and Flottum, K. (eds), *Honey Bee Pests, Predators, and Diseases*, 3rd edn. AI Root Company, OH, pp. 121–141.

8

Principles of good sanitary beekeeping practices

The management of *Apis mellifera* colonies demands good farming practices to promote honeybee welfare, encourage pollination, and ensure safe production of food. Many factors may act as stressors on the colonies (Figure 1.32). Veterinarians involved in the beekeeping sector need to be aware of good sanitary beekeeping practices (GSBPs) (Vidal-Naquet, 2013). Many guides are published worldwide to help beekeepers with their husbandry.

This chapter is not a guide to GSBPs but is intended to help lay the foundations for those practices. Good sanitary beekeeping practices should adhere to the 'hazard analysis and critical control point' (HACCP) principles, a major pillar of veterinary public health (Europa, 2009). This chapter attempts to follow, for the most part, these principles.

The FAO and OIE have together produced a *Guide to Good Farming Practices for Animal Production Food Safety* (OIE and FAO, 2009). Food safety is the final objective of this guide, and it can be seen that this is, in turn, the consequence of good farming practices. Thus, this guide specifies that 'good farming practices should also address socioeconomic, animal health and environmental issues in a coherent manner'. The honeybee *A. mellifera* is often seen as symbolic of biodiversity, a healthy environment as well as being the producer of a safe and natural food.

This chapter considers good beekeeping practices, following and adapting these from the FAO/OIE-recommended good farming practices.

On a farm, from the animal husbandry (beekeeping in apiculture) to the extraction of products, many elements are 'at risk from biological, chemical (including radionuclide) and physical agents' (OIE and FAO, 2009). These agents may impair honeybee health and hive products 'through a wide variety of exposure points' in the management of both honeybee colonies and the food chain, with consequent potential risks for honeybees and consumers (OIE and FAO, 2009; Vidal-Naquet, 2013). Furthermore, the welfare, strength, and health of honeybee colonies are a crucial challenge because of the role bees play as pollinators.

The main hazards (biological, chemical, and physical) that may affect managed colonies, along with the corresponding control points, are presented in Table 8.1. Of course, the list of hazards is unlimited and these tables and this chapter mainly represent how to operate to minimize hazards:

1. Identify the risks.
2. Check the corresponding control points.
3. Manage the risks.

According to the recommendations of the OIE and FAO presented in this chapter, the following headings cover the listed hazards (OIE and FAO, 2009): general honeybee farm management; honeybee health management; veterinary medicines and biological aspects; honeybee feeding and watering; environment and apiaries; and handling honeybee colonies and hive products.

1 The HACCP principles

The European Parliament Regulation covering the hygiene of foodstuffs provides a good

Table 8.1 Hazards and corresponding control points in beekeeping

Hazards	Control points
Biohazards	
Introduction of pathogens and contaminants	Honeybee trade and commercial exchanges
	Renewal of the livestock: queens, package bees, artificial swarms
	Feeding supplement and water
	Records of acquisitions and migratory beekeeping
	Hygiene of visitors and personnel
	Drifting and robbing
	Vehicles, clothing, small materials (hive tools), equipment
	Purchase of second-hand equipment
Transmission of pathogens and contaminants	Apiaries, hives, hive density
	Disease diagnosis (horizontal and vertical transmission)
	Hygiene of visitors and personnel
	Hive bodies, supers, frames, wax
	Vehicles, clothing, small materials (hive tools), equipment
	Drifting and robbing
	Varroa destructor: vector of viruses
Increased susceptibility to pathogens	Management of colonies (including migratory beekeeping)
	Selection
	Colony strength
	Hive and apiary sites
	Feeding supplement and water
	Diagnosis
	Colony density
Miticide resistance (and antimicrobial resistance in the countries where these are permitted)	Diagnosis
	Therapeutic regime
	Record keeping
Foodborne infections and contaminations (in particular in the case of honey supplementation during the overwintering period)	Feeding supplement production, purchase and storage
	Feeding supplement quality
	Feeding supplement choice
	Record keeping
Honeybee colonies not well adapted to conditions of husbandry	Honeybee strain selection
	Record keeping

Hazards	Control points
Chemical hazards	
Chemical contamination hazards in beekeeping management	Cleaning, disinfecting, and sterilizing products used
	Material protection products used
	Hygiene practices
	Feeding supplement and water quality
	Residue control
Chemical contamination of environment, food and water	Agricultural and farming pratices (use of agricultural chemicals and insecticides on livestock) in the area surrounding the apiaries
	Chemical industries in the surrounding environment of the apiaries
	Migratory beekeeping
	Feeding supplement and water quality
	Residue control
Residues of veterinary medicines and drugs used in colonies	Treatment of colonies
	Use of drugs or veterinary medicines without marketing authorization for honeybees
	Sales and prescription controls
	Record keeping
	Residue control
	Quality of feeding supplement and water
Radionuclide pollution	Apiary location
	Foraging sites
	Migratory beekeeping
	Source of feeding supplements and water
Physical hazards	
Injuries and death of bees and in particular the queen	Hive and apiary location
	Migratory beekeeping
	Colony density
	Inspection of the hives, material manipulation
	Material (hives, supers, frames, small material)
	Feeding supplement
	Equipment
	Record keeping

explanation of the HACCP principles (Regulation (EC) No 852/2004 of the European Parliament and of the Council of 29 April 2004 on the hygiene of foodstuffs).

> These principles prescribe a certain number of requirements to be met throughout the cycle of production, processing and distribution in order to permit, via hazard analysis, identification of the critical points which need to be kept under control in order to guarantee food safety:
> - *Identify any hazards that must be prevented, eliminated or reduced to acceptable levels.*
> - *Identify the critical control points at the step or steps at which control is essential.*
> - *Establish critical limits beyond which intervention is necessary.*
> - *Establish and implement effective monitoring procedures at critical control points.*
> - *Establish corrective actions when monitoring indicates that a critical control point is not under control.*
> - *Implement own-check procedures to verify whether the measures adopted are working effectively.*
> - *Keep records to demonstrate the effective application of these measures and to facilitate official controls by the competent authority.* (Europa.eu, 2009)

2 Hazards in beekeeping

As previously noted, honeybees face chemical, biological, and physical hazards. Table 8.1 presents the main hazards and the corresponding control points. This table is adapted for beekeeping from Appendix 1 of the OIE/FAO *Guide to Good Farming Practices for Animal Production Food Safety* (OIE and FAO, 2009). Of course, in theory there is an unlimited number of biohazards, chemical hazards, and physical hazards; however, this table tries to focus on the main ones and on the main control points.

2.1 Biological hazards

Biological hazards are infectious and fungal agents, parasites, pests, and enemies of the hives. These hazards, and their control, have been covered in Chapters 2–7.

2.2 Chemical hazards

Chemical hazards are chemical agents used within the hives (either on the colonies or stored material) and chemical agents affecting bees (mainly foragers on the field), or brought back to the hive by foraging bees or accidentally introduced into the hives. They have been presented in Chapter 2.

2.3 Physical hazards

Physical hazards are the consequence of hive management or accidents, such as hives being knocked over, queens getting crushed during an inspection, or a traffic accident during migratory beekeeping or movement of hives. They may also be the consequence of climate – wind, dampness, dryness, etc.

3 General honeybee farm management

To practice beekeeping, several conditions are necessary. These conditions vary according to country, but all stages from training to regulation should follow GSBPs.

3.1 Training

'Husbandry measures and techniques are ever-changing. Competent Authorities are encouraged to assess training needs amongst stakeholders and promote necessary training' (OIE and FAO, 2009).

Beekeepers should undergo regular training to adapt their husbandry practices to ongoing developments in apiculture. This is especially important given the current health crisis in the beekeeping sector. Thus, according to the OIE and FAO (2009), beekeepers, as farmers and farm managers, should:

- Actively seek and use relevant beekeeping training opportunities for themselves and their workers.

- Be aware of any training courses that may be compulsory in their countries and regions.
- Keep records of all training undergone.

3.2 Legal obligations

Beekeepers should be aware of, and comply with, all local regulations and all legal obligations relevant to honeybee husbandry and food production (OIE and FAO, 2009). Beekeepers should be prepared to undertake:

- Disease reporting. Particular attention must be paid to reporting notifiable diseases and pests to the relevant authorities (see Appendix 2).
- Record keeping.
- Hive and apiary identification.
- Registration of colonies and apiaries (in countries where this is a legal obligation).
- Documentation pertaining to the sanitary organization of the honey house.

3.3 Beekeeping record keeping

Recording data for livestock husbandry, and in particular for colony management and beekeeping practices, is fundamental for understanding health or sanitary problems. Indeed, the entire 'life history' of the colonies, the apiary, and the material management may potentially contain the root cause of any problem that occurs, whether this is physical, chemical, or biological. Hence, the beekeeper should, as far as possible, keep records of the following elements:

- Number of hives and apiaries.
- Introduction of bees within the honey farm: artificial swarms, package bees, and queens. This includes: the origin and date of introduction, the health certificates, and the specific colonies into which these bees were introduced. The recovery of wild swarms should also be recorded.
- Migratory beekeeping and movement of colonies. The routes taken by the colonies to ensure pollination or to produce specific honeys (from lavender, chestnut tree, lime tree, etc.) must be recorded.
- Date, origin, and type of feeding supplements given to the colonies (honey, carbohydrates, and protein supplements).
- Date, origin, and use of veterinary medicinal products (VMPs) within colonies.
- Date, origin, and use of any chemicals (organic acids, miticides without marketing authorization, essential oils, etc.) within colonies.
- Date, origin, and use of any chemical for the cleaning, disinfection, and sterilization of stored hives and supers and frames.
- Date, origin, and use of any cleaning and disinfecting products used on equipment and in the premises and honey house.
- Bee mortalities, colony mortalities, diagnosed or suspected diseases (bacterial, viral, fungal, or parasitic), diagnosed or suspected poisoning. The colonies affected must be recorded. Treatments applied must also be recorded.

3.4 Apiary and colony identification

Identification is an essential element of colony management. It allows traceability and is key to managing colony health and ensuring the safety of the hive products. Knowledge of the origins of colonies is desirable.

The beekeeper should identify:

- The apiary.
- Each hive, with a number or even a specific bar code, allowing traceability and computer tracking of colony management (requeening, feeding, movments, etc.).
- The queens. These should be marked according the international colour code, allowing traceability and making it easier to spot them during hive inspections.

3.5 Hygiene and prophylaxis of diseases

The OIE/FAO *Guide* specifies that:

> Measures aimed at preserving cleanliness, preventing pathogen build-up and breaking possible pathways of transmission are essential in the management of any modern

farming enterprise, regardless of the species or the farming system. (OIE and FAO, 2009)

In modern apiculture, sanitary measures are aimed at maintaining cleanliness but also at preventing the build-up and transmission of pathogens and chemicals. Accumulation of pathogens and chemical residues in hives is a major risk for colonies, and in addition poses a potential risk to consumers of hive products, in particular honey. The selection, management, and maintenance of material is one of the pillars of prophylaxis against diseases and poisoning. A second pillar is management of the colonies and colony health.

3.5.1 Choice of hives and material

The choice of material for hives, supers, frames, wood, and insulation must be adapted to colony health (taking account of the honeybee strain), the aim of the beekeeping (pollination or honey), and the local environment (especially the climate). Hives must remain dry inside and well ventilated to create optimal living conditions for honeybees. Paints, wax, and any protection used on the wood must be harmless for colonies and compliant with regulations covering food-producing animals.

3.5.2 Management of material

In apiaries, the management of hives, supers, and frames should be designed to limit contamination between colonies but also between apiaries. As far as possible, frames and supers should be associated with one hive. Exchanges of frames should be avoided between hives and between supers (Vidal-Naquet, 2013). However, although this is easily manageable in small apiaries, it is much more complicated to restrict these exchanges in honey farms with many colonies and apiaries. However, exchange of material between hives should be done only where necessary and should be restricted as far as possible.

Management of the wood used in the hives is important for the colonies. Over time, wood becomes porous and its thermal insulation properties are reduced; this deterioration creates conditions favourable for diseases and pests. Thus, not only is the choice of wood fundamental, but care for and renewal of wooden items are necessary to minimize the risk of infestation/infection.

Management of wax combs (frames) is also very important, as wax may contain pathogenic agents (e.g. spores of *Paenibacillus larvae* and *Nosema* spp.) and residues of treatments and pesticides accumulated over the years. Very dark wax combs should be removed and changed for new frames with a wax foundation. It is usually accepted that the frames of a hive should be renewed every three years (in a ten-frame Dadant hive, two and if possible three frames should be renewed every three years). Foundations must be done with wax without residues and pathogens; wax from honey cell cappings is the safest to use to make foundations (after extraction of honey, cappings can be be converted into foundations). Old combs should not be converted into wax foundations.

Small tools and clothing (e.g. hive tools, brushes, gloves, beekeeping suits) should ideally be cleaned and disinfected at least after each inspection of a weakened colony.

3.5.3 Maintenance of the material

The maintenance of beekeeping material is a major element of GSBPs. Cleaning and disinfection of removed hives, supers, feeders, frames, and any wooden material before storage or reuse are fundamental.

The maintenance of material is usually performed in winter, when the beekeeping season is over and the colonies are overwintering.

Any damaged wood, and frames removed from diseased colonies (in particular following foulbrood disease and nosemosis), should be removed from the farm and burned.

Otherwise, maintenance of the wood involves:

- Scraping the surface to remove residues of bees, honey, wax, and propolis.
- Disinfection. A blowtorch can remove a lot of pathogens, especially when combined with

subsequent treatment with bleach and acetic acid. Ionization with gamma-rays can also be used to disinfect wood and wax; however, this method is mainly restricted to large honeybee farms.
- Preservation and sterilization of wooden hive parts. Feeders as well as any wooden hive parts may be covered with microcrystalline food-grade hot wax (hot wax dipping procedure). A mixture of microcrystalline wax and paraffin may also be used.

All empty hives must be removed from the apiary, cleaned, disinfected, sterilised, and stored.

Hives, supers, and frames should be stored without any chemical treatment in well-ventilated premises. Supers with frames must be stored stacked in a criss-cross pattern to form a well-ventilated 2 m chimney, open at the top and the bottom to protect them against wax moths.

Management of this material is crucial in beekeeping to limit biochemical and chemical hazards that could adversely affect the strength and health of honeybee colonies.

4 Honeybee colony management

Animal health management lies at the heart of any husbandry. Beekeeping has some unique and particular features due to the biology and physiology of the honeybee. GSBPs must take particular account of these.

If modern closed farming and all-in/all-out systems of food-producing animal husbandry provide general principles for food safety, this approach is not adaptable to honeybee husbandry for one main reason: foraging bees, rather than the farmer, are in charge of the food supply of the colony (according to good beekeeping practice, the beekeeper only provides feeding supplement to avoid colony weakening, e.g. if there is a shortage of blossom, or for overwintering). From the choice and management of the livestock to its renewal, husbandry practices must ensure prophylaxis and early control of diseases.

4.1 Choice and sanitary management of colonies

The beekeeper chooses the honeybee strains to keep in his/her apiary. From making this selection through to honey production, the beekeeper has to manage the colonies based on continuous knowledge of their health status in order to take early appropriate measures should any problems arise.

4.1.1 The choice of honeybee

The choice of the honeybee kept in the apiary is important. The honeybee strains should be adapted to the environmental conditions and to the objectives of the farm (pollination, honey production, royal jelly production, queen rearing, etc.). This is why, in many cases, a local black honeybee exhibiting hygienic behaviour (*Apis mellifera mellifera* in western Europe) is the best choice.

However, according the objectives of the beekeeper as well as the history of the apiary, it may be necessary to practice honeybee selection or to introduce selected queens, artificial swarms, or package bees to create colonies that possess certain desired qualities, such as: gentleness, tranquillity on the combs, hygienic behaviour, low swarming tendency, productivity, and strength for the overwintering period.

4.1.2 Management during the beekeeping season

The apiarist's beekeeping season begins at the end of wintering and lasts until the beginning of the next wintering, and includes periods of colony population growth and decline. Livestock management is of particular importance during this time, and routine inspections of the sanitary status of the colonies are necessary. The main things to consider for sanitary management are as follows:

- Examination of the bee population. Regular assessment of the activity and brood of the colonies is necessary (approximately every 15 days). Examination of the inside of the hive should also be performed regularly, in

particular if the strength of the colony seems to be impaired. This provides the possibility for early management of sanitary troubles (mortality, weakening, poisoning, infectious diseases, etc.).
- Management of the material is important during the beekeeping season, in particular when the bee population increases; installation of the supers on the body of the hives must be done punctually to avoid or limit swarming.
- Management of colonies in the case of migratory beekeeping has to follow some basic rules: the colonies must be prepared for the journey with carbohydrate feeding supplement to limit stress, and the move should be done at night or in the early morning, when all the bees are inside the hive. Of course, transportation regulations must be followed.
- Honey harvesting may be a critical period. The harvest should be performed so as to limit robbing between colonies.
- Monitoring *Varroa* infestation throughout the season allows implementation of integrated pest management to control mite parasitism.

4.1.3 Spring inspection of the colonies

When the overwintering period ends, the queen begins to oviposit and the winter workers begin to rear the new brood. The spring examination of the colonies and the hives is crucial for the forthcoming beekeeping season, in order to maximize pollination activity and honey production. The beekeeper should undertake a meticulous examination of all apiaries and colonies to evaluate the sanitary status of his/her livestock.

The main elements of the spring inspection are as follows:

- Checking all the hives (material and livestock).
- Management of the material. Wooden objects tend to suffer in the winter and must be evaluated. Damaged hives should be replaced and stored in farm premises to be repaired or eliminated. Hive floors have to be cleaned. Frames should be replaced if the wax is too old (i.e. dark in colour). In a hive with ten frames, it is considered that two to three frames should be replaced each year by new ones.
- Evaluation of the colony populations and newly developing broods to assess if the colonies are restarting properly.
- Management of feeding supplement (cf. Chapter 2, section 2.5). Supplementary feeding may be necessary to help the colonies to restart, in particular if the spring is cold and development of vegetation delayed.
- Rejuvenation of the areas nearby and surrounding the hives and apiaries.
- Assessment of the progress of blossomming (and the growth of honeydew plants) in the surrounding area.
- At the beginning of the beekeeping season, *Varroa* infestation of the colonies must be below the threshold of 50 mites per colony. Monitoring *Varroa* infestation may be necessary in colonies selected at random.

4.1.4 Inspection in preparation for overwintering

Examination of the hives at the end of summer/early autumn is crucial for limiting the risks for the colonies during the overwintering period and for the recovery of colony activity the following spring (FERA, 2010).

The main elements of this examination are as follows:

- Checking all the hives (material and livestock).
- Estimating the autumnal population and the presence of young winter bees. Determination of the winter bee population provides an assessment of the strength of the colonies before overwintering.
- A colony that is too weak will not be able to overwinter and should be eliminated. Indeed, this colony may pose a risk as a source of pathogens that can be transmitted to other colonies in the apiary.
- Confirming that the *Varroa* control management methods implemented have been effective. (Control of *Varroa* infestation,

described in Chapter 5, is central to producing a strong brood for wintering.)

- The honey stored, or feeding supplement for the overwintering period, must be rigorously checked. According to the area, the bee strain, and the severity of the local winter climate, it is usually considered that a colony should overwinter with 10–22 kg of honey or equivalent sugar supplement to avoid any sugar deficiency. If honey is used for overwintering, it must be produced by the colony (or by the apiary) and not one brought in, which could be a source of pathogens or chemicals.

During the winter, the beekeeper should visit the hives and apiaries (and check inside if the weather and the temperature permit) to monitor the colonies and to manage feeding if necessary (for example, an unusually severe winter will require more feeding than usual). In some regions, it might be desirable to transfer the colonies to areas with a less cold winter.

4.2 Addressing biohazards

4.2.1 Veterinarian

The beekeeper should establish a 'working relationship' with a veterinarian competent in honeybee pathology. Of course, such veterinarians are quite rare but it would be an asset if a network of honeybee veterinarians could develop in every country, as has begun to happen in France, within the framework of the 'One Health' principle.

The expertise of the vet will allow the achievement of clinical examination and diagnosis in the case of overt disease, outbreak, suspicion of poisoning but also the achievement of sanitary audit for a better sanitary management of the apiary (Vidal-Naquet, 2013).

The presence of veterinarians competent in honeybee pathology is a necessity as specified in the *Guide to Good Farming Practices for Animal Production Food Safety* (noting that honeybees are indeed animals that produce food) (OIE and the FAO, 2009) and the book *Bee Health and Veterinarians* (OIE, 2014):

Owners or managers of livestock should:

- Establish a working relationship with a veterinarian to ensure that animal health and welfare and disease notification issues are addressed.
- Seek veterinary assistance to immediately investigate any suspicion of serious disease.

This is why competent authorities and veterinary schools and faculties should develop courses on honeybee pathology for students and for post-graduate training of veterinarians.

4.2.2 'Hospital apiary'

In some cases, diseased colonies with the potential to recover may be deemed worth saving. They should be isolated from the apiary, if not affected by a notifiable disease that forbids hive movement. Placing these hives in an isolated apiary may allow the colonies to recover while limiting the risk of transmitting biological pathogens.

The beekeeper should kill any colonies that are too weak or potentially pose a danger to the other colonies of the apiary.

4.2.3 *Varroa* infestation control

All beekeeping practices must consider disease prophylaxis and colony health. In the European Union, the use of VMPs in the beekeeping sector is limited; only a few miticides are authorised for treating bees.

The use of miticides is currently necessary to control *Varroa* infestation. The use and choice of acaricides should be based on express knowledge of the mite infestation and take into account the risks the treatment may pose to apiaries. The IPM method is a good sanitary beekeeping practice which may limit miticide resistance.

In other countries (e.g. the US and Canada) antibiotics are permitted in the prevention and control of foulbrood diseases and nosemosis. The use of antibiotics is not considered a good sanitary beekeeping and veterinary practice (cf. Chapter 4). However, in countries where they are permitted, control and/or prevention of infectious diseases with antibiotics must be undertaken carefully and scientifically because of the risks of antibiotic resistance and the presence of residues in the products of the hive. The use of antibiotics in a colony should be done in association with the shaking bee method (also called the shock swarm method).

4.2.4 Renewal of the honeybee livestock

The renewal of honeybee colonies (by the introduction of artificial swarms, package bees, and queens into the apiary) is a potential biohazard for the existing colonies. The sanitary status of any honeybee livestock introduced into an apiary should be known and certified. Quarantine measures before introduction may be necessary because of sanitary risks (pathogenic agents, parasites, pests). Introduction of honeybee livestock from certain countries may require that samples be sent to a reference laboratory to test for exotic pests and parasites (*Aethina tumida*, *Tropilaelaps* spp.).

Livestock renewal may be performed within the honey farm by the process of artificial swarming from a colony of the apiary. The sanitary hazard is then limited, because there is no risk of introducing pathogenic agents, parasites, or pests from foreign livestock.

Renewal of livestock according to GSBP involves the following:

- Renewal of queens (re-queening). It is considered that in managed colonies, the queen should ideally be replaced every year, and at most every two years. Artificial queen rearing or re-queening by supersedure may be undertaken within the honey farm to avoid introducing pathogens, parasites, or pests. The introduction of a purchased queen requires a certificate of health, even if the risk of introducing pathogens is lower than when introducing foreign artificial swarms or package bees. The choice of queen should be considered carefully, taking into account the genetic features the beekeeper wishes the colony to possess (adaptation to the local environment, honey production, pollination activity, docility, lower tendency to swarm, hygienic behaviour, etc.).
- Producing artificial swarms. Creating artificial swarms provides a means to renew and increase the livestock. This method requires careful consideration and should be performed only on strong colonies.
- Introduction of foreign artificial swarms or package bees. Artificial swarms or package bees are potential biohazards as they pose the risk of introducing pathogens into the apiary. This risk can be considered significant. The beekeeper may quarantine these artificial swarms and package bees. Traceability and sanitary certification are necessary.
- Recovering a (wild) swarm. Recovering a swarm from a tree, for example, constitutes a biohazard for the apiary. A recovered swarm should be isolated from the apiary if possible and a one-shot miticide (e.g. oxalic acid or formic acid) applied to control *Varroa* infestation and avoid infestation of the colonies in the apiary.

4.3 Addressing chemical hazards

Chemical hazards are a major risk for honeybees and are considered by many stakeholders in the beekeeping sector as mainly responsible of the current sanitary crisis.

Chemical hazards may come from the honey farm (management of the material, control of *Varroa* infestation) or the environment (crops, pesticides, and industrial chemicals):

- Crops are frequently treated against insect pests. Because bees are also insects, and feed in particular on crops, these pesticides pose a major hazard to bees, and hence threaten pollination. Phytosanitary products may endanger the health of the colonies (see Chapter 2).
- Because bees are food-producing insects, beekeepers must take measures to protect not just the health and strength of the colonies but also the health of the consumers of hive products.

Thus, dealing with chemical hazards requires the following GSBPs:

- The beekeeper should use within the hives only those chemicals or VMPs authorised for use on honeybee colonies, in particular when controlling *Varroa* infestation. Chemicals, etc., used within the hives should be officinal substances. For example, the organic acids (oxalic acid, formic acid, lactic acid) currently utilised in preparations for *Varroa* control management ought to be purchased from a pharmacist or veterinarian and not from a paint shop as often occurs.
- The beekeeper should use only authorised cleaning, disinfecting, or sterilizing products on stored material.
- The beekeeper should be familiar with the vegetation and crops that his colonies forage on and pollinate. Beekeepers can sometimes chose where hives are located, and should avoid risky areas.
- The beekeeper should also be aware of, and should evaluate, any use of anti-parasitic chemicals by neighbouring farms.
- Asking neighbouring farmers to share information about their chemical (on crops) and anti-parasitic (on animals) practices should help to minimize chemical hazards.

4.4 Addressing physical hazards

Beekeeping practices always present risks for honeybee colonies. These practices should respect the welfare and safety of the bees:

- The beekeeper should have sufficient practical experience to be able to inspect the colonies in the hives.
- The beekeeper has to manage hives in such a way as to limit losses due to physical hazards. Handling, opening, and transporting (migratory beekeeping) should be performed with the utmost care to protect the colonies within the hives. The queen, in particular, must be protected when any handling is performed.
- The biology and physiology of the honeybee should be considered when opening the hives for examination or for any management. Draughts and cold must be avoided because these may harm bees but more importantly damage the brood.

5 Veterinary medicine products

The beekeeper should be aware of and respect the legislation concerning the use of VMPs and drugs in apiculture. As already mentioned, in the EU, the only VMPs sold officially are miticides. In certain countries, some VMPs are prescription drugs.

VMP use in terms of GSBPs involves the following considerations:

- The beekeeper should use only VMPs officially sanctioned for use on honeybees.
- The use of other active ingredients, e.g. organic acids, must be done according to the prevailing sanitary and public health legislation (officinal substances, prescription, preparation method, etc.)
- Currently, the use of antibiotics is forbidden in the EU, though these are authorised in some other countries.
- The beekeeper must be aware of potential risks to him/herself and other apiary workers and must take all necessary protective measures.
- The use of VMPs must be done in accordance with the veterinary prescription and/or the instructions supplied.
- Details of treatments must be recorded in writing, and should include: origins, use, batch number, date of administration, doses, identification of the colonies treated.
- Storage of VMPs must follow legislation and sanitary regulation.
- The treatments applied must not be harmful to the health of the colonies.
- Treatments against the mite *Varroa* must be applied according to a carefully considered strategy.
- Treatments must not be applied to the hive during honey-flow and honey production.

- The treatments (strips, sponges, and other carriers) should be applied for a given time and then removed punctually from the hive.
- Drug carriers must be destroyed according to the regulations concerning VMP waste disposal.

6 Honeybee colony supplementary feeding

The food resources of honeybee colonies are nectar, honeydew, pollen, and water. However, supplementary feeding of managed colonies may be necessary in some circumstances to limit the risk of starvation or deficiency, which can cause colony weakening and collapse. Water is crucial for colonies (homeostasis of the nest, brood rearing, etc.), especially as it is not stored in the nest as pollen and honey are.

Supplementary feeding may be performed in three main circumstances: in the case of starvation or risk of deficiency ('emergency' feeding), to stimulate colony activity ('speculative' or stimulating feeding), or to replace honey removed from the hive ('surrogate' feeding) (G. Therville-Tondreau, personal communication, Nantes, 2013) (cf. Chapter 2, section 2.5).

The beekeeper should:

- Acquire feeding supplements from suppliers who follow good manufacturing practices (OIE and FAO, 2009).
- Ensure a high-quality water supply at or close to the apiary.
- Avoid handling, which could be a source of chemical or biological contamination, and can result in fermentation of the feeding supplement.
- Make sure that the composition of the feeding supplements is tailored to suit the needs of the colony.
- Use honey from the colony or the apiary if using honey as a feeding supplement. The use of other honeys must be avoided due to the risk of chemical and biological (spores of *Paenibacillus larvae* in particular) contamination.
- Honey containing melezitose should not be used for overwintering because it tends to crystallise. Colonies overwintering on honey containing melezitose have a greater risk of collapsing during the winter or during the following spring as crystallization of the melezitoze may induce dysentery in winter workers (Imdorf *et al.*, 1985).
- Use feed that is suited to the needs of the colony and the time of the year. Usually, in winter and early spring, when the weather is cold, candy is the food of choice. In spring, when the weather is better and the colony begins to restart, syrup should be used.

7 Hive and apiary environment

The location of the apiary and the situation of the hives in an apiary are both crucial to the health of the colonies.

7.1 Location of an apiary

The beekeeper should:

- Ensure he/she has easy access to the apiary.
- Ensure that the apiary and the spaces around the hives are suitably maintained.
- Ensure that the hives are protected against any dampness in the air or from the soil, and are positioned carefully with respect to the wind (the entrance of the hive must be protected from the prevailing winds to avoid physical hazards, and to allow the bees to fly out freely). According to the area and the strain of bee, it may be necessary to move the hives to overwinter in a region with more clement weather.
- Protect as far as possible the apiary against pests and predators.

7.2 The apiary within the environment

The beekeeper should:

- Ensure the presence of natural food resources. He/she should know the vegetation and crops found in the areas surrounding the apiaries.
- Ensure the presence of a high-quality water supply.
- Ensure the quality of the vegetation (during the flowering and blossoming period) and the presence of water in any location to where hives are moved (in the case of migratory beekeeping).
- Limit as far as possible any risks of confinement within the hive (which favours a number of diseases, e.g. European foulbrood disease and nosemosis).
- Know, if possible, the farming practices and the use of pesticides on crops near his/her apiary. Discussion between farmers and beekeepers about the use of phytosanitary products by the farmer may limit the risks of poisoning. Of course, it is hoped that use of pesticides on fields, orchards, or vineyards will be rational and proportionate.
- Know, if possible, the practices being followed by neighbouring beekeepers, particularly with respect to *Varroa* control management; in general, awareness of the possible presence of diseased colonies nearby is important because robbing and drifting are the two main natural routes of transmission of infectious and parasitic diseases of the honeybee.

8 Handling of honeybee colonies and hive products

8.1 Addressing biohazards

The beekeeper should:

- Ensure the (good) sanitary status of his/her colonies if the farm produces honeybees intended for sale.
- Ensure that the honeybees (package bees, artificial swarms, queens) intended for sale are fit to travel and are transported in the best sanitary conditions possible.
- Ensure optimal sanitary conditions for honey extraction from the frames.
- Ensure that any contamination by pathogenic agents in the honey and products of the hive intended for sale is as low as possible.
- Ensure optimal conditions for the packaging and storage of the honey and products of the hive to maintain their quality.
- Keep records of the honeybees (package bees, artificial swarms, queens) leaving the honey farm and their destination.
- Keep records of the products of the hive leaving the honey farm and their destination.

8.2 Addressing chemical hazards

The beekeeper should:

- Fully respect any legislation on maximum residue levels (MRLs).
- Ensure that no colony has been treated during the honey flow and that drug carriers have been removed from the hives according to the specified schedule.
- Ensure that no colony has been treated with illegal substances or veterinary medicines, such as antibiotics, in countries where these VMPs are forbidden in apiculture.

8.3 Addressing physical hazards

The beekeeper, as a producer of honeybees (queens, package bees, artificial swarms) and/or honey, should:

- Respect the welfare of honeybee colonies during their husbandry and transportation.
- Ensure of the quality of the transportation material (hives, hive nucleus, queen trays).
- Ensure the preservation of the quality and safety of the products of the hive during transportation.

9 General sanitary practices for honey extraction and production

Even if honey is considered a low-risk food product, good sanitary practices must be applied throughout its extraction from the frames and subsequent processing (ADAPI, 2003).

European regulation defines within its 'hygiene package' the food safety objectives to be achieved, leaving the food operators, and in particular honey producers and the honey industry, responsible for adopting the safety measures to be implemented in order to guarantee food safety (Europa.eu, 2009). Honey producers and honey business operators have to apply the principles of the hazard analysis and critical control points (HACCP) system introduced by the Codex Alimentarius (the code of international food standards drawn up by the United Nations Food and Agriculture Organization). The basic principle of the production of honey in the honey house is walking-forward logic (Vidal-Naquet, 2013).

Beekeepers have to respect the physicochemical criteria of honey defined by the regulation.

Council Directive 2001/110/EC of 20 December 2001 (reproduced in Appendix 5) relating to honey specifies the legal definition and physical and chemical characteristics of honey as follows:

> Honey is the natural sweet substance produced by *Apis mellifera* bees from the nectar of plants or from secretions of living parts of plants or excretions of plant-sucking insects on the living parts of plants, which the bees collect, transform by combining with specific substances of their own, deposit, dehydrate, store and leave in honeycombs to ripen and mature.

The fructose, glucose, and sucrose content of honey are defined, as well as moisture (in general not more than 20%), the electrical conductivity, free acid content, diastase activity, and hydroxymethylfurfural (HMF) content. In general, HMF must be not more than 40 mg/kg, except in baker's honey. In Europe, honeys of declared origin from regions with tropical climate and blends of these honeys: not more than 80 mg/kg.

References

ADAPI, DDSV13, GDSA13 (2003) *Guide des bonnes pratiques d'hygiène dans les mielleries adaptées.* Available at: www.beekeeping.com/articles/fr/GBPH_mielleries.doc (accessed 15 September 2014).

Europa.eu (2009) Food Hygiene. Available at http://europa.eu/legislation_summaries/food_safety/veterinary_checks_and_food_hygiene/f84001_en.htm (accessed 15 September 2014).

FERA: The Food & Environment Research Agency (2010) Preparing honey bee colonies for winter. Available at: https://secure.fera.defra.gov.uk/beebase/downloadNews.cfm?id=79 (accessed 14 September 2014).

Imdorf A., Bogdanov, S., and Kilchenmann, V. (1985) Du miel de miellat cristallisé dans les hausses et les corps de ruches – comment réagir? Centre Suisse de Recherches Apicoles. Available at: http://www.agroscope.admin.ch/imkerei/00302/00307/index.html?lang=fr&download=NHzLpZeg7t,lnp6I0NTU042l2Z6ln1ae2IZn4Z2qZpnO2Yuq2Z6gpJCDeHt4fWym162epYbg2c_JjKbNoKSn6A-- (accessed 14 September 2014).

OIE, FAO (2009) *Guide to Good Farming Practices for Animal Production Food Safety*. FAO and OIE, Rome.

Vidal-Naquet, N. (2013) Les bonnes pratiques apicoles. In SNGTV (ed.), *Proceedings of the Journées nationales des GTV.* Nantes, pp. 773–781.

9

Honeybee veterinary medicine and practice

It is currently quite unusual for a beekeeper to summon a veterinarian in the event of sanitary trouble, disease, suspicion of poisoning, or colony collapse as is done in other husbandry sectors. However, veterinarians competent in bee pathology are able to use diagnostic and clinical skills that can prove an asset to beekeepers (Barbançon *et al.*, 2014).

The first part of this chapter deals with the clinical examination of an apiary. The second part considers the sanitary audit of an apiary that veterinarians may perform, and how this may help beekeepers with their apiary management.

In honeybee veterinary medicine, certain features of *Apis mellifera* have to be taken into account compared to other reared species:

- Honeybees are insects and not mammals.
- *Apis mellifera* is a social insect; although the individual is the honeybee, the unit is the colony as a super-organism.
- *Apis mellifera* is the only managed or reared species for which the food is not brought and controlled by the farmer.
- Honeybees are food-producing reared animals.

1 Clinical examination of colonies and elements of semiology

Veterinary practitioners acquire during their studies and their practice an approach to clinical examination and diagnosis when faced with any diseased animal, whatever the species. This diagnostic procedure is strict; overlooking any step runs the risk of reaching a wrong final diagnosis (Roy, 2011). This is also the case for honeybee veterinary medicine. However, the usual means of clinical examination (temperature taking, auscultation, palpation, etc.) are not practicable in this insect species. A method adapted for the honeybee must be developed (Roy, 2011), as described here.

One element does not change compared to veterinary medicine for other species: clinical examination always begins by collecting anamnesis and recording the symptoms observed.

The intervention of a practitioner in the field may occur:

- If symptoms are observed in bees and/or brood, colony weakening or collapse occurs, production decreases, or poisoning is suspected.
- At the request of sanitary authorities.
- At the request of insurance companies.
- To undertake an epidemiological study as part of a surveillance system.
- To prevent diseases.
- In the framework of a sanitary audit that can be performed in a honeybee farm as in other animal-rearing farms.

Preliminary remark

The management of the visit, in particular removing and resetting the frames in the hive during the visit, must be under the control of the beekeeper. The veterinarian should observe how the beekeeper practises bee husbandry and be alert to any clinical signs. Another reason is that when opening a hive, although some workers may unfortunately be crushed, it is vital that the queen not be harmed.

1.1 Conditions for a good clinical examination

Visiting the hives must be done during the hottest hours of the day. The clinical examination must be performed in a coordinated manner, step by step, and as quickly as possible to avoid disorganization and weakening of the colony.

1.2 Anamnesis (medical history)

Listening to the client beekeeper is essential in order to gather as much information as possible. Unfortunately, the data gathered are often sparse and superficial and sometimes mistaken (Roy, 2011).

The anamnesis must be as detailed as possible:

- Date of occurrence or first observation of the symptoms and their evolution.
- Migratory routes (crops pollinated, migratory beekeeping, etc.).
- Frequency and dates of inspections of the apiaries and colonies.
- *Varroa* control method used.
- Water access characteristics (distance, standing water, flowing water, etc.).
- Features of the farm: traditional beekeeping, organic beekeeping, extensive or intensive beekeeping, honey production, pollination activity, etc.
- Crops and flora in the surrounding environment, but also weather (not only at the moment of the clinical exam but also for the past weeks and months).
- Apiculture environment. It is important to assess the density of the apiaries in the surrounding environment. Furthermore, during the season, migratory beekeeping may lead many beekeepers to put their hives in the same area for pollination or production of monofloral honey (e.g. in areas surrounding lavender fields in the south of France).
- The epidemiological context: knowledge of any problems in nearby colonies, if available, should be an important point of the anamnesis. Is there a greater probability of the colonies being faced with an infectious or toxicological threat due to local beekeeping and farming (phytosanitary product use) practices?

1.3 Initial external examination

On arrival on site, observation of the environment, of the general activity of the bees on the apiary and in front of each hive, the appearance of the hives, the activity at the hive entrance, and the soil on the front of the hive represents the first step of the clinical examination.

1.3.1 The environment

Watching and observing carefully the apiary environment and surrounding area provides information that should be taken into account when making the clinical examination and performing the diagnosis (Figure 9.1):

- Observing the location of the apiary gives information on water and food resources, prevailing winds, the potential presence of enemies of the hives, and potential physical

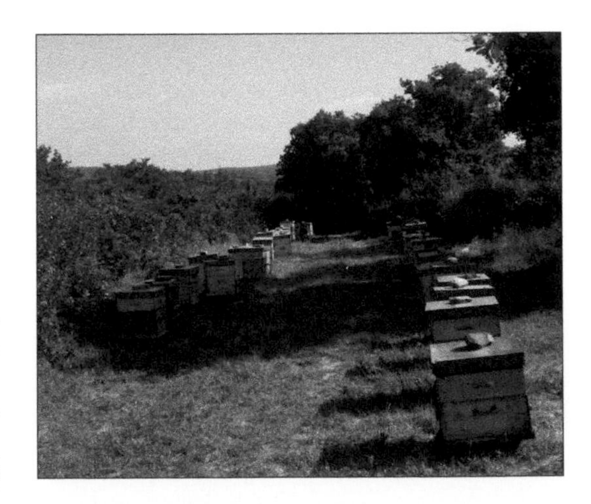

Figure 9.1 Apiary surroundings. Observing the apiary surroundings, the apiary maintenance, and the placement of the hives provides much information for a clinical examination. (© Nicolas Vidal-Naquet.)

risks (vibrations when close to a road or a railway, etc.).

- The forest, floral, and agricultural environment provides vital information. For example, cereal crops, canola, sunflowers and maize crops, vineyards, orchards, etc., are treated with particular phytosanitary products so knowing the local crops provides an appreciation of the 'toxic risk' faced by the colonies. When preparing the visit, observation of a satellite view (e.g. Google Maps) of the apiary location and on average 3 km around may provide interesting information (e.g. a nearby industrial area). 3 km is considered the maximum distance for foraging flights.
- Maintenance of the immediate environment and access to the apiary must be evaluated. Poorly maintained surroundings are not good sanitary beekeeping practice and may be evidence of inadequate husbandry.

1.3.2 Appearance of the hive

The appearance of the hives, and their placement, must be considered as important elements in the clinical examination:

- Choice of hive, e.g. Dadant, Langstroth, and Warré models. Usually beekeepers in areas with cold winters use a relatively large-volume hive which can store a high quantity of honey. However, the space available to the bees within a hive must be matched to the size of the colony.
- Hive maintenance: paint or woodstain, protection against pests and enemies, renewal of damaged hives, etc.
- Hive placement: suitable placement may help to estimate the risk of drifting.
- Measures to protect hives from dampness (e.g. by using a hive stand).
- An apiary with the same kind of hives allows the strengths of different colonies to be compared.

1.3.3 Examination of the alighting board and the front of the hive

The alighting board is a surface at the front of the hive where the bees land and take off. Observation of the alighting board and the front of the hive is important for the following reasons (Figures 9.2 and 9.3):

- Assessment of the number of bees entering and leaving the hive provides a measure of the colony activity.
- The alighting board and the area in front of the entrance should be searched for the presence of predators, enemies, and pests of the colonies, e.g. hornets hovering in flight waiting for forager bees.
- To check for the presence of unusual or abnormal features, including:

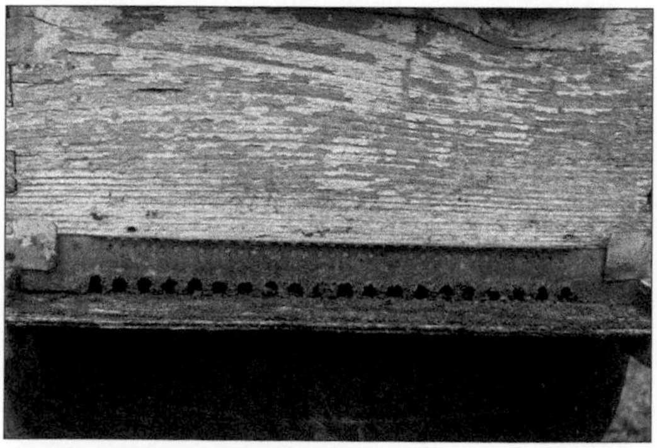

Figure 9.2 Alighting board of a hive with a collapsing colony, showing a high level of faeces and debris. (© Nicolas Vidal-Naquet.)

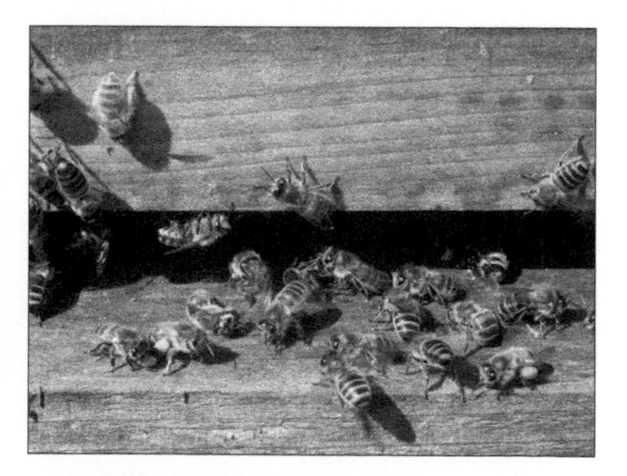

Figure 9.3 Alighting board of a highly active hive. (© Nicolas Vidal-Naquet.)

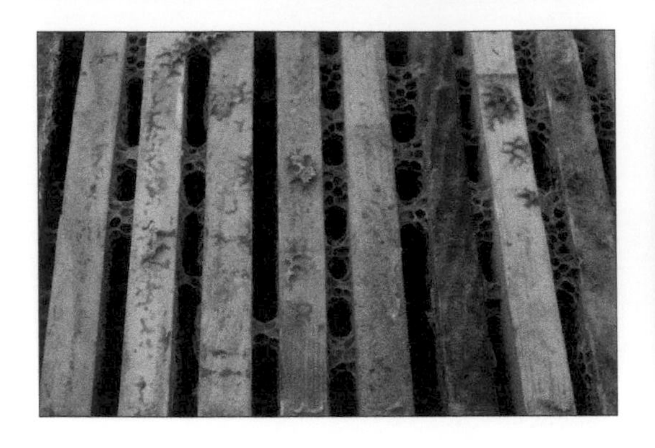

Figure 9.4 A hive of a collapsed colony with no bees. (© Nicolas Vidal-Naquet.)

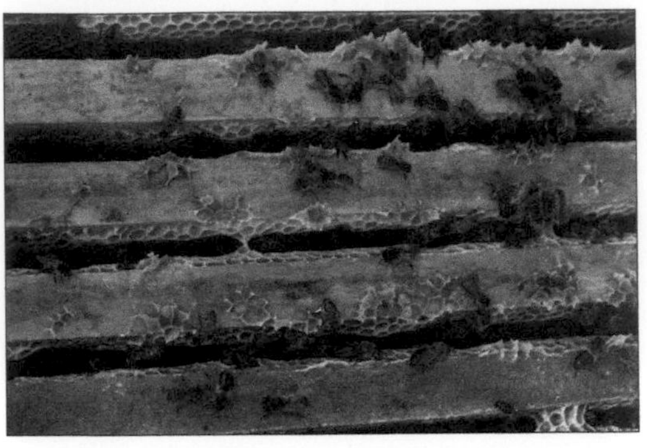

Figure 9.5 A hive of a weakened colony with few bees. (© Nicolas Vidal-Naquet.)

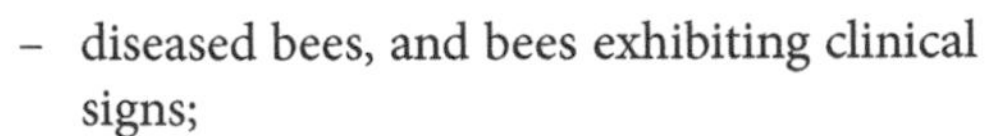

  - diseased bees, and bees exhibiting clinical signs;
  - dead bees;
  - brood mummies;
  - faeces;
  - waste (it must be taken into account that some scavengers, e.g. lizards, birds, and ants, feed on dead bees, waste, etc.).
- Examination of the soil in front, under (if a mesh-floor is used inside the hive), and around the hive can provide much information on the health status of the colony: dead bees (a few dead bees are usually observed in healthy colonies but a carpet of dead bees is suggestive of an impairment of colony health), mummies, crawling bees unable to fly, etc.

Before opening the hive, the percussion of the hive body provides information on the presence of the colony, which typically makes a humming sound. A stethoscope may be used to listen to the activity inside a hive. The weight of the hive can be evaluated by cautiously and slightly lifting the hive; this is particularly important before the overwintering period to evaluate the honey resources.

This first 'external' examination gives an appreciation of the assets, hazards, and risks of the environment and the status of the hives, and provides an initial picture of the vitality of the colonies (Roy, 2011).

When examining a colony, it is important to remember that some bees may be not found: foraging bees may be away on foraging sites (though there is usually a permanent toing and froing of foragers) or may have died during foraging or have been unable find their way back to the hive.

1.4 Clinical examination of the colony

A digital camera is helpful to enable a better examination of the frames (number of bees, abnormalities, evaluation of brood quality and quantity, etc.) on a computer screen. The clinical examination will encompass all living and non-living elements of the hive. It has to be well structured and quickly implemented

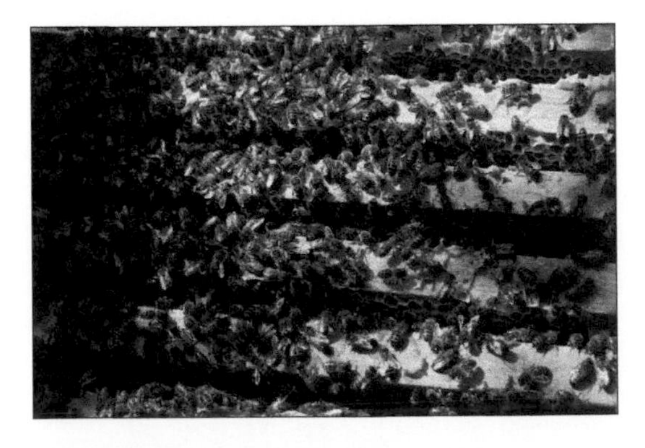

Figure 9.6 A hive of a healthy and strong colony. (© Nicolas Vidal-Naquet.)

(15 minutes for a full examination of a hive is considered sufficient by many practitioners).

1.4.1 Examination when opening the hive

When opening the hive, the first point to notice is the presence or not of propolis: the outer cover and inner cover may be glued by the propolis – this is a defence behaviour of the colony.

When the covers are removed, the following points should be checked:

- Usual or unusual behaviour (aggressiveness) of the colony.
- The inter-comb spaces occupied by bees must be numbered, allowing an estimation of the population strength:
  - In the season, all the frames covered by bees and all the inter-comb spaces occupied by bees indicate a strong colony.
  - Weakened colonies may present only a few bees or a few inter-comb spaces occupied by bees.
- The smell of the hive. The usual odour of a hive is that of the wax. If a foul or vinegar smell is detected, a disease of the brood may be suspected.
- The presence of other insects within the hive, e.g wasps, moths, hornets, ants, and beetles. Although the presence of some ants is often considered usual in colonies, the presence en masse of these insects or other predators and enemies may be a sign of a weakened colony or a colony with weak defensive behaviour (Roy, 2011). At the present time, the search for the small hive beetle has to be done inside the hives.

1.4.2 Examination of the adult bees

After opening the hive, the beekeeper carefully removes the frames from the hive. The first step of the internal examination is to estimate the number of workers. This is mainly a subjective method done using a trained eye, though the Liebefeld method is an interesting quantitative approach (see section 1.4.6 below).

With practice, a trained eye will detect any abnormalities among the worker bees:

- Physical symptoms: body deformities, asymmetric wings, abnormal wing wear (K-wings), hairless bodies, changed body colour, size of the body, distended abdomen, etc.
- Parasitic symptoms: presence of phoretic *Varroa* on the thorax and abdomen of the bees.
- Neurological symptoms: aggressive or limp and weak bees, trembling and crawling bees, bees moving slowly, bees with shaking wings, bees unable to fly.
- Behavioural and social symptoms: bees fighting with guards; clusters of bees in front of the hive. However, each strain and each colony has its own behavioural features which must be taken into account.
- Digestive symptoms: elongated probosces, constipation (distended abdomen), signs of dysentery on the combs and hive.

The veterinarian and beekeeper should seek out the queen when examining a hive. However, not too much time should be devoted to finding her:

- The queen may be affected by certain problems, such as body size and wing abnormalities.
- If the queen is present and the colony broodless, the queen is probably infertile.

1.4.3 The frames and the brood

The frames are wooden structures, within which a foundation sheet is laid on which the cells are constructed (to prevent uncontrolled construction within the hive). Its examination is fundamental. During the visit, all the frames and the 'non-living' elements of the hive body must be carefully examined:

- The frames should be quite easy to remove from the body of the hive. If they are not, this may be caused by a recent propolis foraging activity or because of a lack of hive surveillance by the beekeeper.
- The wax and the cells: colour and consistency are elements to check. New wax is white to yellow. Older waxes become black and may contain residues and pathogenic agents.

- Pollen and honey stored must be evaluated. The quality and amount of pollen (variety of colours, pollen cells range area) and honey (aspect, consistency) stored can be estimated. The stored amount will depend on the time of the year when the visit takes place (and on the production status of the colony).
- A check should be made for the presence of the signs of pests in the wood (cavities, crevices) or the observation of silken thread (a sign of wax moths).

Removing the frames from the hive must be done in a defined order, starting with the peripheral frames (containing food reserves and on which stand mainly foragers) and moving on to the more central frames with brood (on which stand mainly inside bees, i.e. nurses, workers, cleaning workers, etc.).

The most important aspect of the frame examination is the scrupulous and careful observation of the brood. This is a key part of the clinical exam. According to Roy (2011), this examination can be regarded as corresponding to mammalian cardiac auscultation. In a healthy colony, in the season, the worker brood is well developed, regular, and divided over several frames. The different stages of the worker brood may be observed: uncapped brood with eggs and larvae apparent, and capped brood. The condition of the brood is a testament of former health troubles of the colony or can reveal existing problems.

The brood will give information on the laying activity of the queen. The presence of numerous eggs and young larvae indicate recent oviposition activity by the queen.

Conversely, a lack of eggs will correspond to a very recent laying arrest (less than 3 days) and a lack of larvae of a definite age (e.g. 5 days) will correspond to a laying arrest 8 days previously. This can be linked to meteorological conditions, strong honey flow, requeening, etc.

The clinical examination of the brood should include the following:

- Number of frames with brood.
- Distribution of the brood on a comb: homogeneous or heterogeneous (irregular pattern).
- The brood shapes: concentric circles with larvae of the same age indicate regular queen laying. Deviations from this pattern can be ascribed to meteorological conditions, strong honey flow, former or present diseases, re-queening, etc.

The brood surface must be compared to the worker population. Indeed, it is fundamental to estimate if there are enough bees to rear the brood (see section 1.4.6 below):

- A colony lacking a worker brood during the season has no future, even if some bees remain.
- Abnormalities of the brood observed are various and all must be checked and listed as precisely as possible:
  - The brood may have a mottled or scattered appearance.
  - The brood may present an unpleasant smell (vinegar-like, foul).
  - The capped brood may be concave or convex and punctured.
  - The presence of dead larvae, coloured larvae, viscous larvae, of scales, etc.
  - The presence of mummies.
  - The presence of caterpillars burrowing tunnels inside the brood.
  - The appearance of some uncapped pupae in a small linear tunnel (bald brood)
- The presence of drone brood may be observed. It is usually present in spring and summer when queens are reared by colonies. The drone brood under normal conditions represents a small percentage of the total area of the brood comb.
  - A colony with only drone brood is usually a queen-less colony (or a colony with a diseased unfertile queen). The worker bees begin to oviposit male haploid eggs. The future for such a colony is bleak.
- The presence of queen cells may be the consequence of preparation to swarm, replacement of the queen by supersedure,

or replacement of the queen by emergency queen cells. The location and structure of the queen cells may provide information about the cause of queen rearing. The nature of these cells can also be a consequence of beekeeping practice (requeening by supersedure, artificial swarm, etc.).

1.4.4 The floor of the hive

Significant information can be obtained from the floor of the hive. Diseased bees, dead bees, pests, and predators may be observed. It is necessary to check the cracks and crevices in the wood to search for potential hidden predators.

1.4.5 Health status, weakening, mortality, collapse

Defining the health status of a honeybee colony is not easy.

The evaluation of the health status of a colony must take into account:

- The state of the food stored: honey, pollen.
- The size and quality of the brood.
- The size of the colony and the distribution of the population.
- The behaviour of the bees.

This will depend on the season (a colony is smaller when overwinterwing or at the end of the wintering period), the honeybee sub-species and strain, and on factors such as swarming, queen-less colonies, etc.

What defines a colony as being in good health?

Defining whether a colony is in good health is not easy, though the following four points provide a good indication:

- There is no clinical sign of disease.
- The brood/adult ratio is in line with the expected evolution of the colony and the time of year (there must be enough workers to rear the brood).
- There is foraging activity and production of honey and beebread.
- The total quantity of pollen and honey stored surrounding the brood is estimated to be matched to the needs of the colony.

Colony weakening

The definition of weakening is also not entirely straightforward, though 'a lack of strength of a beehive' is one general description (European Union Reference Laboratory for Honeybee Health, 2011). Weakening is linked to an unexpected decrease in bee population density and dynamics (as distinct from normal seasonal variations). Weakening may be the consequence or the cause of a reduction in brood (surface and/or brood-comb frames) and/or due to honeybee disorders and/or depopulation. Weakening is combined with a decrease or cessation of honey production.

Two types of weakening need to be considered (European Union Reference Laboratory for Honeybee Health, 2011):

- Weakening with apparent abnormal and recent adult honeybee individual mortality (>1% of the population of the colony) observed in the close surroundings of the hive (in particular in the front of the hive entrance).
- Weakening without apparent adult honeybee individual mortality with or without abnormal clinical signs or behaviour at the adult level and/or brood level. (In the frame of a clinical examination, this kind of weakening is somehow difficult to appreciate, in particular because the medical history of the colony is often not well known. The colony strength must be compared to the other colonies in the apiary. One question must be borne in mind: is the colony declining or is its health status improving?)

Mortality

Colony mortality clearly occurs when the colony itself dies. However, a colony may also be considered as dead if all the factors essential to its viability are missing (very few bees, no brood, no queen, no food stored, etc.).

In the frame of anamnesis, colony mortality must be characterized by when during the year it occurs, as well as by the rate of colony loss within an apiary:

- Winter mortality of honeybee colonies. 'Winter mortality of honeybee colonies is a normal annual seasonal phenomenon in apiaries' (AFSSA, 2008). Depending on climate and region, the average normal winter mortality is reported to be 10%. Above this rate, the winter mortality is an abnormal phenomenon.
- Colony mortality during the beekeeping season. Mortality during the season is not a 'normal phenomenon in an apiary'(AFSSA, 2008).

The mortality of a colony should be also characterized by the circumstances in which it occurs:

- Following a period of weakening or progressive depopulation with or without apparent cause.
- Colony collapse refers to a 'quick loss of bees leading to its total destruction' (AFSSA, 2008). In the US, this is termed colony collapse disorder (CCD) (cf. Conclusion).

Mortality of adult bees

When considering colony weakening or colony mortality, but also if the colony seems to be of normal strength, any diseased and dead bees must be characterized in particular by their appearance, number, and location. The presence of dead bees, usually in front of the hive, is normal due to population renewal during the beekeeping season. The daily mortality rate for all bees in a colony is estimated as being about 1% of the whole population. This corresponds to about 400–500 honeybees for colonies containing 40,000–50,000 bees (EFSA, 2012). Bee mortality can also be evaluated using collection cages; however, this is mainly done under experimental conditions or as part of a surveillance network.

A search must be made for dead bees both outside and inside the hive. The level of mortality must be defined, from insignificant to severe and to complete.

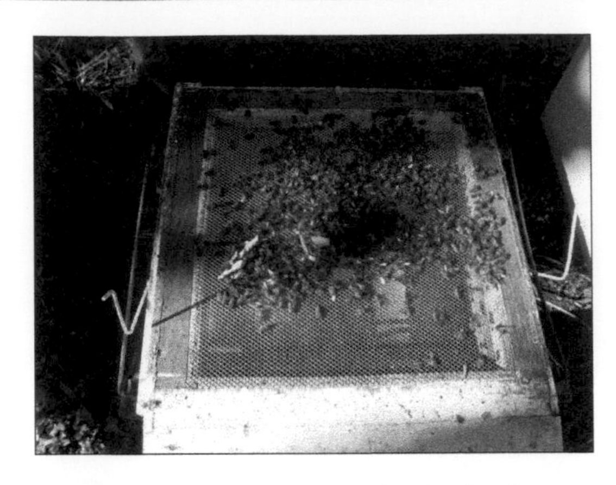

Figure 9.7 The mesh-floor of a dead colony. Note the presence of many dead bees on the floor. In this case, the colony had died of famine during overwintering. (© Nicolas Vidal-Naquet.)

The appearance of the dead bees may help to determine whether death was a recent event or had occurred some time previously (folded legs under the body, hairless cadavers, and very light weight suggest that death occurred long before the date of the visit) (C. Roy, Nantes, 2013, personal communication).

1.4.6 A method to evaluate the strength of the colony: the Liebefeld method

Although the trained eyes of a beekeeper or a veterinarian with experience in the beekeeping sector can estimate the strength of a colony, the bee population, and the brood-rearing activity of nurse workers, it may be interesting to obtain as objective a measurement as possible in order to compare this to expected values.

Correct application of the Liebefeld method (Imdorf *et al.*, 2010) during an inspection may be used to evaluate population, brood, and brood-rearing activity (Roy, 2011). If performed throughout the season, this method can be used to monitor annual colony development, and can provide indicators on the population dynamics of the colony.

The Liebefeld method provides the following information:

- A quite accurate evaluation of the population of workers and the size of the brood.
- An accurate evaluation of the brood nursing activity. The number of workers must be in proportion to the scale of brood rearing in order to allow an efficient turnover of the colony population.
- Comparison with expected values with regard to the strain reared, the time of the year, and other factors, e.g. the environment.

The evaluation of the number of bees will depend on the kind of hive, and should be performed under favourable meterological conditions:

- Dadant model: a fully recovered frame face (including the wood) is assumed to have 1,400 bees and a surface area of 11 dm^2.
- Langstroth model: a fully recovered frame face (including the wood) is assumed to have 1,100 bees and a surface area of 8 dm^2.
- Usually, on 1 dm^2 surface area of comb, there are 130 bees and up to 400 if the bees have their heads inside the cells.
- In European honeybee strains and in natural conditions, there are on average 850 worker cells per dm^2 of comb (Winston, 1987). Wax foundations are embossed with 750–800 cells per dm^2.
- The evaluation must take into account the bees standing on the walls of the hive: 500–3,000 bees during the season.

The evaluation of the brood surface should be performed on the same frame for which the bee population has been estimated. The areas with uncapped brood and capped brood must be evaluated by measuring their respective surface areas.

These measures give the following information:

- An estimate of the whole population at the time of the visit and a possible comparison with expected values for managed colonies (depending on the time of the year, the strain reared, and also on local factors).

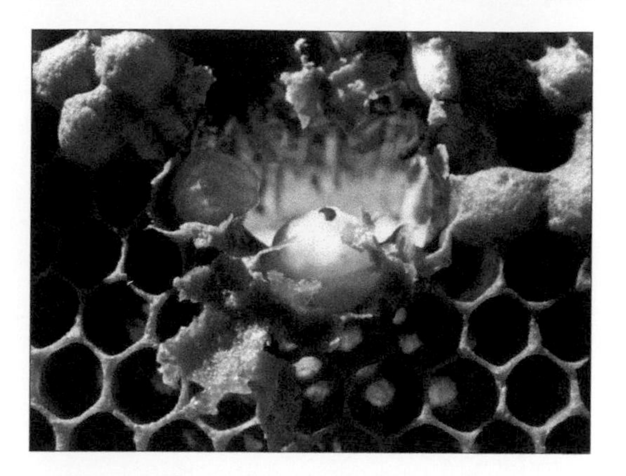

Figure 9.8 Manual uncapping of drone brood cells may reveal the presence of *Varroa*. (© Nicolas Vidal-Naquet.)

- Evolution of the colony population if the beekeeper monitors the colony throughout the season.
- The brood-rearing activity of the colony, which is one of the most important parameters to know. It can be evaluated from the number of uncapped brood cells per 100 bees (the ratio of the number of uncapped brood cells/number of bees). When the brood rearing is maximum, this number is often more than 100%, meaning that, on average, one bee is in charge of more than one uncapped brood cell (but all the bees are not nurses) (Imdorf *et al.*, 2010). Thus when there are many uncapped brood cells, a lot of bees are needed. If the ratio of the number of uncapped brood cells to the number of bees is too high, there will be a great risk of a lack of nurses when the colony activity is maximum.

1.5 Testing and sampling

1.5.1 Tests in the field

Some tests may be performed in the field to evaluate brood health and adult health:

- The brood. Uncapping some brood cells enables inspection of the larvae and pupae to evaluate their colour, odour, consistency (using the matchstick test to detect American foulbrood disease), and the possible presence of the mite *Varroa* inside the capped cells (this should be performed by uncapping drone brood) where its reproductive cycle occurs. Because of the whitish colour of honeybee larvae and pupae, the mites appear more easily than the phoretic *Varroa* on adult bees. In the field, it is also possible to estimate *Varroa* infestation by counting a sample of 50–100 drone larvae by uncapping the brood with a honey uncapping fork (see Chapter 5).

- *Varroa* infestation level may also be assessed in the field by sampling adult honeybees using the icing-sugar method, which keeps the bees alive (see Chapter 5).
- Some test kits are designed for ease of use in the field. If American or European foulbrood disease is suspected, or if the diagnosis is in doubt (e.g. in the case of suspected American foulbrood from an inconclusive matchstick test – see Chapter 4, section 1.3.2), an ELISA test may be performed. This allows immediate sanitary management if a positive result is obtained.
- In the case of early spring colony weakening, the digestive tracts of a sample of workers should be analysed to evaluate the colour: the digestive tract is revealed by pulling and removing the abdomen from a bee (ch. Chapter 6, section 3.3). A normal digestive tract is coloured yellow to reddish due to the pollen. A whitish-coloured digestive tract may be the consequence of Type-A nosemosis.
- Adults can also be dissected to isolate the thorax and thereby highlight the tracheal tract inside. Inspection using a binocular loupe may show the presence (or not) of *Acarapis woodi*.

1.5.2 Sampling for laboratory testing

Laboratory tests are often needed for a diagnosis, and implementation of 'good sampling practices' is essential to achieve as precise results as possible (Franco *et al.*, 2012).

As in all species, sampling must be done according to a number of factors:

- Disease or poisoning is suspected.
- Aims of the diagnosis: is the testing for an unnotifiable or notifiable disease, as part of an an insurance claim, or to analyse chemicals if poisoning is suspected?
- Cost. Who is paying for the tests – the beekeeper, the sanitary authorities, the insurance company? Analysis of chemical residues and PCR tests are expensive and beekeepers are often little inclined to spend money on these.

Preparations for sampling must be made before the visit (Appendix 3): cardboard boxes, Eppendorf tubes, brown wrapping paper, glass containers, and plastic bags must be brought.

Dispatch of samples must be made according to the regulations covering the sending of biological material.

1.5.3 Laboratory analysis for diagnosing apiculture problems

The laboratory analysis results alone do not constitute the diagnosis. They must, as in other species, be interpreted according to the anamnesis and the clinical examination. Moreover, as the honeybee is a social insect characterized in particular by a perpetual turnover of the population, the interpretation of results must be adapted to this species.

Several methods, already described in the chapters of this book that cover diseases, may be used in the apiculture sector for diagnosis (Franco *et al.*, 2012; OIE, 2014):

- Identification and counting using a microscope, culture of pathogenic agents, PCR, mass spectrometry, biochemical tests, and antibody-based techniques are the main techniques used for analysis of pathogenic agents.
- The Quick Easy Cheap Effective Rugged Safe (QuEChERS, Fellbach, Germany) method allows extraction of chemicals from the matrices. Analyses of extracts are then performed with liquid chromatography with tandem mass spectrometry (LC-MS/MS) and/or gas chromatography time-of-flight

(GC-ToF) (Johnson, 2010; Wiest *et al.*, 2011; Lehotay, 2012).

1.5.4 Field and laboratory tests as prophylactic methods against overwintering colony weakening or collapse

The clinical examination of healthy colonies in combination with laboratory testing may be interesting as a prophylactic method against colony collapse or weakening in summer and autumn. Before the overwintering period, the degree of *Varroa* infestation and the DWV load are considered as highly predictive markers for honeybee colony weakening or mortality during winter (Dainat *et al.*, 2012). The evaluation of the honey resources or sugar supplement of the managed colonies for overwintering is also an important factor to consider.

1.6 Conclusion of the clinical examination

All the data produced by the clinical (and laboratory) examination will be analysed to reach a diagnosis and to propose to the beekeeper solutions to enhance the health and strength of his/her colonies. In the field of the honeybee pathology the anamnesis is a crucial element of the diagnosis as many human, environmental, weather, climatic, floral, agricultural factors may influence the health and strength of the managed colonies.

The conclusion of a clinical examination is a probable or positive diagnosis with the help of laboratory analysis if necessary. The quality of the results will depend on how long the beekeeper waited to call for help after noticing the problem: the sooner the beekeeper initiates the clinical examination process, the more useful the results will be. Once the diagnosis has been made, appropriate management can be decided. However, in many cases, management begins before waiting for the laboratory results, if these are needed.

A diagnosis of health problems within a honeybee colony demands a reasoned sanitary approach (Roy, 2011):

- In the case of suspicion or positive diagnosis of a notifiable disease, the relevant authorities must be warned and will have to take sanitary measures.
- If a colony is affected, the health of the other colonies of the apiary must be checked. The sooner the weakened colony can be examined, the sooner and easier the diagnosis will be done.
- If an apiary is affected, neighbouring apiaries should be monitored. If an apiary is affected, two factors need to be considered as a priority: the beekeeping practices and the surrounding environment. The management of material and bees may be the cause of contamination between the hives of an affected apiary. Environmental features may also be responsible of the troubles of an entire apiary. Thus it is important to know the health of neighbouring apiaries both for diagnosis as well as for prevention.
- If all the apiaries of a honeybee farm are affected, the sanitary beekeeping practices have to be re-evaluated. A sanitary audit of the honeybee farm will reveal these practices.

2 Sanitary audit of husbandry in apiculture

Beekeeping is an animal husbandry with the particularity that the beekeeper may be a landless farmer and the honeybee *A. mellifera* is a social insect with particular features, notably the food resources are provided by the environment and not by the farmer.

Beekeepers tend to manage sanitary problems with their colonies by themselves or within the beekeeping 'community'. The intervention of a veterinarian (usually an official veterinarian or more often a beekeeping technician) in a honey farm is usually the consequence of acute problems.

The sanitary crisis facing the beekeeping sector has been responsible for major economic damage, in particular in large beekeeping farms with many hives and apiaries.

As in other forms of husbandry in the 1970s and 1980s (Ragon, 2009), apiculture has become aware of the need for a global analysis, taking into account the honeybee, beekeeping practices, the environment, the weather, food and water resources, and any other elements acting on colonies (Figure 1.32).

Programmes taking an overall view of cattle farms have been performed since the 1970s in the US and the 1980s in France (Ragon, 2009). In beekeeping farms, sanitary audits based on veterinary practice have been developed since the end of the 2000s (L'hostis and Barbançon, 2009, 2013; Barbançon *et al.*, 2014). A sanitary audit of a beekeeping farm has the following objectives (L'hostis and Barbançon, 2013):

- To identify hazards, risks, and finally problems occurring in the honeybee farm and their consequences. Particular attention has to be paid to chemical hazards.
- To find and provide, as far as possible, appropriate solutions to these troubles.

This sanitary audit is mainly a matter of prevention, even when performed during a sanitary crisis. Unlike mandatory surveys at the request of sanitary authorities, the sanitary audit is and should remain a step that beekeepers take voluntarily (Ragon, 2009). If mandatory, beekeepers should understand in a positive way the help that such an approach may bring to improve their practices, to improve the sanitary status of their colonies, and hence to improve the production of their honey farms.

According to the Group of Medicine of the Populations of VetAgro Sup in Lyon, France, performing a sanitary audit of a husbandry is based on three pillars (Commun, 2011; Le Sobre and Commun, 2013):

- Analysis of documents: record keeping, production assessments.
- Observation and examination of the livestock (honeybee colonies).
- Analysis and observation of beekeeping practices.

This approach must take into account factors predisposing to colony weakening, disease, poisoning, and anything that can impair the production of a beekeeping farm. Because of their environmental dependence managed honeybee colonies are, more than other reared species, confronted with a range of factor that can contribute to of disease. Every element, every hazard (see Chapter 8) that might impair the balance of a colony must be evaluated when performing a sanitary audit. However, a sanitary audit is much more than simply an analysis of the biochemical, chemical, and physical hazards developed in Chapter 8. A guide to beekeeping practices is a matter for beekeepers; a sanitary audit is performed by veterinarians to help the beekeeper improve his/her husbandry management, taking into account every factor that might impair livestock health and production.

Once the audit has been performed, a report will be produced. At each step, this report will evaluate the key points, the weaknesses of the beekeeping farm, and in particular the predisposing factors of disease or weakening in the colony. The report will propose, as a conclusion, elements, practices, and solutions to limit the risks evaluated.

For beekeepers, a sanitary audit will help them to understand as far as possible the possible troubles facing their honey farms, improve their beekeeping practices if necessary, and enhance the health and productivity of their livestock.

For the veterinary profession, this approach may help veterinarians competent in honeybee veterinary medicine to increase the involvement of their profession in the beekeeping sector in order to bring to bear their know-how regarding animal health.

This section has presented some of the main elements to record within a sanitary audit. However, a sanitary audit must be adapted to each honey farm according to the type of beekeeping being undertaken. After the presentation of these elements, various points are presented for inclusion in the audit report.

Appendix 4 presents a table listing a practical method for performing a sanitary audit. This table attempts to be exhaustive but will certainly need to be augmented and adapted according to the needs of particular regions/countries and beekeeping industries.

2.1 When should a sanitary audit take place?

A sanitary audit may take place:

- At the request of a beekeeper as a preventative approach to assess his/her husbandry practices in order to improve his/her sanitary beekeeping practices and productivity.
- At the request of a beekeeper when sanitary problems occur, such as infectious disease, suspicion of poisoning, high mortality level, unexplained falls in production, etc.
- When mandated by sanitary authorities. In this case, the audit will not be a proactive and voluntary step taken by the beekeeper but may rather be seen as a constraint, with the intrinsic negative effects created by such a demand.

2.2 Analysis of documents and data from the honey farm

All factors must be analysed, bearing in mind the question: is this a key point, a risky point, or a weak point for the honeybees and thus for the beekeeping farm and its produce?

2.2.1 Honey farm data: workers, farm, and produce

The factors to record and analyse in terms of the human aspects of the farm and its productivity are the following:

- The activity type: is the beekeeper a professional or a leisure beekeeper?
- The history of the beekeeping farm: how old is the farm?
- How many people work on the beekeeping farm and what is their training and professional experience in beekeeping?
- Is accurate and sufficient record keeping performed? What kind of information is reported therein (management, sanitary data, productivity data, etc.)?
- Does the record keeping conform to agricultural and sanitary regulation (legislation)?
- The produce of the beekeeping farm is an important element to consider. Indeed, these products are witness to the activity and productivity of the livestock of the honey farm, and especially to the strength of the colonies:
  - Do the colonies serve to pollinate crops on a commercial basis?
  - What are the products of the hive harvested by the beekeeper: honey, pollen, royal jelly, propolis, wax, venom? What is the productivity, in terms of both quality and quantity?
  - What are the characteristics of the farm's honey production: quality and quantity of monofloral honeys, polyfloral honey, honeydew honey?
  - Production of live bees. Does the beekeeper produce package bees, nuclei (a small hive of bees, usually covering from two to five frames and used primarily for starting new colonies, or rearing or storing queens), queens for trade or only for renewing his/her colonies?

2.2.2 Data concerning the livestock and the apiaries

The data on livestock and apiaries should usually be recorded. The analysis of these data should be done during this first step of the sanitary audit.

- Livestock features:
  - Present livestock data:
    - ► Total number of colonies.
    - ► Number of colonies for pollination activity.
    - ► Number of colonies for honey production.
    - ► Number of colonies for pollen production.
  - Colonies and queen-rearing activity:

    - ▸ Number of artificial swarms produced each year.
    - ▸ Destination of the artificial swarms, i.e. whether these are traded or used to renew or increase the number of colonies.
    - ▸ Number of queens reared each year whether these are traded or used for requeening the colonies of the farm.
  - Evolution of the livestock over the past three years.
  - Mode of maintaining or increasing the honey farm's livestock, i.e. renewal of the livestock by colony division (producing artificial swarms), but also sometimes by gathering 'wild' swarms.
  - Does the beekeeper purchase honeybees (queens, package bees, nuclei on frames) for renewal of or increasing his/her livestock?
- Features of the apiary sites:
  - Are the apiaries sedentary?
  - Does the beekeeper practice migratory beekeeping? What are the features and the routes of the migratory beekeeping?
  - Are the apiaries easily accessible?
- The environment of the apiaries and hives:
  - Are the apiaries within a dense apicultural area? Are there many other hives and apiaries in the vicinity?
  - What are the environmental features of the apiaries area within a 3 km radius (including while migratory beekeeping)? Cereal crops, arboriculture, forest, mountain, fields with hedgerows, urban, etc.
  - Is the environment potentially toxic for insects and in particular honeybees (evaluation of the use of phytosanitary products on crops, insecticides in farms, presence of chemical industry in the neighbouring area)?
  - Meteorological features of the areas in which the apiaries are located, including areas used for migratory beekeeping.
  - Presence of water?
  - Relationships with the farmers and knowledge of their phytosanitary product use.

2.2.3 The sanitary and colony health data

The beekeeper's record-keeping must include sanitary and health data. These data provide crucial information for a sanitary audit.

- Mortality and collapse of colonies must be recorded, as well as their circumstances and features.
  - Time of the year (winter or early spring summer, autumn) when the troubles occur.
  - Rate of winter losses.
  - Rate of beekeeping season losses.
  - Causes of the losses if known.
- Occurrence and sanitary status towards notifiable and other infectious diseases in the past few years. Have laboratory analyses been performed? What were the results?
- Occurrence of poisoning or suspected poisoning in the past few years?
  - Symptoms observed.
  - Mortality.
  - Were laboratory analyses performed? What were the results?
- Management of *Varroa* infestation. Because *Varroa destructor* (and 'honeybee parasitic mite syndrome') is one of the main causes of winter mortality and weakening, knowledge of *Varroa* control management is an important part of the data to analyse:
  - How is control of mite infestation performed?
  - Which method is used to monitor mite infestation within the colonies?
  - Which veterinary medicines or drugs are used within the colonies, and at which time of the year?
  - Origins of veterinary medicines, drugs, or other substances used in mite control?
  - What are the technical methods used to control *Varroa* mite infestation?
  - Is *Varroa* infestation control managed by an integrated pest management scheme?

After having recorded these data, a visit to the colonies has to be made. It is also possible to analyse beekeeping practices before this visit to make the most of the time spent on the farm (L'hostis and Barbançon, 2013).

2.3 Apiary visits and examination of the hives

When performing a sanitary audit of a beekeeping farm it is necessary to visit in person (L'hostis and Barbançon, 2013). A visual evaluation of the apiary environment and the location and placement of the hives within the apiary, as well as examining the hives themselves, is fundamental.

Not all the colonies have to be examined; rather, a random selection of colonies should be analysed. This will give a sufficient idea of the sanitary context of the husbandry and of the beekeeping practices being used.

The examination of colonies and of the apiary site has been described previously. If necessary, sampling for analysis should be undertaken.

An inspection of the premises where the material is stored and the honey house where the honey is extracted and where hive products (honey, pollen, propolis, wax, venom) are packaged and stored must also be performed.

2.4 Analysis of beekeeping practices

Beekeeping practices should be analysed by considering point by point the biohazards, chemical hazards, and physical hazards described in Chapter 8. However, in the context of a sanitary audit, some points are particularly important to check and analyse.

2.4.1 Hive management

The choice of hives, and of the material used (wood or plastic), is the first step in the beekeeping analysis. Within the hive, are mesh-floors and queen excluders used?

Renewal, cleaning, and disinfection of hives and supers should be recorded.

The placement of the hives within the apiary is an important feature to study: are the hives protected from damp and wind? Is there enough sun for the colonies?

2.4.2 Frames and wax management

Management of the frames is an important element to analyse. Indeed, the frames represent the structure of the nest of the colony. The combs wired within the frame are the site of brood rearing and honey and pollen storage. The origin of the wax foundations as well as the renewal of the combs must be recorded.

The storage practices used for hives, supers, and frames have to be evaluated.

2.4.3 Small equipment

It is also important to analyse the management of the small equipment used in beekeeping. Maintenance and disinfection of hive tools, as well as honeybee suits, veils, and gloves, should be evaluated.

2.4.4 The livestock

The features of the livestock (honeybee colonies) must be appreciated: the strain of *A. mellifera* reared in the honey farm is a crucial element of beekeeping practice. The methods of selection and the choice of characteristics selected have to be evaluated (if selection is performed on the honeybee farm).

- Is the honeybee a local black bee or an introduced black bee?
- Has the honeybee sub-species or strain reared been introduced from another country because it possesses certain characteristics deemed favourable (e.g. Caucasian honeybee, Buckfast honeybee, Ligustica honeybee)?
- What is (are) the origin(s) of the honeybees introduced into the apiaries?
- Is re-queening practised in the colonies?
- Are the queens produced on the farm or are they introduced from elsewhere? From where were they purchased? When were the queens produced?
- What is the frequency of re-queening? What are the reasons for requeening? What are the selection objectives and criteria?

- Is drone rearing performed in the apiary?

2.4.5 Inspections by the beekeeper of the hives and apiaries during the beekeeping season

Regular routine inspections of the colonies are essential for optimal control of the colonies' strength, health, and productivity. Recording the number and the method of inspections undertaken as part of the audit is a necessity:

- How many times are the colonies visited each year?
- How long do these visits last?
- What steps are taken during these inspections?
- Is the weight of the colonies monitored throughout the year?

2.4.6 Visits before overwintering and before the beekeeping season

The overwintering period is a critical period for honeybee colonies, and it is commonly assumed that a beekeeper should examine his/her colonies before and after overwintering:

- Is an end of summer/autumn visit performed?
- How is this visit performed? Are all the colonies and all the frames examined? Is particular attention paid to the rearing by the colonies of winter bees?
- Before overwintering, does the beekeeper monitor the *Varroa* infestation level?
- If a colony is considered to be too weak to overwinter, what decision does the beekeeper take about this colony?
- Is a spring visit performed?
- How is this visit performed? Are all the colonies and all the frames examined?
- At the beginning of the beekeeping season, does the beekeeper monitor the *Varroa* infestation level?

2.4.7 Management of colony feeding

The provision of feeding supplements is a necessity for managed colonies. As described in Chapter 2, section 2.5, many kinds of supplement are available depending on the objective of the feeding. It is necessary to evaluate the feeding practices of the beekeeper, i.e. the timing, the quantity distributed, and the objective of feeding. Details of the feeding supplements should be evaluated: origins, traceability, methods of storage, analysis (in particular to define the level of HMF, which is toxic to bees) (see Chapter 2, section 2.5).

2.5 Sanitary audit report

2.5.1 Evaluation of hazards, key points, and points to improve

The audit should be performed by a veterinarian competent in honeybee veterinary medicine. Indeed, wide-ranging and thorough knowledge of honeybee biology and pathology provides an appreciation of the risks and hazards, and enables these to be ranked in order of importance. This knowledge will improve the husbandry practices of the beekeeper, and, as a consequence, the sanitary status of his/her farm, and the quality and quantity of the products and/or the pollination activity of the farm.

Hence, once the audit has been performed, it is necessary (L'Hostis and Barbançon, 2013):

- To identify the risks, hazards, and critical points.
- To determine if those risks and hazards may immediately and/or in the future endanger the colonies and the production of the honey farm.
- To rank the critical points in order to appreciate the most important risks and hazards.

Analysis of the risks and hazards provides a list of key points and weak points of the husbandry. This list allows general recommendations to be made as part of the conclusion of the audit.

2.5.2 The audit report

The audit report combines an analysis of the paperwork, examinations performed, and beekeeping practices. The conclusions and recommendations of the audit are the ultimate goal of this approach to beekeeping practice. If possible, the audit should ideally be written immediately, firstly to keep the positive momentum from the visit, and secondly to implement the proposed corrective measures as soon as possible.

The report can be divided in four parts (L'Hostis and Barbançon, 2013):

- Factual elements of the husbandry management.
- Sanitary status of the honey farm (including the health status of the colonies) and results of laboratory tests (if performed).
- Diagnosis: the key findings regarding the husbandry and hence the points to improve must be clearly explained to the beekeeper.
- Proposed improvements, listed in order of priority. These measures must take into account the features of the honey farm, their ease of implementation, and the ability of the beekeeper to apply them. It may be necessary to spread out the suggested measures according to their expected impact and according to the time of the year. The human factor must be taken into account and diplomacy should be used by the veterinarian to present and explain the reasons for the measures proposed. Explaining why and how is essential to gain the beekeeper's approval for these measures.

The measures proposed are mainly medical measures and sanitary measures. Medical measures in Europe mainly concern control of *Varroa* infestation. Sanitary measures concern beekeeping practices, such as the location of the apiaries, the site of the hives, and the management of the colonies and material.

Once performed and explained, the audit must be followed by discussion between veterinarian and beekeeper about implementation of the proposed management. Some control points – e.g. the rate of winter mortality (L'Hostis and Barbançon, 2013) – should be defined to establish the implementation and efficiency of the sanitary audit. A second visit may be performed to review the sanitary situation.

2.6 Second visit after auditing

This visit can be performed in the months following the audit. The objective of this 'control' visit is to check (L'Hostis and Barbançon, 2013):

- The feasibility of the measures proposed.
- The correct implementation of these measures.
- The efficiency of these measures.

The efficacy of the measures taken depends on the correct and complete implementation of the audit recommendations (if no other stressor is weakening the colonies).

The aim of the audit is to consider the husbandry as a whole. Each honey farm has its own features and the measures proposed must be adapted to each one. Analysing beekeeping practices by means of an audit allows many aspects of the honey farm to be improved.

A veterinarian competent in honeybee veterinary medicine is the most appropriate professional to perform this audit due to:

- Knowledge of honeybee biology and pathology.
- Familiarity with clinical examination and diagnosis.
- Professional experience.
- Having an overall knowledge of the sanitary management of husbandry.

References

AFSSA Report (2008) Mortalités, effondrements et affaiblissements des colonies d'abeilles. [Mortality Collapse and Weakening of Bee Colonies.] Agence Française de Sécurité Sanitaire des Aliments.

Barbançon, J.M., L'Hostis, M., and Vidal-Naquet, N. (2014) Good veterinary practices in beekeeping. In Ritter, W. (ed.), *Bee Health and Veterinarians*. OIE, Paris, pp. 187–192.

Commun, L. (2011) Structurer sa visite en médecine des populations: le trépied d'observations. *Le Point Vétérinaire*, 321–355.

Dainat, B., Evans, J.D., Chen, Y.P., Gauthier, L., and Neumann, P. (2012) Predictive markers of honey bee colony collapse. *PLoS ONE*, 7(2): e32151. doi:10.1371/journal.pone.0032151

European Union Reference Laboratory for Honeybee Health (2011) Guidelines for a pilot surveillance project on honeybee colony losses. Available at: http://ec.europa.eu/food/archive/animal/liveanimals/bees/docs/annex_i_pilot_project_en.pdf (accessed 11 November 2014).

Franco, S., Martel, A.C, Chauzat, M.P., Blanchard, P., and Thiéry, R. (2012) Les analyses de laboratoire en apiculture. In SNGTV (ed.), *Proceedings of the Journées nationales des GTV.* SNGTV, Nantes, pp. 859–867.

Imdorf, A., Ruoff, K., Fluri, P. (2010) *Le développement des colonies chez l'abeille mellifère.* Station de recherche Agroscope Liebefeld-Posieux ALP, Berne.

Johnson, R. (2010) Honeybee Colony Collapse Disorder. Congressional Research Service. CRS Report for Congress. 7-5700. Available at: http://cursa.ihmc.us/rid=1JJM69DXL-27XB9CC-12CF/bees.pdf (accessed 31 August 2014).

Lehotay, S.J. (2006) Quick, Easy, Cheap, Effective, Rugged, and Safe (QUECHERS) approach for determining pesticide residues. *Methods in Biotechnology. Pesticide Protocols*, 19: 239–261.

Le Sobre G. and Commun, L. (2013) Audit d'élevage en référé: étude des documents et constatations en ferme. *Le Point Vétérinaire*, 337: 44–50.

L'Hostis, M. and Barbançon, J.M. (2009) Pour un réseau sanitaire renforcé. *Abeilles et Cie*, 130: 30–33.

L'Hostis, M. and Barbançon, J.M. (2013) *Conception et intérêts des audits sanitaires en apiculture.* In Barbançon, J.-M. and L'Hostis, M., and Ordonneau, D. (eds), *Journée Scientifique Apicole*, Aix-les-bains, pp. 79–96.

OIE (2014) Manual of Diagnostic Tests and Vaccines for Terrestrial Animals 2014. Apinae. Section 2.2; Available at: http://www.oie.int/en/international-standard-setting/terrestrial-manual/access-online/ (accessed 24 August 2014).

Ragon, I.R. (2009) Mise en place du bilan sanitaire volontaire en élevage bovin, l'exemple de la loire (42). Thèse pour l'obtention du grade de Docteur Vétérinaire, Ecole Nationale Vétérinaire de Lyon.

Roy, C. (2011) La semiologie en apiculture. In SNGTV (ed.), *Proceedings of the Journées nationales des GTV.* Nantes, pp. 915–922.

Wiest, L., Buleté, A., Giroud, B., Fratta, C., Amic, S., Lambert, O., Pouliquen, H., and Arnaudguilhem, C. (2011) Multi-residue analysis of 80 environmental contaminants in honeys, honeybees and pollens by one extraction procedure followed by liquid and gas chromatography coupled with mass spectrometric detection. *Journal of Chromatography A*, 1218(34): 5743–5756.

Winston, M.L. (1987) *The Biology of the Honeybee.* Harvard University Press, Cambridge, MA.

Conclusions

Colony collapse disorder (CCD): one reality, several causes?

Environmental problems, poisoning, infectious diseases, parasitic diseases, pests, and predators, combined with inadequate beekeeping practices, are able to affect colony health, creating the conditions for colony weakening and/or collapse and the economic consequences this entails. In 2006, US beekeepers reported significant (30–90%) losses of colonies in their apiaries (USDA, 2014). (Some winter losses are usual; 5–15% is considered acceptable, depending on the region.) A name was given by scientists to the clinical signs observed with these greater colony losses: colony collapse disorder or CCD. However, more recently CCD has begun to be considered as no different to other colony losses (van Engelsdorp and Pettis, 2014).

Symptoms usually attributed to CCD

The characteristic symptoms described in CCD-affected colonies are (Ellis *et al.*, 2010; van Engelsdorp *et al.*, 2009; van Engelsdorp and Pettis, 2014):

- A rapid loss of worker bees, though the capped brood remains intact.
- The absence of any adult bees in the hive or the apiary. Sometimes a very few bees may remain alive in or around the hive.
- Robbing bees and the usual pests (e.g. the wax moths and the small hive beetle) show little interest in the honey and pollen stored in the affected hives (delayed kleptoparasitism).

Some symptoms of weakened colonies are often related to CCD (Ellis *et al.*, 2010):

- Not enough worker bees to rear the brood present in the colony.
- The affected colony is only composed of young workers.
- The queen is present.
- Bees are not interested in the food provided by the beekeeper.

Current thinking on the causes of CCD

Some questions about CCD remain: if the clinical signs of collapse are similar or close in several colonies, is there one underlying cause of the 'outbreaks' of CCD? Is CCD different to other colony losses?

Among field biologists and researchers, CCD is supposed to be the consequence of many factors, which may or may not be acting together. Terms and expressions such as 'multifactorial causes', 'interaction between stressors', 'several factors acting in concert' are widely used. In the first descriptive epizootiological study published in 2009 (van Engelsdorp *et al.*, 2009), 200 quantifiable variables were compared between affected colonies and controls. The conclusion was that:

- No single pathogen or parasitic agent was found with sufficient frequency to conclude it was involved in CCD.
- No evidence of a single (or more) pesticide in CCD-affected colonies and apiaries. Residues of pesticides (insecticides, acaricides, herbicides, fungicides, etc.) and their metabolites have been found in samples from both CCD-affected and unaffected colonies.

- According to van Engelsdorp *et al.* (2009), 'bees in CCD colonies had higher pathogen loads and were co-infected with more pathogens than control populations, suggesting either greater pathogen exposure or reduced defences in CCD bees'.

All research attempts to highlight a single cause of CCD have failed.

Thus, it is possible to assume that though the symptoms are similar, the causes are probably not the same in each case of CCD outbreak. The biology and physiology of the honeybee may explain the similar symptoms observed in some cases and the causes can be supposed to be diverse. Furthermore, according to van Engelsdorp and Pettis (2014), 'there is little doubt that the attention this phenomenon has received has helped highlight long-held concerns over bee health'.

CCD and colony losses in general, irrespective of the cause, are complex disorders that probably involve many stressors. Veterinarians qualified in honeybee pathology, whether serving as practitioners, laboratory researchers, or officials working in association with biologists, agronomists, researchers, etc., are vital for a better understanding of colony weakening and loss.

References

Ellis, J.D., Evans, J.D., and Pettis, J. (2010) Colony losses, managed colony population decline, and Colony Collapse Disorder in the United States. *Journal of Apicultural Research*, 49(1): 134–136.

USDA (2014) Honey Bees and Colony Collapse Disorder. Available at: http://www.ars.usda.gov/News/docs.htm?docid=15572 (accessed 3 September 2014).

van Engelsdorp, D. and Pettis, J.S. (2014) Colony collapse disorder. In Ritter, W. (ed.), *Bee Health and Veterinarians*. OIE, Paris, pp. 157–159.

van Engelsdorp, D., Evans, D.E., Saegerman, C., Mullin, C., Haubruge, E., Nguyen, B.K., Frazier, M., Frazier, J., Cox-Foster, D.L., Chen, Y., Underwood, R., Tarpy, D.R., and Pettis, J.S. (2009) Colony collapse disorder: a descriptive study. *PLoS ONE*, 4(8): e6481.

Appendix 1

Average values and typical features of the biology of honeybee colonies and beekeeping techniques

	Values/features	Source
Individual values		
Lifespan of summer worker bees	15–38 days	Winston, 1987
Lifespan of spring and autumn worker bees (intermediate seasons)	30–60 days	Winston, 1987
Lifespan of overwintering bees	170–243 days	Imdorf, 2010
Lifespan of drones (spring–mid-summer)	21–32 days	Winston, 1987
Average lifespan of a queen	<4 years (re-queening each year or every two years becomes a necessity in managed colonies)	Winston, 1987
Size of a worker bee	14–15 mm	Winston, 1987
Size of a queen	18–20 mm	Winston, 1987
Size of a drone	19 mm	Winston, 1987
Weight of a worker bee (emergent)	81–151 mg	Kerr and Hebling, 1964
Weight of a (European) worker bee before swarming, engorged with nectar	130 mg	Winston, 1987
Weight of a drone (emergent)	196–225 mg	Winston, 1987
Weight of a queen (emergent)	178–292 mg	Winston, 1987
Maximum wax production of wax-producing bees	3 mg of wax/day	EFSA, 2012
Nectar foragers: volume of nectar the crop can hold	40–70 mm3	Louveaux, 1958
Pollen foragers: amount of pollen carried in the pollen basket	4.2–15 mg	Louveaux, 1958; Winston, 1987; EFSA, 2012
Propolis foragers: amount of propolis carried in the pollen basket	30 mg/trip (300 mg/day)	EFSA, 2012
Water foragers: amount of water carried in each water foraging flight	30–58 μl/ trip (1.4–2.7 ml/day)	EFSA, 2012
Foragers: duration of a foraging flight for nectar	30–80 mn (highly variable depending on flowers visited, etc.)	EFSA, 2012
Number of foraging trips of nectar foragers	10 trips/day (highly variable depending on flowers visited, etc.)	EFSA, 2012
Foragers: duration of a foraging flight for pollen	10 mn (highly variable depending on flowers visited...)	EFSA, 2012

	Values/features	Source
Number of foraging trips of pollen foragers	10 trips/day (highly variable depending on flowers visited, etc.)	EFSA, 2012
Water foragers: number of foraging trips	5 trips/h and a total of 46 trips/day	EFSA, 2012
Drones: number of mating flights per day	3-5 mating flights (drones die following a successful mating flight)	EFSA, 2012
Drones: duration of mating flights	30–60 min	EFSA, 2012
Colony values		
Number of drone cells/dm^2	520	Winston, 1987
Number of worker cells/dm^2 (wild nests)	857	Winston, 1987
Inner cluster temperature during hibernation (average)	20°C	Winston, 1987
Nest temperature during brood rearing	30–35°C	Winston, 1987
Nest temperature dangerous for brood rearing	>36°C	Winston, 1987
Clustering limit temperature threshold	<18°C	Winston, 1987
More compact clustering temperature threshold	<14°C	Winston, 1987
Assumed maximum natural daily mortality within a colony during the season	1% of the colony population per day	EFSA, 2012
Development of colonies in central Europe (key values)		
Population at the beginning of hibernation in Central Europe	8,000–15,000	Imdorf, 2010
Usual (normal) winter bee losses (central Europe)	2,000–3,000	Imdorf, 2010
Population at the end of hibernation (central Europe)	5,000–13,000	Imdorf, 2010
Population peak in summer (central Europe)	25,000–40,000	Imdorf, 2010
Young bees reared per season (central Europe)	130,000–200,000	Imdorf, 2010
Development of the castes		
Development of the queen		
Egg stage	3 days	Winston, 1987
Larval stage	5.5 days	Winston, 1987
Pupal stage (capped brood)	7.5 days	Winston, 1987
Emergence	16 days after ovipositing	Winston, 1987
Development of the worker		
Egg stage	3 days	Winston, 1987
Larval stage	6 days	Winston, 1987
Pupal stage (capped brood)	12 days	Winston, 1987
Emergence	21 days after ovipositing	Winston, 1987
Development of the drone		
Egg stage	3 days	Winston, 1987
Larval stage	6.5 days	Winston, 1987
Pupal stage (capped brood)	14.5 days	Winston, 1987
Emergence	24 days after ovipositing	Winston, 1987

	Values/features	Source
Queen reproduction features		
Occurrence of mating flight after emergence	5–13 days after emergence, an orientation flight occurs; mating flights occur subsequently (and require good weather)	Philippe, 2007; Texas A&M University, 2014
Number of copulations required	7–17	Winston, 1987
Number of spermatozoa in the spermateca after mating flight(s)	Up to 7 million	Dade, 1977
Daily queen laying ability during the season	On average 1,500 eggs/day	Winston, 1987
Annual queen laying ability	175,000–200,000	Winston, 1987
Beginning of queen ovipositing after mating flight(s)	2–4 days	Philippe, 2007
Characterization of female larval stages		
Stage L1 (1st larval instar) uncapped	Head diameter 0.33 mm Weight 0.1–0.5 mg	Rembold *et al.*, 1980
Stage L2 uncapped	Head diameter 0.47 mm Weight 0.35–1.5 mg	Rembold *et al.*, 1980
Stage L3 uncapped	Head diameter 0.70 mm Weight 1.3–6 mg	Rembold *et al.*, 1980
Stage L4 uncapped	Head diameter 1.05 mm Weight 4.2–32 mg	Rembold *et al.*, 1980
Stage L5 uncapped and LS after capping	Head diameter 1.58 mm Weight 27–280 mg	Rembold *et al.*, 1980
Characterization of female pupal stages		
Pw	White-eyed pupa, unpigmented cuticle	Piulachs *et al.*, 2003
Pp	Pink-eyed pupa, unpigmented cuticle	Piulachs *et al.*, 2003
Pr	Red/brown-eyed pupa, unpigmented cuticle	Rembold et al., 1980
Pb	Brown-eyed pupa, unpigmented cuticle	Piulachs *et al.*, 2003
Pbl	Brown-eyed pupa, light pigmented cuticle	Piulachs *et al.*, 2003
Pbm	Brown-eyed pupa, intermediate pigmented cuticle	Piulach *et al.*, 2003
Pbd	Brown-eyed pupa, dark pigmented cuticle	Piulachs *et al.*, 2003
Pha	Pharate adult (pupa looks like adult)	Piulachs *et al.*, 2003
Feed consumption and requirements		
Individual food intake of adult honeybees + exposure to bee products		
Nurse/brood attending bees consumption (sugar in nectar or/and honeydew honey stored in the hive)	34–50 mg/bee/day (April–October, in temperate countries)	EFSA, 2013
Nurse/brood attending bees consumption (pollen from beebread)	≥6.5–12 mg/bee/day (beebread)	EFSA, 2012

	Values/features	Source
Wax-producing bees (sugar in nectar or/and honeydew honey stored in the hive)	18 mg/bee/day	EFSA, 2012
Wax-producing bees (contact exposure with pollen from flowers)	5–10% pollen in wax and propolis	EFSA, 2012
Forager needs of sugar for flight (sugar in nectar or/and honeydew honey stored in the hive)	8–12 mg/h	EFSA, 2012
Pollen forager consumption (sugar in nectar or/ and honeydew honey stored in the hive)	≥10–16 mg/bee/day	EFSA, 2012
Nectar or honeydew forager consumption (sugar in nectar or/and honeydew honey stored in the hive)	≥32–128mg/bee/day	EFSA, 2012
Water forager (sugar in nectar or/and honeydew honey stored in the hive)	72–110 mg/bee/day	EFSA, 2012
Forager consumption (pollen from beebread)	0 mg/bee/day	EFSA, 2013
Pollen forager exposure to pollen from contact exposure with flowers	150–300 mg/bee/day	Winston, 1987; EFSA, 2012
Propolis forager exposure to propolis – contact exposure	30–300 mg/bee/day	EFSA, 2012
Volume of water carried by a water forager in her crop (droplets on leaves, axils, puddles in field, surface water) (contact and oral exposure)	30–58 µl/trip;1.4–2.7 ml/bee/ day	EFSA, 2012
Drone consumption (sugar in nectar or/and honeydew honey stored in the hive)	21–90 mg/bee/day	EFSA, 2012
Drone consumption (pollen from beebread)	0.36 mg/bee/day, only on the first days after emergence	EFSA, 2012
Virgin queen needs for mating flights (sugar in nectar or/and honeydew honey stored in the hive)	42–81 mg/bee/day	EFSA, 2012
Queen consumption (sugar in nectar or/and honeydew honey stored in the hive)	42–81 mg/bee/day	EFSA, 2012
Individual food intake of winterbees		
Consumption for thermoregulation when overwintering (sugar in nectar or/and honeydew honey stored in the hive)	8.8 mg/bee/day in temperate region to maintain a temperature at 15–20°C in the center and 5–8°C in the periphery of the cluster	EFSA Journal, 2012
Intake when foraging at the end of winter (sugar in nectar from flowers, honeydew from plants)	32–128 mg/bee/day	EFSA Journal, 2012
Intake when foraging at the end of winter (contact exposure with pollen from flowers)	150 mg/bee/day	EFSA Journal, 2012
Consumption when brood rearing at the end of winter (pollen from beebread)	6.5–12 mg/bee/day	EFSA, 2012
Consumption when brood rearing at the end of winter (sugar in nectar or/and honeydew honey stored in the hive)	34–50 mg/bee/day	EFSA Journal, 2012
Worker larvae food needs		
Sugar (sugar in nectar or/and honeydew honey stored in the hive)	59.4 mg/larva/5 days	EFSA Journal, 2013
Pollen (pollen from beebread)	1.5–2 mg/larva/5 days	EFSA Journal, 2013

	Values/features	Source
Drone larvae food intake		
Sugar (sugar in nectar or/and honeydew honey stored in the hive)	98.2 mg/larva/6.5 days	EFSA, 2013
Pollen (pollen from beebread)	2.04–2.72 mg/larva/6.5 days	EFSA Journal, 2013
Food needs to rear one worker bee		
Pollen	125–145 mg	Rosov, 1944; Winston, 1987
Honey	142 mg	Rosov, 1944
Colony requirements (annual)		
Honey	60–80 kg per year	Winston, 1987
Pollen	15–55 kg per year	Winston, 1987
Water	20–42 litres/colony/year and during summer up to 20 litres/week/colony or 2.9 litres/day/colony (highly variable)	EFSA, 2012
Evaluation of the brood and adult bees		
Dadant hive – number of bees on a full frame	1,400	Imdorf *et al.*, 2010
Dadant hive – surface area of a frame side (dm^2)	11	Imdorf *et al.*, 2010
Langstroth hive – number of bees on a full frame	1100	Imdorf *et al.*, 2010
Langstroth hive – surface area of a frame side (dm^2)	8	Imdorf *et al.*, 2010
Number of bees per dm^2 of frame area	130	Imdorf *et al.*, 2010
Number of bees per dm^2 of frame area when all the bees have their heads inside cells	up to 400	Imdorf *et al.*, 2010
Number of bees per cluster (size 12 cm × 6 cm × 3 cm)	750	Imdorf *et al.*, 2010
Number of worker cells/dm^2 (wild nests)	857	Winston (1987)
Number of worker cells/dm^2 (embossed wax)	750 on average – may vary according to practice	
Number of drone cells/dm^2	520	Winston, 1987
Honey requirement for overwintering	18–22 kg	FERA, 2010
Re-queening requirement	Every one or two years	

Sources

Dade, H.A. (1977) *Anatomy and Dissection of the Honeybee* (rev. edn 2009). International Bee Research Association, London.

EFSA Journal (2012) Scientific opinion on the science behind the development of a risk assessment of plant protection products on bees (*Apis mellifera*, *Bombus* spp. and solitary bees). Available at: http://www.efsa.europa.eu/fr/efsajournal/doc/2668.pdf (accessed 18 September 2014).

EFSA Journal (2013a) Conclusion on the peer review of the pesticide risk assessment for bees for the active substance clothianidin. Available at: http://www.efsa.europa.eu/en/efsajournal/doc/3066.pdf (accessed 5 November 2014)

EFSA Journal (2013b) EFSA Guidance Document on the risk assessment of plant protection products on bees (*Apis mellifera*, *Bombus* spp. and solitary bees). Available at: http://www.efsa.europa.eu/fr/efsajournal/doc/3295.pdf (accessed 30 October 2014).

European Union Reference Laboratory for Honeybee Health (2011) Guidelines for a pilot surveillance project on honeybee colony losses. Available at: http://ec.europa.eu/food/archive/animal/liveanimals/bees/docs/annex_i_pilot_project_en.pdf (accessed 11 November 2014).

FERA: The Food & Environment Research Agency (2010) Preparing honey bee colonies for winter. Available at: https://secure.fera.defra.gov.uk/beebase/downloadNews.cfm?id=79 (accessed 14 September 2014).

Imdorf, A., Ruoff, K., and Fluri, P. (2010) *Le développement des colonies chez l'abeille mellifère*. Station de recherche Agroscope Liebefeld-Posieux ALP, Berne.

Kerr, W.E. and Hebling N.J. (1964) Influence of the weight of worker bees on division of labor. *Evolution*, 18, 267–270.

Louveaux, J. (1958) Recherches sur la récolte du pollen par les abeilles (*Apis mellifica* L.). *Annales des abeilles*. 1(4): 197–221.

Philippe, J.M. (2007) *Le guide de l'apiculteur*. Edisud, Aix-en Provence.

Piulachs, M.D., Guidugli, K.R., Barchuk, A.R., Cruz, J., Simoes, Z.L.P., and Bellés, X. (2003) The vitellogenin of the honey bee, *Apis mellifera*: structural analysis of the cDNA and expression studies. *Insect Biochemistry and Molecular Biology*, 33: 459–465.

Rembold, H., Kremer, J-P., and Ulrich, G.M. (1980) Characterization of postembryonic developmental stages of the female castes of the honey bee, *Apis mellifera* L. *Apidologie*, 11(1): 29–38.

Rosov, A.S. (1944) Food consumption by bees. *Bee World*, 25: 94–95.

Texas A&M University (2014) Honey bee biology. Available at: https://insects.tamu.edu/continuing_ed/bee_biology/ (accessed 12 July 2014).

Winston, M.L. (1987) *The Biology of the Honeybee*. Harvard University Press, Cambridge, MA.

Appendix 2

Diseases notifiable to the OIE and European countries

	AFB	EFB	Varroosis	Nosemosis	Tracheal acariosis	Brood mycosis	Virosis	*Aethina tumida*	*Tropilaelaps* spp.
OIE	Yes	Yes	Yes	No	Yes	No	No	Yes	Yes
Austria	Yes	No	Yes	No	No	No	No	Yes	Yes
Belgium	Yes	Yes	Yes	No	Yes	No	No	Yes	Yes
Bulgaria	Yes	Yes	Yes	Yes	No	No	No	Yes	Yes
Czech Republic	Yes	Yes	Yes	No	No	No	No	Yes	Yes
Denmark	Yes	Yes	Yes	No	Yes	Yes	No	Yes	Yes
Estonia	Yes	Yes	Yes	Yes	Yes	No	No	Yes	Yes
Finland	Yes	No	No	No	No	No	No	Yes	Yes
France	Yes	No	Yes	Yes (*N. apis*)	No	No	No	Yes	Yes
Germany	Yes	No	No	No	No	No	No	Yes	Yes
Greece	Yes	No	No	No	No	No	No	Yes	Yes
Hungary	Yes	Yes	Yes	No	Yes	No	No	Yes	Yes
Ireland	Yes	Yes	No	No	No	No	No	Yes	Yes
Italy	Yes	Yes	Yes	Yes	Yes	No	No	Yes	Yes
Kosovo	Yes	Yes	Yes	Yes	No	No	No	No	No
Lithuania	Yes	Yes	Yes	Yes	Yes	No	No	Yes	Yes
Norway	Yes	Yes	Yes	Yes	Yes	Yes	No	Yes	Yes
Poland	Yes	Yes	Yes	No	Yes	No	No	Yes	Yes
Portugal	Yes	Yes	Yes	Yes	Yes	Yes (*A. apis*)	No	Yes	Yes
Romania	Yes	Yes	Yes	Yes	Yes	Yes	Yes	Yes	Yes
Slovakia	Yes	No	Yes	No	No	No	No	Yes	Yes
Slovenia	Yes	No	No	No	No	No	No	Yes	Yes
Spain	Yes	No	Yes	No	No	No	No	Yes	Yes
Sweden	Yes	No	Yes	No	Yes	No	No	Yes	Yes
UK	Yes	Yes	No	No	No	No	No	Yes	Yes

Cyprus, Latvia, Netherlands: no data found.
AFB, American foulbrood disease; EFB, European foulbrood disease.

Sources

Chauzat, M.-P., Cauquil, L., Roy, L., Franco, S., Hendrikx, P., and Ribière-Chabert, M. (2013) Demographics of the european apicultural industry. *PLoS ONE*, 8(11): e79018. doi:10.1371/journal.pone.0079018.

OIE (2014b) OIE Listed Diseases. Avalaible at http://www.oie.int/en/animal-health-in-the-world/oie-listed-diseases-2014/ (accessed 29 April 2014).

Appendix 3

Sampling

Sampling for chemicals

Matrix sampled	Quantity of sample to take	Packaging	Storage temperature
Honey	250 g	Glass container sealed and enveloped in a plastic bag	4°C
Royal jelly	20 g	Glass container sealed and enveloped in a plastic bag	–20°C
Wax and propolis	20 g	Cardboard or paper packing	4°C
Fresh pollen (pollen balls)	50 g	Cardboard or paper packing	–20°C
Beebread	50 g (20 cm^2 of beebread cells)	Cardboard or paper packing	–20°C
Bees	50 g (on average 500 bees)	Cardboard or paper packing (plastic must be avoided for bees)	–20°C
Plants	10 litres of flowering plants	In jar, wrapped in brown paper	–20°C

Sampling for laboratory testing and diagnosis of pathogenic agents

Matrix sampled	Quantity of sample to take	Packaging	Storage temperature
Adult bees: alive, with clinical symptoms or recently died	>20 bees Suspected Acarapidosis: >200 bees *Nosema apis* infestation level: >60 bees (older ones if possible) *Varroa destructor*: >300 inside bees	Brown wrapping paper, cardboard packing – plastic containers are not recommended	At room temperature if delivered the same day; otherwise –20°C
Brood	Square 10 cm × 10 cm with at least diseased 15 larvae and/or pupae	Cardboard box or stiff plastic box	At room temperature if delivered the same day; otherwise –20°C
Brood	Larvae or any symptomatic element	Eppendorf-type tube	At room temperature if delivered the same day; otherwise –20°C
Parasites, pests, suspicion of invasive pests (eggs, larvae, insects, acarians, etc.)	Several specimens if possible	Cardboard box for insects or screwtop tube	–20°C

The best way to sample is for the veterinarian to contact the selected laboratory before sampling and sending the matrix.

Adapted from Franco, S., Martel, A.C., Chauzat, M.P., Blanchard, P., and Thiéry, R. (2012) Les analyses de laboratoire en apiculture. In SNGTV (ed.), *Proceedings of the Journées nationales des GTV.* SNGTV, Nantes, pp. 859–867.

Appendix 4

Veterinary beekeeping sanitary audit guide

Date of the audit			

Purpose of the sanitary audit | | | **Observations**

	Yes	No	Observations
Prevention approach	☐	☐	
Sanitary troubles affecting the colonies	☐	☐	
Suspicion of intoxication	☐	☐	
Compulsory audit demanded by authorities	☐	☐	

If sanitary trouble:

Date of occurrence of the troubles, symptoms		
Date of the last symptom-free visit		
Number of apiaries affected		
Number of colonies affected		
Rate of mortality		
Mortality in the same apiary		
Other		

Description of the symptoms and troubles

Production

Is the production affected?	☐	☐	
Which production?			
In which proportion?			

General data of the honey farm – features and objectives

Field	Evaluation		Observations
Beekeeper			
Name and address of the beekeeper			
Kind of activity	Yes	No	
Professional	☐	☐	
Leisure	☐	☐	
Semi-professional	☐	☐	
Professionals			
How many professionals?			
Training			
Visitors to the farm			
Trainee beekeeper	☐	☐	
Beekeepers	☐	☐	
Honey farm features			
Production for trade:			
Pollination activity	☐	☐	
Honey	☐	☐	
Pollen	☐	☐	
Propolis	☐	☐	
Wax	☐	☐	
Royal jelly	☐	☐	
Package bees	☐	☐	
Artificial swarms	☐	☐	
Queens	☐	☐	
Production			
Pollination activity	☐	☐	
Honey production (and quantity)	☐	☐	
Honey production/hive			
Local honey	☐	☐	
Features of local honey			
Pollen production	☐	☐	
Pollen production/hive			
Wax production	☐	☐	
Royal jelly production	☐	☐	
Propolis production	☐	☐	
Data recording			
Recording			
Record keeping	☐	☐	
Computerized system	☐	☐	
Data capture frequency			
Data capture features			
Sanitary troubles	☐	☐	
Husbandry data	☐	☐	
Production data	☐	☐	
Other			
Remarks and information			

General data of the honey farm – livestock and environment

Livestock

Number of colonies

Producing honey
Producing pollen
In pollination activity

Breeding

Swarms produced/year
Queens produced/year

Breeding method

Division	☐	☐
‘Wild swarm’ collection	☐	☐

Introduction after purchase of bees (and number)

Queens	☐	☐
Artificial swarms on frames	☐	☐
Package bees	☐	☐

Apiary site

Sedentary?	☐	☐
How many?		
Number of colonies/apiary		
Migratory beekeeping?	☐	☐
How many?		
Number of colonies/apiary		
Collective migratory sites		

Accessibility of the apiary(ies):

By car	☐	☐
On foot	☐	☐
Distance		

Apiary environment

Beekeeping activity in the vicinity:

Nearby apiaries	☐	☐
How many?		
Relationship with neighbouring beekeepers?	☐	☐

Features of the apiary site

Risk of moisture	☐	☐
Shaded site	☐	☐
Sunny site	☐	☐

Landscape type (within a 3 km radius)

Cereal crops	☐	☐

Arboriculture	☐	☐
Forest	☐	☐
Bocage landscape	☐	☐
Urban	☐	☐
Mountain	☐	☐
Other	☐	☐
Chemical environment		
Is the environment toxically risky?	☐	☐
Pesticides and chemical industry	☐	☐
Pesticides used on crops	☐	☐
Insecticides used on nearby cattle husbandry		
Meteorological features		
On the sedentary apiaries		
On the migratory apiaries		
Water resource		
Running water	☐	☐
Stagnant water	☐	☐
Watering place	☐	☐
Water renewal frequency	☐	☐
Distance		

Conclusions

	0	1	2
Livestock	☐	☐	☐
Location	☐	☐	☐
Environment	☐	☐	☐

0 = Inadequate; 1 = Satisfactory; 2 = Very satisfactory

Observations

General data of the honey farm – sanitary aspects

Field	Evaluation Yes	Evaluation No	Observations
Colony losses	Yes	No	
Annual mortality			
Annual mortality rate			
Mortality rate in sedentary apiaries			
Mortality rate in migratory apiaries			
Winter losses? How many?	☐	☐	
Season losses? How many?	☐	☐	
How are these losses evaluated?			
Infectious and fungal diseases			
Infectious diseases			
American foulbrood	☐	☐	
European foulbrood	☐	☐	
Type-A nosemosis	☐	☐	
Type-C nosemosis	☐	☐	
Paralysis	☐	☐	
Deformed wing virus disease	☐	☐	
Sacbrood disease	☐	☐	
Chalkbrood	☐	☐	
Others	☐	☐	
Implementation of the shock swarm technique			
Destruction of colonies due to outbreaks			
Number of colonies destroyed			Main result
Laboratory test results	Attached annex		
Intoxications			
Global surrounding poisoning risk	☐	☐	
Mortality due to suspected poisoning	☐	☐	
Mortality due to confirmed poisoning	☐	☐	
Laboratory test results	Attached annex		Main result
Relationship with sanitary authorities			
Control by officials	☐	☐	Date
Current sanitary measures	☐	☐	
Causes of these measures			
Sanitary status towards notifiable diseases			
American foulbrood			
Type A Nosemosis			
Aethina tumida			
Tropilaelaps clareae			

Conclusions

Observations

	0	1	2
Colony losses	☐	☐	☐
Infectious and fungal diseases	☐	☐	☐
Intoxications	☐	☐	☐
Notifiable diseases	☐	☐	☐

Control of *Varroa* infestation

Field	Evaluation Yes	Evaluation No	Observations
Year Y–2			
Evaluation of Varroa infestation (when)			
Monitoring natural mite fall	☐	☐	
Drone brood uncapping method	☐	☐	
Monitoring total mite drop	☐	☐	
Monitoring phoretic *Varroa* on adults	☐	☐	
Frequency of evaluation of infestation			
Treatment strategy	☐	☐	
Integrated pest management	☐	☐	
Biotechnical methods implemented			
Veterinary medicine products (VMPs)			
VMPs used			
Alternation of treatments			
Other drugs used			
Oxalic acid	☐	☐	
Formic acid	☐	☐	
Lactic acid	☐	☐	
Others	☐	☐	
Are these drugs pharmaceutical products?	☐	☐	
Efficacy of the treatment			
Infestation rate at the end of the season			
Infestation rate in spring			
Year Y–1			
Evaluation of Varroa infestation (when)			
Monitoring natural mite fall	☐	☐	
Drone brood uncapping method	☐	☐	
Monitoring total mite drop	☐	☐	
Monitoring phoretic *Varroa* on adults	☐	☐	
Frequency of evaluation of infestation			
Treatment strategy	☐	☐	
Integrated pest management	☐	☐	
Biotechnical methods implemented			
Veterinary medicine products (VMPs)			
VMPs used			
Alternation of treatments			
Other drugs used			
Oxalic acid	☐	☐	
Formic acid	☐	☐	
Lactic acid	☐	☐	
Others	☐	☐	
Are these drugs pharmaceutical products?	☐	☐	

Efficacy of the treatment

Infestation rate at the end of the season

Infestation rate in spring

Year Y

Evaluation of Varroa infestation (when)

Monitoring natural mite fall	☐	☐	
Drone brood uncapping method	☐	☐	
Monitoring total mite drop	☐	☐	
Monitoring phoretic *Varroa* on adults	☐	☐	
Frequency of evaluation of infestation			
Treatment strategy	☐	☐	
Integrated pest management	☐	☐	
Biotechnical methods implemented			
Veterinary medicine products (VMPs)			
VMPs used			
Alternation of treatments			
Other drugs used			
Oxalic acid	☐	☐	
Formic acid	☐	☐	
Lactic acid	☐	☐	
Others	☐	☐	
Are these drugs pharmaceutical products?	☐	☐	
Efficacy of the treatment			
Infestation rate at the end of the season			
Infestation rate in spring			

	0	1	2	**Observations**
Year Y–2	☐	☐	☐	
Year Y–1	☐	☐	☐	
Year Y	☐	☐	☐	

Field examination

Field	Evaluation	Observations
Visual appreciation of the apiary location		
Apiary access		
Apiary maintenance		
Hive location and maintenance		
Moisture protection		
Risks of drifting and/or robbing		

Clinical examination of colonies	Yes	No	Precise description
Alighting board and front of the hive			
General observations			
Evaluation of activity			
Presence of predators	☐	☐	
Presence of symptomatic bees	☐	☐	
Neighbourhood affected	☐	☐	
Unusual aggressive behaviour	☐	☐	
Dead bees, diseased bees, others			
Dead adult bees	☐	☐	
Dead larvae and pupae	☐	☐	
Aspect			
Faeces	☐	☐	
Waste	☐	☐	
Examination when opening the hive			
General aspect of the wood (frames, hive body, super, feeder)			
Number of intercomb spaces occupied by bees			
Behavioural features when opening the hive			
Smell	☐	☐	
Presence of other insects or pests	☐	☐	
Examination of the adult bees			
Physical symptoms	☐	☐	
Neurological symptoms	☐	☐	
Behavioural symptoms	☐	☐	
Digestive symptoms	☐	☐	
Phoretic *Varroa*	☐	☐	

Examination of the queen			
Size	☐	☐	
Abnormalities of the wings	☐	☐	
Other	☐	☐	
Examination of the brood			
Surface and number of brood combs			
Presence of eggs	☐	☐	
Presence of larvae (uncapped brood)	☐	☐	
Presence of capped brood	☐	☐	
Appearance of the brood			
Appearance of the cappings			
Presence of punctured cappings			
Smell of the brood			
Evaluation of the population (value or approximate evaluation)			
Adult bees			
Brood reared			
Adult bees/brood			
The floor of the hive			
Description of elements found on the floor			
Sampling			
Adult honeybees	☐	☐	
Brood	☐	☐	
Wax	☐	☐	
Pollen	☐	☐	
Honey	☐	☐	
Other (plants, water, etc.)	☐	☐	
Laboratory tests requested			
Day of sending			
Date of receipt			
Results			

Remarks and observations

Beekeeping practices – material and premises

Fields	Evaluation		Observations
Hives			
Kind	Yes	No	
Dadant 10-frame	☐	☐	
Langstroth	☐	☐	
Warré	☐	☐	
Voirnot	☐	☐	
Other	☐	☐	
Material			
Wood	☐	☐	
Plastic	☐	☐	
Other	☐	☐	
Mesh floor	☐	☐	
Queen extruder	☐	☐	
Feeders	☐	☐	
Maintenance			
Modality			
Frequency			
Cleaning	☐	☐	
Disinfection and sterilization	☐	☐	
Storage	☐	☐	
Location of the hive in the apiary			
Protection against damp (hive stand)	☐	☐	
Protection against wind	☐	☐	
Other observations			
Supers			
Cleaning	☐	☐	
Disinfection and sterilization	☐	☐	
Methods of disinfection and sterilization			
Method of storage			
Protection against moths			
Frames			

Renewal

How many per year and per hive

Becoming of old frames

Wax

Origin

Quantity of wax purchased each year

Reutilization of cappings of honeycombs ☐ ☐

Is old wax reutilized to make new embossed wax foundations?

Frame cleaning

By bees on the apiary ☐ ☐

By bees on another apiary ☐ ☐

Small materials

Hive tools

Number

One used for all the apiaries ☐ ☐

Disinfection between apiaries? ☐ ☐

Tissues

Gloves ☐ ☐

Beekeeping suit ☐ ☐

Cleaning and disinfection ☐ ☐

Sanitation of premises and honey house

Observation and evaluation ☐ ☐

Conclusions

	0	1	2
Hives	☐	☐	☐
Super and frames	☐	☐	☐
Small material	☐	☐	☐
Sanitation of premises	☐	☐	☐

Observations

Beekeeping practices – livestock

Fields	Evaluation		Observations
Honeybee strain – selection – genetics	Yes	No	Method of selection if necessary
Honeybee			
Local black honeybee	☐	☐	
Introduced black honeybee	☐	☐	
Buckfast	☐	☐	
Other	☐	☐	
Origins of the honeybees			
Morphometry			Selection objectives and criteria
Queens			
Reared on the farm	☐	☐	
Purchased	☐	☐	
Renewal (frequency, cause)			
Period of rearing			
Drones			
Apiary drone rearing			
Feeding colonies			
Kind of feeding supplement and period			Period of use
Syrup	☐	☐	
Candy	☐	☐	
Honey	☐	☐	
Protein supplement	☐	☐	
Other	☐	☐	
Features			
Origins			
Traceability			
Storage methods			
Objectives			
Spring stimulation (speculative feeding)	☐	☐	
Rearing (artificial swarm production) (speculative feeding)	☐	☐	

Overwintering preparation (and surrogate feeding)	☐	☐	
Emergency feeding needed in the past year?	☐	☐	
Methods of supplement distribution			
Systematic	☐	☐	
After evaluation of the needs (weight of the hive)	☐	☐	
Duration			
Repetitive small quantities dispensed (spring stimulation)	☐	☐	
Volume/colony			
Visits to the apiaries during the season			
Frequency			
<2 per year and per colony	☐	☐	
2–5 per year and per colony	☐	☐	
>5 per year and per colony	☐	☐	
Duration			
<2 mn per colony	☐	☐	
2–5 mn per colony	☐	☐	
>5 mn per colony	☐	☐	
Objectives			
Simple monitoring of the alighting board	☐	☐	
Examination hive opened	☐	☐	
Examination of all the frames	☐	☐	
Spring and autumn visits			
Summer/autumn visit before wintering	☐	☐	
All hives/frames/colonies examined	☐	☐	
Spring visit before the season	☐	☐	
All hives/frames/colonies examined	☐	☐	
Management of weakened colonies before overwintering	☐	☐	
Migratory beekeeping			
Aim of migratory beekeeping?			
How is migratory beekeeping performed?			
Routes?			
When?			
'Welfare' of the bees?			
Feeding before transportation?	☐	☐	

Conclusions

	0	1	2
Honeybees	☐	☐	☐
Feeding supplements	☐	☐	☐
Visits during the season	☐	☐	☐
Visit before overwintering (autumn)	☐	☐	☐
Visit before season (spring)	☐	☐	☐
Migratory beekeeping	☐	☐	☐

Observations

Elements of an audit in the case of intoxication (complement to field visit)

Fields	Evaluation Yes	Evaluation No	Observations
History			Name and adress
Report from the beekeeper			
Date and time of the observation			
Date and time of the last symptom-free visit			
Number of dead colonies			
Number of weakened colonies			
Contacts already taken			
Sanitary authorities	☐	☐	
Beekeeping technician	☐	☐	
Person delegated	☐	☐	
Person authorized	☐	☐	
Environment			
Considered at risk	☐	☐	
Crop(s) suspected			
Other pesticide, drug, or chemical source suspected			
Clinical symptoms			
Mortality			Provide precise descriptive features
Number of colonies affected			
Are the colonies affected in the same apiary	☐	☐	
Proportion of colonies affected in the apiary(ies)			
Number of apiaries affected			
Distance between apiaries			
Are neigbouring apiaries affected?	☐	☐	

Dead bees			
Present?	☐	☐	
Larvae, pupae, adults?			
Aspect			
Estimated rate/colony			
Dead bees on the alighting board	☐	☐	
Dead bees on the floor	☐	☐	
Dead bees on the soil in front of the hive	☐	☐	
Dead bees in the surrounding environment	☐	☐	
Diseased bees (description) – cf. 'Clinical examination' above			Provide precise descriptive features
Examination of the frames			
Presence of brood	☐	☐	
'Normal' brood	☐	☐	
'Abnormal' brood	☐	☐	
Population of inside bees	☐	☐	
Normal adult/brood ratio	☐	☐	
Honey	☐	☐	
Pollen	☐	☐	
Sampling – cf. Sampling rules			
Honey	☐	☐	
Pollen	☐	☐	
Dead bees	☐	☐	
Diseased bees	☐	☐	
Asymptomatic bees	☐	☐	
Brood	☐	☐	
Other (plants, water, etc.)	☐	☐	

Remarks and observations

Sources

Roy, C. and Vilagines, L., Personal communication, 2014

L'Hostis, M. and Barbançon, J.M. (2013) Conception et intérêts des audits sanitaires en apiculture. In J.-M. Barbançon, M. L'Hostis, and D. Ordonneau (eds), *Journée Scientifique Apicole*, Aix -les-bains, pp. 79–96.

Le Sobre, G. and Commun, L. (2013) Audit d'élevage en référé: étude des documents et constatations en ferme. *Le Point Vétérinaire*, 337: 44–50.

Index